Deadly Choices

DEADLY CHOICES

Coping
with Health Risks
in Everyday Life

JEFFREY E. HARRIS, M.D., Ph.D.

BasicBooks
A Division of HarperCollinsPublishers

Designed by Ellen Levine

93 94 95 96 ◆/RRD 9 8 7 6 5 4 3 2 1

Library of Congress Cataloging-in-Publication Data

Harris, Jeffrey E.
    Deadly choices : coping with health risks in everyday life /
Jeffrey E. Harris.
        p. cm.
    Includes bibliographical references and index.
    ISBN 0–465–02889–6
    1. Health—Decision making.   2. Health behavior.
    3. Health risk assessment. I. Title
    RA776.9.H37   1993
    613—dc20
                                                    92–56173
                                                        CIP

For Johanna, Zoe, and Luke

Contents

Preface

Day after day, the latest research findings of medical scientists make instant news stories. We, the consuming public, read and hear the stories. *Oat bran lowers blood cholesterol. Bald men get more heart attacks. French people get fewer heart attacks. Vasectomy causes prostate cancer. A low blood cholesterol can be dangerous. Too much iron causes heart attacks. Eating nuts prevents heart attacks. New diet pills suppress appetite. Vitamin E prevents soreness after a workout. Margarine causes heart attacks.*

The scientists' findings are synthesized by blue-ribbon panels of experts, whose reports also make news stories. We read and hear these stories, too. *Commercial diets may not work. Value of mammography under age fifty doubted.* The panel reports are praised and denounced by professional and trade organizations. Having commissioned the expert reports and tested the political waters, government officials issue recommendations. We read and hear the advisories, the guidelines, and the warnings. *Use latex condoms. Eat five portions of fresh fruits and vegetables daily. Get a Pap smear.*

We go to our physicians for advice and treatment. Some of us worry about our weight. Others worry about getting in shape, or getting breast cancer, or menopause, or AIDS. Our perspectives are different. But we all ask our doctors the same questions: *What do these latest medical findings, blue-ribbon reports, and government advisories mean for me? Whom do I believe? How do I choose?* Our doctors give their views. Sometimes they tell us to ignore what we have read, or to wait and see. Sometimes they don't know what to say.

Then we go home and decide. Every day, day after day, we choose. We eat hamburgers. We forget to take a pill. We try an aerobics class. We have sex. We make our imperfect choices.

For the past nineteen years, I, too, have read the medical stories, heard the government warnings, and asked my doctor for advice. I, too, have made my own choices. But I have also seen things from the other side. As a scientist, I have published research articles, given press interviews, served on expert panels, and helped make public policy. As a physician, I have tried to help my patients, one by one, make up their minds. And I have seen my scientific colleagues and medical friends go home and make up their own minds, too.

I have seen the two sides moving farther and farther apart. With each new medical "discovery," the consuming public grows increasingly hard-nosed and wary. My own patients have grown so skeptical that they reject the latest health pronouncements out of hand. They see the media, the scientific establishment, and the government as creating a standard of perfection that no one can adhere to. *Eat no more than 30 percent of calories in the form of fat. Get regular aerobic exercise, sufficiently intense to elevate your heart rate to 60 percent of maximum, for at least twenty minutes three times per week. Take at least four milligrams of folic acid daily to prevent your future baby from having spina bifida or other neural-tube defects.*

My patients see critical questions of life and death framed in sweeping terms that have little personal relevance. They ask me: *Why should I get a mammogram, when my mother didn't have breast cancer? Why should I eat fresh fruits and vegetables, when my cholesterol is already low and my electrocardiogram is normal? Why should I worry about cholesterol, when I know I'm going to die of cancer? Why should I use condoms, when I'm certain my girlfriend doesn't have AIDS?* When they read and hear the health messages, they see words that have lost their ordinary meanings, or that never had any meanings: *good cholesterol, risk factor, polyunsaturated fat, aerobic exercise, yo-yo dieting.*

I understand these reactions. I, too, react with cynicism and confusion when I hear the latest medical news story, even though I *think* I know more. But the scientific establishment doesn't seem to understand. Bewildered and dismayed, the blue-ribbon panels issue more reports, documenting that people aren't following their recommendations. *Americans continue to be sedentary. They continue to be overweight. They continue not to use condoms. They aren't checking with their doctors about high blood cholesterol.*

As a physician, I can only do so much. I cannot follow my patients home. Still, there must be a way to close the gap, to bring the message down to the personal level. That's why I wrote this book.

This is not a comprehensive manual of medical advice. Don't expect to find low-fat recipes, or price lists of arthritis medicines, or instructive pictures on how to stretch various muscle groups. If you're leaving tomorrow for an equatorial country, you will not find out here what shots you need to get. I cannot solve your specific medical problems. Nor can I cover every controversial issue. Instead, I have focused on a few of the most important ones: heterosexual behavior and AIDS, exercise, weight-control, cholesterol, smoking, and breast cancer.

My goal is to help you, the consuming public, to decode the messages from the scientific establishment, the media, and the public health officials. I have tried not to be patronizing. You will not be lectured on the ten easy steps to enlarge your biceps and trim your waistline in just weeks, while you sit there passively. Instead, I want readers to get involved, to think about the choices they make every day. There is a lot of scientific information in the pages that follow. But there is also a bigger picture, a philosophy, a way of thinking, which is just as important.

Nor is this a book about public policy. I do not take the scientific establishment or the public health officials or the media to task. As you will read, there are good reasons why they do what they do. I may have some ideas from time to time on how better to communicate, to recommend, and to warn, but I am not trying to reform the world. I just want to help.

I cannot always offer the final answers. Medical science is no monolith. There are multiple viewpoints. Science isn't always right. There are false leads, contradictory data, even lies. Science doesn't stay put, either. Scientists change their minds. Just when we most need to know, science becomes tentative, contemplative, unpunctual. Science postpones while the rest of us keep our appointments. When there is genuine debate, I do my best to consider opposing positions. When the case is closed, I'll say so. And when I think I've got the right answer, I'll stick my neck out. I'll speculate.

I'm writing about the real choices that people have to make—not artificial decisions by nonexistent perfect medical consumers who adhere to every guideline and warning. Since I can't write a book for and about everyone, I have chosen to tell a half-dozen different stories. The stories are fictitious composites of thousands of real stories I have heard. In each story, somebody faces a choice. Sometimes the choice has obvious life-and-death consequences. Other times the consequences are distant but just as deadly. I dissect each choice. I try to get to the essence of the problem. What is learned from one choice I try to apply to the next. If there is any compliment that you, as reader, can bestow upon me, it is that you see yourself somewhere in the pages that follow.

Acknowledgments

Among the people whom I am about to thank, most will disagree with something I have to say in this book. A great many have not read drafts of the manuscript. A few may be surprised that they are being thanked at all.

I thank Martin Kessler of Basic Books for waiting ages for me to write this book and, when I finally got started, for his unflagging confidence in my abilities until the very end. I thank Linda Carbone at Basic Books for carefully reading every paragraph, asking questions, and making suggestions. I thank Jane Judge at Basic Books for swiftly and efficiently moving the manuscript through production.

I thank the Massachusetts General Hospital, where I trained as an intern and a resident, for permitting me to practice on its medical staff for the past nineteen years. I thank my patients, who must unfortunately remain unnamed, but with whom I have spent thousands of hours talking about the issues in this book, trying out new ways to explain my ideas, and, most of all, just listening. Among my colleagues in our internal medicine group practice who have helped me along the way, I thank Gregg Meyer, Larry Ronan, Jim Dineen, Al Mulley, Jim Richter, Nancy Rigotti, Carol Ehrlich, Peter Slavin, Lauretta Salerno, John Allen, Barbara Chase, Sharon

Folleytar, Cheryl Fargo, Linda Lambros, Maria Marzullo, Erica Weed, Rosaria Carter, Tracy Cardinal, Quintina Palmer, Joan McGrath, Phoebe Matthews, Norma Soto, Rita Rizzo, Debra Smith, and, most of all, John Stoeckle, our beacon.

I thank my students and colleagues at the Massachusetts Institute of Technology, especially in the Economics Department, where I have taught everything from mathematical statistics to health economics. While this book focuses on medical issues, my economics colleagues will not help but see their influence upon my thinking. During the fall of 1992, my department head, Peter Temin, gave me a valuable sabbatical semester, for which I am grateful. Among my present and past MIT colleagues, I want particularly to thank Irving London (who once asked me to accompany him to Paris, and he knows the rest), Jean-François Lacronique (who invited me back again), Henry Farber (with whom I learned about survival analysis), Bill DuMouchel (who made me a Bayesian at heart), and my secretary, Helen Dippold.

I am grateful to those professional colleagues who have sought my advice as an expert scientist and economist in both government and the private sector, including Marc Edell, Don Shopland, Roger Baker, and John Pinney. Among the many scientific colleagues with whom I have talked, corresponded, or heard lectures over the past few years, I want to acknowledge the influence of Joseph Catania, Michael Criqui, Daniel Kopans, Richard Doll, Ralph Paffenbarger, George Blackburn, John Foreyt, Howard Raiffa, Paul Lachance, David Gordon, Xavier Pi-Sunyer, JoAnn Manson, Thomas Wadden, Kenneth Arrow, Steven Blair, William Evans, Walter Willett, Samuel Lesko, Hollis Kowaloff, and David Herzog. I, not they, take responsibility for what I say.

I have spent many hours outside the academic, medical, and governmental worlds, tossing around the many questions that pervade this book. Among the many people who listened to my ideas, or who contributed in their own way, I thank Bobby English, Kerry Murtaugh, Mark Kitsis, Tom Moore, Piero Melia, Dan Sacco, Pat Carney, Peter Groark, and fellow members at Middlesex Health and Fitness. I thank Ed Lang, Joanne Hallisey, Jane Leung, Dave Gabbe, Patrick Wentland, Geert Kinthaert, Jody Kosinski, Mike Powers, Jack McMahon, Norm Gallant, Dick Ring, John Chadis, and fellow members at the Bay State Speedskating Club. I thank Jeannette Neill, Jim Viera, and Christien Polos at the Jeannette Neill Dance Studio. I thank Julius Kaiser and Cecilia Colledge at the Skating Club of Boston. Alan and Carol Spielman and sons Daniel and Darren are to be thanked for special reasons.

Finally, I thank Johanna, Zoe, and Luke Harris for enough things to fill a hundred books, but most of all for reminding me, one day at a time, that they knew I could do it.

1

The Margarine Battle Book

Introduction

For two and a half years, I had a dull headache at breakfast time. It didn't happen every morning, and it always went away by lunch. I wouldn't call it a migraine. It wasn't even a splitting headache. I couldn't figure out what caused that vague feeling of fullness behind my eyes at about 6:45 A.M. Finally, I made the diagnosis.

The exact date eludes me, but my symptom began during the summer of 1990. My wife and I had always gotten up early, to drink coffee and read the newspapers. Then we'd awaken the two children, and our family would have breakfast together. I was forty-two years old, and I had just sworn off scrambled eggs. I was trying to lower my blood cholesterol level by eating a double portion of oatmeal every morning. At first, I thought that my headache was an egg withdrawal reaction. I resumed eating scrambled eggs, and even tried a cheese omelette, but with no relief. We had switched to filtered coffee because of its purported cholesterol-lowering effect. But a temporary return to the pot-brewed variety left my symptom unchanged. Anyway, the oat bran craze seemed to be fading. A few months earlier, new research studies had failed to confirm its salutary influence on blood cholesterol levels. So I stopped the oatmeal. But the headaches still came. A toasted English muffin, dabbed with margarine, turned my vague sensation of fullness into a distinct throb. Had I been more perceptive, I would have realized that the margarine-induced exacerbation of my symptom was a clue to its etiology.

I shall spare you my long list of false leads. For a time, the headache eased. Then, one evening in March 1993, while I was cleaning out my junk drawer under the kitchen counter, I decided to sort through my pile of news clippings. I am a physician, and my patients continually ask me about the latest medical breakthroughs. Trying to keep up, I made a habit of cutting out newspaper articles, which I would file away in a drawer next to the dish towels. I glanced at a headline near the bottom of the pile: THEORY LINKS "GOOD CHOLESTEROL" TO BREAST CANCER.[1] Forget it, I thought to myself. Women who drink alcoholic beverages have higher breast cancer rates and, coincidentally, higher "good cholesterol" levels. It's just a theory, anyway. The clipping was dated June 12, 1990. That was about the time I started to watch my cholesterol. I felt vaguely queasy.

I pulled out another clipping, dated August 16, 1990. The headline read: MARGARINE, TOO, IS FOUND TO HAVE THE FAT THAT ADDS TO HEART RISK. My left eyelid twitched. "Margarine, the spread millions use instead of butter in hopes of preventing heart disease, contains fatty acids formed during processing that actually increase coronary risk," wrote the science reporter. "These fats, called trans monounsaturated fatty acids, were shown in a well-designed Dutch study to raise blood levels of a harmful form of cholesterol and to lower levels of a form that protects against heart disease."[2] Then it happened. Directly behind my left eye, then the right, came the fullness. My headache was back.

I next found a clipping from January 1, 1991, entitled VASEC-TOMIES AND PROSTATE CANCER: A LINK? I began to read: "Two studies suggest that vasectomies might slightly increase the risk of developing prostate cancer, but the researchers caution that the findings are highly tentative and that other factors may be at work."[3] It is ironic, I thought, how this story was downplayed two years earlier. By February 1993, two new reports of higher prostate cancer rates in previously vasectomized men would make the front page and the evening news.[4] While the late-1990 studies suggested that vasectomy might "slightly increase" cancer risk, the 1993 studies showed increases of 50 percent or more. In 1990, the experts said that men with vasectomies appeared to have more cancer merely because they had more checkups with their urologists, who in turn found more cancers. In the 1993 studies, this explanation had not held up. Researchers were now speculating that prostate cancer might be related to decreased prostatic fluid or suppressed immune reactions after a vasectomy. According to an expert quoted in the earlier clipping, "men who had undergone the procedure should not be alarmed." Not be alarmed? I'd certainly be alarmed. My headache had eased.

As I went through my pile of newspaper clippings, I gradually became aware that my headache was exacerbated only by reading specific subjects. Articles entitled ELECTRIC CURRENTS AND LEUKEMIA SHOW PUZZLING LINKS IN NEW STUDY (February 8, 1991) and ELECTROMAGNETIC FIELDS ARE BEING SCRUTINIZED FOR LINKAGE TO CANCER (April 2, 1991) had almost no effect. The same went for MAJOR U.S. STUDY FINDS NO MISCARRIAGE RISK FROM VIDEO TERMINALS (March 14, 1991), and U.S. OVERESTIMATES PERIL OF RADON IN HOMES, NEW STUDY SAYS (March 29, 1991). INNER-EAR DAMAGE LINKED TO JARRING HIGH-IMPACT AEROBICS (December 6, 1990) made only my left eye twitch. Then I came upon CHOLESTEROL CURB URGED FOR CHILDREN OVER 2 (April 9, 1991). The clipping began: "Government health officials recommended for the first time yesterday that children over two years old adopt a low-fat, low-cholesterol diet to prevent heart disease later in life."[5] I felt the throbbing again.

I flipped ahead a full year, trying to confirm the pattern. Reading through PANEL CRITICIZES WEIGHT-LOSS PROGRAMS (April 2, 1992), I felt absolutely fine. Then I found VITAMIN C LINKED TO HEART BENEFIT (May 8, 1992). People who took daily supplements of Vitamin C got fewer heart attacks, said a study. Of course, people who took one supplement could also have taken other antioxidants, such as Vitamin E and beta-carotene, which the body turns into Vitamin A. The latter idea was supported by an earlier clipping (November 14, 1990) entitled VITAMIN A TYPE MAY LOWER RISK OF HEART TROUBLE. Nowhere was there a single incriminating word about cholesterol. I was thinking about how Vitamin C supplements became popular in the late 1960s, just when coronary death rates started falling, when I picked up a clipping entitled HIGH LEVEL OF IRON TIED TO HEART RISK, dated September 8, 1992.[6] This one said that the key to coronary heart disease was iron. Phooey to cholesterol, it said. I felt ill.

I was getting near the top of the pile. An article entitled NOW WHAT? U.S. STUDY SAYS MARGARINE MAY BE HARMFUL (October 7, 1992) described a new Agriculture Department study that seemed to confirm the Dutch study of August 1990. "It's a nightmare," said a specialist in oils. "It's a really nasty thing when you try to explain it. There's total confusion for consumers." In support of the USDA's new findings, the reporter cited the preliminary results of a Harvard study of 85,000 nurses, which had been presented at a scientific meeting the previous June. According to the Harvard researchers, "Intakes of margarine, cookies and cake—major sources of trans isomers—were significantly associated with a higher risk of coronary heart disease."[7] Neither the USDA nor the Harvard study had been published in a peer-reviewed scientific journal. But if these new findings turned out to be correct, then the newly proposed food labels that distinguished only between total fat and saturated fats would go down the drain.[8] After all, trans fats were in some imitation cheeses, frozen fish sticks, ready-made frostings, candies, fast-food french fries, and chicken nuggets. They wouldn't be classified as saturated fats, but they would raise a person's cholesterol, just as saturated fats do—at least most saturated fats. Well, no publication yet. Then I remembered a story I had clipped from the newspaper only a few days before. I hadn't even filed it yet. HARVARD STUDY LINKS MARGARINE TO HIGHER HEART DISEASE RISK, dated March 5, 1993.[9] The pale blue kitchen walls were moving in on me.

I was reasonably capable of blocking out or dismissing any news story on cancer, weight control, exercise, sexually transmitted diseases, birth defects, arthritis, fertility, or menopause. But any mention whatsoever of saturated fat, trans fat, cholesterol, margarine, or heart attacks rendered me instantly symptomatic. And any combination of articles made me claustrophobic.

I had finally made the diagnosis: My headache was precipitated by acute exposure to information.

My experience in the kitchen was hardly the first time I had thought about the ceaseless barrage of health news. Nor was I the first person to realize that the American psyche has been under siege by a well-equipped army of scientific experts, government officials, public health specialists, corporations, and journalists, whose heavy-duty arsenal consists simply of words. Many writers, in fact, had complained about the constant artillery fire of medical stories, government pronouncements, and product claims. So had my patients. Yet no one seemed to have a realistic, practical solution to the problem.

More than a few commentators made a farce of the whole thing. "The right thing to do," wrote one local columnist, "is to pay no attention to this manipulative nonsense and eat a decent breakfast, like Eggs Benedict with Canadian bacon and real Hollandaise or the pastrami hash served at the Bostonian Hotel."[10] Some columnists juxtaposed stories about absurd hazards, such as eyeball injuries from toothpicks or genital trauma from the misuse of vacuum cleaners.[11] The implication was that ordinary people who expressed even a modicum of genuine concern about the latest medical news were self-righteous, overwrought, fanatical "health nuts."[12] As Russell Baker wrote, when we smell sizzling hamburger fat in the restaurant air, we might be inhaling sidestream cholesterol.[13]

Most of my patients adopted a purely defensive strategy, dismissing all medical news stories out of hand. "Don't believe it," became their new mantra of rejection. Who could blame them? The oat bran juggernaut of 1989, crushed by two new studies published in January 1990,[14] was rehabilitated by still newer studies in February and April 1991.[15] When a patient who has been trying to get into shape reads that inner-ear damage has been *linked* to jarring high-impact aerobics, her instant reaction is: Childhood leukemia was *linked* to electric power lines and home hair driers. Miscarriages were *linked* to radiation from computer terminals.

This is not simply a case of cognitive dissonance. True, some scientific findings may upset long-held personal beliefs. But the columnists and my patients were voicing suspicion and incredulity for another reason. If one medical study can be reduced to an absurd joke, if another study is later retracted, if yet another is overridden or contradicted, then *every* new study must be wrong. It's a spillover effect. The problem is that *every* new study isn't a joke. It matters whether margarine raises heart disease risk. It matters whether a high blood level of the so-called good cholesterol enhances breast cancer risk. It's conceivable that vasectomy does raise prostate cancer risk. It's conceivable that Vitamin C supplements do lower heart disease risk. This is serious business, inescapably serious business.

Some authors have suggested various strategies that I would describe collectively as "priority scoring": Don't worry about small risks. Go after the big ones first. Focus on those risks that you can actually reduce, and not on those that are unavoidable or immutable. As attractive as these ideas may appear, they give us little practical guidance. Heart disease and cancer are the major killers in America, and when they don't kill, they still cause pain and suffering. Even a small increment or reduction in these big risks can matter. A sensible reader cannot instantly reject the news about margarine and heart disease, or about antioxidants and heart disease, on the grounds that heart disease constitutes a small risk or that the use of margarine and vitamin supplements is beyond our control. The fact that a person may already have taken other sensible risk-reducing measures, such as controlling blood pressure or quitting smoking, does not eliminate her need to make decisions about margarine or vitamins. One cannot simply ignore the news stories on vasectomy and prostate cancer, because prostate cancer is no small risk for American men, striking over 130,000 annually.[16] One can choose whether to have a vasectomy and, once it's done, whether to have it undone. It's not beyond our control.

The admonition to ignore small risks doesn't tell us how to gauge health risks, or how small is small enough. Is the risk of leukemia from hair driers unquestionably small? It may very well be, but that's a problem for experts in mathematical risk assessment. It's not the sort of calculation that a reasonably intelligent lay reader is prepared to make on the back of the newspaper five minutes before the kids will be getting up. What's more, a negligible risk for one person may be a significant risk for another. AN ASPIRIN EVERY OTHER DAY IS FOUND TO REDUCE MIGRAINES, ran an October 3, 1990, headline from my pile of clippings. Is the risk of migraine small? It depends on your gender, for one thing. (Women have migraines about three times as often as men.) Is the risk of ulcers or bleeding problems from aspirin small? That sounds like a question only one's doctor could answer after a full medical evaluation. ASPIRIN FOUND TO AID SOME PREGNANCIES, said another article

from my pile, dated June 14, 1991.[17] How much might a low
dose of aspirin, taken daily during the last six months of pregnancy, reduce the risk of delivering a dangerously small baby?
Answering that question requires a highly individualized
assessment of one's underlying risk of having a premature
newborn.

In another article, dated January 31, 1991, a medical expert
"ranked the value of the various recommendations in preventing particular diseases, based on thousands of studies among
people around the world."[18] For breast cancer, a triple check-
mark (meaning "highly effective") was given to a low-fat diet,
and a single check-mark (meaning "somewhat effective") was
assigned to a high-fiber diet. This priority scoring certainly
jibed with my January 18, 1990, clipping entitled REDUCING FAT
MAY CUT RISK OF BREAST CANCER. But after reading FIBER IS LINKED
TO REDUCED BREAST CANCER RISK on April 3, 1991, a lay reader
might wonder whether a high-fiber diet shouldn't get two
checks. And after reading BIG NEW STUDY FINDS NO LINK BETWEEN
FAT AND BREAST CANCER on October 21, 1992, which also
reported that a high-fiber diet afforded no protection, the
same reader might very well toss the entire scoring system in
the can.[19] Of course, it's not that a priority-scoring strategy is
such a bad idea. The real problem is how to update the scores
when new information comes in. There's just no simple formula or rule for doing that.

Still other commentators have offered various strategies
that I would place under the rubric of "information management." These are basically simple rules of thumb for deciding
when the ordinary lay reader should pay serious attention to a
news story. Unfortunately, none of these rules constitutes a
genuine substitute for critical thinking. One oft-repeated dictum, for example, is that the source of the report matters. The
public should attach more weight to a study published in a
peer-reviewed scientific journal (especially if there is an editorial in the same issue) than to an unpublished report that came
out of a medical meeting or a news conference. Corollaries to
this rule are that studies from Harvard deserve more attention
than those from Podunk, and that research sponsored by government grants counts more than industry-sponsored studies.[20]

That's fair enough. The February 8, 1991, story on electric

currents and leukemia was based on a preliminary summary of
a study distributed by an industry group; and the April 2, 1991,
story on electromagnetic fields was based on a draft report
from a government agency. But the news story on Vitamin C
and heart disease that appeared on May 8, 1992, came from a
study that was supported by government grants, conducted by
a research team at UCLA, and published in a peer-reviewed
scientific journal. The late-1990 wave of vasectomy-prostate
cancer studies was likewise published in a peer-reviewed journal.[21] And the 1993 wave of vasectomy studies, which appeared
in the *Journal of the American Medical Assocation,* even merited
an editorial.[22] The first study on margarine and cholesterol,
published on August 16, 1990, appeared in the *New England
Journal of Medicine,* and the editorialist, who held that butter is
still worse than margarine and that consumers should reduce
all fats, didn't exactly trash the Dutch researchers.[23]

There is no simple rule by which an intelligent lay reader
can automatically assign "credibility points" to a news report.
Anyone who seriously thinks that Harvard research should get
more points than UCLA research is advised to contemplate
whether the Agriculture University in Wageningen is the
Dutch equivalent of Harvard or Podunk, taking into account
that the lead author was a fellow of the Netherlands Heart
Foundation. The November 14, 1990, news story on beta-
carotene and heart disease came from Harvard research, but it
was based upon only a preliminary presentation at a scientific
meeting. That doesn't mean it should be discounted. The
October 7, 1992, news story on margarine cited an unpublished USDA study, as well as a preliminary report of a Harvard study of 85,000 nurses that had thus far been presented
only at a medical meeting. I discounted the latter only to find
it published in the *Lancet* a few months later. The two 1991
research studies that rehabilitated oat bran both acknowledged "support" by the Quaker Oats Company.[24] One was published in the *American Journal of Public Health* (along with an
editorial) and the other in the *Journal of the American Medical
Association.* One simply cannot use the fact of company support—technical or financial—to destroy their credibility.

Next in line after credibility scoring is "publication counting." Readers are advised not to heed a new research finding
until it is retested and independently confirmed. Science is

fickle. We should wait for scientists to make up their minds.[25] I
have often wondered how ordinary consumers are to apply
this dictum without a personal computer, a high-speed
modem, and a free on-line account at the National Library of
Medicine. So far, four studies have found a relation between
vasectomy and prostate cancer, while three studies have been
negative. Anyone who merely kept count of publications
wouldn't have the slightest notion of what to do next. In 1991,
many experts recommended a low-fat diet to prevent breast
cancer. Then, in October 1992, a new research study appeared
to contradict the low-fat diet–breast cancer hypothesis. The
issue is not whether the pro-low-fat publications have a 500-
plus batting average, but whether the most recent contra-low-
fat study was a home run.

A more sophisticated information management strategy is
to suspend belief of any medical finding that derives from "epidemiology." This rule is embodied in the well-worn but insidi-
ous proposition that statistical association cannot prove cause
and effect. All the studies of vasectomy and prostate cancer
were epidemiological. No researcher randomly assigned large
numbers of human subjects to vasectomy or no-vasectomy. The
men in these epidemiological studies made their reproductive
decisions themselves, not as part of an experiment but in the
natural course of their lives. To reject these epidemiological
studies with pat slogans about statistics is to abandon critical
judgment. When experts say that "other factors may be at
work," they are obligated to name those factors. They cannot
hide behind unsupported assertions that men with vasectomies have different sexual habits than other men, and that
these unspecified differences in sexual habits somehow affect
their cancer risks. No formula or rule of information management can extricate us from the genuine possibility that vasectomy might increase one's cancer risk.

Of course, there is a much simpler strategy: stalling. This is
actually a common feature of the check-who-paid-for-it, ignore-
Podunk, wait-for-peer-review, look-for-confirmation, and beware-
epidemiology approaches. The main difference is that it isn't
necessary to give a specific excuse for stalling. After all, people
with high blood cholesterol levels don't die from heart attacks
overnight. They have time to wait and see what happens. The
problem with this approach is that waiting is not a viable alter-

native for everyone in all circumstances. You have to decide whether to have a vasectomy. You have to decide whether to buy an electric hair drier. You have to decide whether to take high-impact aerobics. You have to decide whether to enroll in a commercial weight-loss program. You have to decide whether to have sex with someone.

One cup of filtered coffee, one bowl of oatmeal, and one pat of margarine are not going to change my coronary risks. Nor are ten of each. But at some point, they'll begin to matter. I started to worry about my cholesterol at age forty-two. The news stories about cholesterol in children suggested that I should have started to worry about it forty years before. Now I am forty-five years old. Can I still wait? At some point, I have to face the fact that the cumulation of my lifetime dietary choices matters.

Quite apart from these strategies, one can take refuge in fatalism. This is perhaps the second favorite approach of my patients. Cousin Cornelius did everything right. He watched his cholesterol. He stopped smoking. He went walking and jogging. And he got some weird blood cancer in his sixties. So there. But Cornelius may have stayed vigorous enough to tolerate multiple bouts of chemotherapy, radiation, and bone marrow transplantation. In a genuine sense, his efforts paid off. His quitting smoking helped to cure his cancer. Of course, Cornelius might still die after a second bone marrow transplant. But that's no excuse not to try one's best.

If there is a common element to all these strategies, it is best summarized by the word *skepticism*. My patients who flatly reject the latest studies are, in a sense, only the most extreme skeptics. But where is the line between skepticism and escape? Are all the commentators and columnists, with all their suggested approaches for dealing with the glut of medical information, actually telling us no more than to run away from it?

For a time, I thought I had the answer. After all, this well-equipped army of scientific experts, government officials, corporations, and journalists basically had only one weapon in its arsenal: words. The problem, so I thought, had to be in the words themselves. The important medical questions of our day were couched in a strange language that prevented us from seeing the answers clearly. In the translation from scientific parlance to ordinary discourse, important words had lost their meaning, had an entirely misleading import, or never had a meaning. If one could reframe the issues properly, redefine the words properly, then everything would be cleared up.

Without doubt, language matters. People would make better decisions if they knew what "good cholesterol" and "saturated fat" and "antioxidant" and "coronary heart disease" actually meant. But my idea turned out to be, at best, only partly right. One cannot keep redefining every misleading word every time the newspapers or TV specials publicize another medical breakthrough. It is not simply a matter of sending lay readers to science journalism seminars. Most serious journalists have already been to these seminars, and they are still struggling with difficult questions about the best way to communicate. If tomorrow night, after you've finished this book, some serious-looking reporter on the evening news described a new study to the effect that sleep causes colon cancer—with eight to nine hours producing a 50 percent increase in risk, and nine-plus hours doubling the risk—I wouldn't be there to tell you what the words mean.

The answer, I came to understand, had to be an attitude, a philosophy, a way of thinking. So I started out with a basic proposition. Some will label me a highfalutin existentialist. Others will brand me one of those low-life economists. The basic proposition is this: We cannot escape our choices. Some risks of everyday living are unavoidable. Others are avoidable, or at least reducible. But our decisions are unavoidable. We do not and cannot know everything. We make mistakes. But we have to choose.

Some of our personal health choices may have immediate, life-threatening consequences. Others have distant consequences. But in the end, they are all matters of life and death. When we decide whether to have sex, we face the distant, deadly risk of death from HIV. When we decide what to eat, day after day, the consequences of our choices add up, and those consequences can, in the end, be just as deadly.

The answer, I came to understand, is not to dodge the mortar fire of medical information but to confront it, to charge into battle, to attack. That's how my headache went away.

In the chapters that follow, ordinary people will make choices in the course of their everyday lives. Their stories are fictitious

composites of thousands of stories that I have heard. But they
are nonetheless real people. They did not all go to medical
school or get a Ph.D. in biochemistry. They're not all experts
in anything. They've read the newspapers, watched the
evening news, talked to their friends, and checked with their
doctors. In every case, we catch them as they are about to
make a decision. Our heroes don't attend medical consensus
conferences, or perform a computerized biomedical literature
search, or take a jet to consult a world authority. They don't
ponder epidemiology, or decide whether a researcher is credible, or verify that a medical study has been replicated. They
just choose.

Their choices are not easy. In fact, some of their choices are
unthinkable, even unbearable. But they make them anyway.
Someone named Dinah will decide whether or not to have
unprotected sex with a man named Caleb. The consequences
of this absolutely ordinary choice include the possible transmission of the deadly AIDS virus. The consequences may be
unthinkable, but the choice is real. Someone named Ruth will
decide whether or not to have a double mastectomy to prevent
possible breast cancer. Her sister and mother already have
breast cancer, and a cousin has ovarian cancer. She has no
alternative but to decide. We shall not dodge Ruth's choice
either.

Not every choice will seem so momentous. Stephen will
decide, after ten minutes of a bench-stepping aerobics class,
whether or not to continue. Eve will decide whether or not to
stay on the telephone line while she waits for a sales representative from a commercial weight-loss program. Gideon will
decide what to order for lunch and dessert at a French restaurant. Andrew will decide whether or not to try, once more, to
quit smoking. None of these mundane choices is a matter of
immediate life and death. But all are, in the long run, deadly.

These decision makers are all different. They all have special circumstances. They each see themselves as special,
unique. And they are. That is one important reason why we
need to examine their decisions in context. To ask whether
the latest medical stories on margarine or vasectomies or Vitamin C or oat bran are credible or actionable is to ask questions
out of context. Without individual facts, without concrete
details, the issues become vapid, stale, lifeless. When it comes

to diet and cancer, or diet and heart disease, the question is not what *one* should eat, but what *Gideon* should eat, what *I* should eat, what *you* should eat.

There will not necessarily be a correct answer. Even after we thoroughly dissect each choice, even after we examine the relevant facts, even after we show empathy and compassion for our decision makers, there will be room for disagreement. The medical experts may not agree with me. You may not agree with me. And even when we all agree on the best choice, our heroes sometimes do the wrong thing. That's because they are real people. They are imperfect.

Ruth's decision about preventive mastectomy may seem like a once-in-a-lifetime choice. It is and it isn't. If she decides not to have an operation, she will decide again tomorrow. She will decide whether it's worth staying on a low-fat diet in an attempt to prevent cancer, or having regular mammograms, or taking antioxidants, or undergoing prophylactic chemotherapy with tamoxifen. Dinah will decide whether to have sex with Caleb. If they continue to see each other, she will decide again tomorrow, and next week, again and again. Whatever Gideon has for lunch on a particular Friday afternoon, there will be saturated fat and monounsaturated fat and trans fat in every lunch of every afternoon. Our heroes' choices are recurrent. They add up. Their consequences accumulate. What will matter for Stephen, in the end, is not whether he finishes one aerobics class but how many years he persists with his attempts to stay physically active.

We are all different. The warnings and advisories and health messages that we receive day after day are meant for us all collectively, but for none of us individually. They apply only to a fictitious, representative person. What is true for this nonexistent typical person may not necessarily be true for us. When Eve decides whether to enroll in a weight-loss program, she doesn't care whether the average person drops out after a month, or how many pounds the average person loses, or what the average person's chances are of weight regain. She wants to know her own chances. She doesn't want to know whether diets do or do not work for the average person. She wants to know what weight-loss strategy will work for her. To answer these questions, Eve may need to learn more about herself. She may need to make several tries until she finds the way.

This is not an easy task. It will be no easier for Andrew to find the best strategy to quit smoking. Since we are all different, we cannot always adhere to standard procedure. We have to navigate, to find our own way.

When we make our choices, we weigh benefits against costs. We balance the good against the bad. Sometimes the benefits so outweigh the risks that our choices are unequivocal. Andrew's decision about his cigarette smoking is not whether to quit, for that isn't a decision at all. The real issue is how to quit. For Gideon, the choice is different. He will eat the beefsteak that his colleague James orders for him. He will then be faced with a choice of dessert. Yes, the steak does contain cholesterol and saturated fats. No, Gideon hasn't necessarily made an egregious error. Perhaps there were superior choices on the menu. But Gideon does not eat cholesterol and fat and protein and carbohydrates and selenium. He eats food. Food is a complicated mixture with many chemical components. Gideon's choice is not about eating only good food. It's about eating food that contains more good than bad.

Will Dinah live happily ever after with Caleb? Will Eve manage to control her weight? Will Gideon prevent coronary heart disease? Will Stephen keep exercising and drop dead from a heart attack anyway? Will Ruth contract breast cancer anyway? Might Andrew still end up with emphysema? Or get hit by a car crossing the street? In the final analysis, none of our heroes' lives are under their full control. Plain luck matters. They can do the right things and still die grisly, premature deaths. Or they can make massive errors and get away with it. They cannot foretell the future, but they can make reasonable forecasts. In fact, in Ruth's choice, forecasting is exactly what she most needs to do. Ruth will have to speculate about the status of breast cancer diagnosis and treatment over the next decade. She has no choice but to do so. Whatever happens to our decision makers, they do not shirk.

In *The Butter Battle Book, by Dr. Seuss*, the Yooks eat their bread with the butter side up, while the Zooks eat theirs with the butter side down. The book ends with Grandpa Yook telling his grandson to "Be patient. . . . We'll see. We will see. . . ."[26]

In a sense, you are about to read *The Margarine Battle Book*, or at least *Son of Butter Battle*. No, I did not give away the punch line on Vitamin C and heart disease. I really didn't commit myself on margarine. For that matter, I've got a lot of explaining to do. What, exactly, is a trans fatty acid and a saturated fatty acid? What is good cholesterol? What, come to think of it, is coronary heart disease? Does a low-fat, high-fiber diet, in fact, offer no protection against breast cancer?

This book will not be just about on which side of my English muffin the margarine goes. For example, the best way to avoid HIV is to abstain or to engage in protected sex. Everyone knows that, right? Then why doesn't everyone do it?

2

The Deadliest Choice
Sex and HIV

I am not the surgeon general of the United States Public Health Service. But if I were, I would feel duty-bound to introduce a chapter on the heterosexual transmission of AIDS with the following pair of warnings:

WARNING: HIV, the deadly virus that causes AIDS, can infect any human being. Any person who has been infected by HIV can transmit the virus to his or her sex partner. HIV-infected people may look perfectly normal. They may be unaware of their infection, or they may not reveal it even if they know.

WARNING: To avoid contracting HIV, don't have sex with anybody. Failing this, have sexual intercourse only with one permanent partner who is proven to be uninfected and who, in turn, continues to have sex only with you. Failing this, the inserting male partner must wear a properly lubricated, intact latex condom along the entire length of his penis from the onset of his erection until after his complete withdrawal. A new latex condom is required for each and every sex act.

I do not have a teenage son or daughter, not yet. But if I were advising my adolescent child on sex and AIDS, I would send basically the same message as the surgeon general. To be sure, I would add some words about unintended pregnancy and sexually transmitted diseases other than AIDS. I would point out the pitfalls in too hastily equating sex with love. I would explain how alcohol and street drugs can alter judgment and self-control. I would talk about integrity and self-worth, about sex and personal responsibility. Still, the bottom line would be much the same. Sex is natural and important, but it's also a risky enterprise. Don't have sexual intercourse, I'd tell my teenager, until you're grown up and have chosen a permanent partner whom you are certain is uninfected and loyal to you. If, for any reason, this no-sex rule is broken, then use a latex condom each and every time.

So much for preliminaries. The remainder of this chapter contains subject matter that I would dare not broach as a parent or, in loco parentis, as a public health official. In what follows, I speak to you as an adult.

I am innocent of plagiarism. I did not lift the foregoing warnings from a government publication. The drafting is mine. Most surgeons general, in fact, have not been so explicit about condom use. Nor am I guilty of setting up a straw man. The words in the boxes, along with the optional special message to teens, constitute the standard American prescription on sex and HIV.

This standard message has many variations. At one extreme, federal health officials have withheld grant funds from organizations whose educational materials did not pass an "obscenity test" or did not promote abstinence above all else.[1] At the other, the November 1992 issue of *Cosmopolitan,* in a special section on "What Women Should Know About AIDS," acknowledged that most of us cannot be absolutely sure about our partners' promises of sexual fidelity or not sharing needles, so if you have sex, use a latex condom. Even a negative antibody test is no guarantee against recent HIV infection, *Cosmo* explained, because it can take up to six months for the fact of infection to show up as a positive blood test. The man should also wear a condom during mouth-to-penis sex, *Cosmo* noted, because it is possible to become infected orally.[2] The December 1991 issue of *Newsweek*, in a cover story on "Safer Sex," urged women receiving oral sex to use a dental dam, a flat latex device that is hand-held over the vagina.[3] Magic Johnson, however, in his 1992 book, noted that the latex in dental dams is not the same kind of latex used in latex condoms, but that the use of some kind of barrier during cunnilingus or anilingus, even household plastic wrap, is better than no barrier at all.[4]

All these variations and subthemes, however, do not belie the basic consensus: Sexual abstinence prevents HIV transmission. Failing that, practice permanent mutual monogamy with a proven-negative partner. Failing that, use condoms. This hierarchy of choices is implicit in virtually every message transmitted by TV newscasts, magazine features, newspaper editorials, celebrity videos, and public service advertisements.

But the message is defective. A disturbing, nearly unspeakable question has been left unanswered: *If not abstinence, then monogamy. If not monogamy, then condoms. If not condoms, then what?*

The standard American prescription on sex and HIV is starkly framed in black and white, as if there were no reasonable middle ground between chastity and protected sex, no room for judgment on the part of thinking adults, no nuances, no shades of gray. There is zero risk and there is positive risk. Any course of action other than complete abstinence, total monogamy, or absolute adherence to condoms entails a positive risk. And a positive risk is bad, unmentionable, unthinkable, because HIV is deadly.

Yet all over America, night after night, ordinary, well-meaning heterosexual men and women are violating the sharp-line prescriptions. They're taking their chances without knowing absolutely everything about their partners, without total insistence on zero risk, without knowing for sure. Some of these rule breakers are, no doubt, taking unreasonable risks. Others, perhaps, are not. One way or another, the plain fact is that the vast majority are not coming down with HIV, and they know it. What's worse, they know that the basic American decision-making paradigm on sex and AIDS is an illusion, a fantasy, a shadow backlit from a perfect platonic world. These men and women aren't misinformed. They're not out of the loop. They hear the message. They understand the message. They ignore the message.

They ignore it not because they are bad people, or immoral people, but because they are fallible people. Having heard the message, they go home, close their doors, and decide whether, with whom, and how to have sex. Looming over their decisions is the risk of contracting a viral infection with the deadliest of consequences. The consequences are deadly, but the choice is, ironically, mundane. These people cannot and do not expect to erase every scintilla of risk. In the ordinary course of everyday life, they—all of us—routinely face distant death as best as they can.

If we are breaking the surgeon general's rules—and I shall shortly convince the diehard skeptics that this is doubtless true—then how should we think about our sexual choices? If we do not absolutely toe the mark, do we have any other options? The media, the public health authorities, the scientific experts, the socially responsible corporations, and the charitable foundations cannot tell us. To do so would be to suggest the unsuggestable, to broach the unbroachable. The senders of the mainstream message on sex and HIV are trapped into a corner. They are compelled to give us advice that seems distant, sometimes irrelevant, to our everyday conduct. But we, the decision makers, are not trapped. We have choices. The transmitters are slaves, but the receivers are free men and women.

I am not downplaying the heterosexual transmission of human immunodeficiency virus in the United States or any other nation. I do not deny that heterosexually transmitted HIV infection abounds in certain sub-Sarahan African countries and is spreading rapidly in some parts of Asia and South and Central America. In fact, the apparently low proportion of heterosexual AIDS cases in the United States is a misleading result of the very high numbers of infections transmitted by man-to-man sex and by needle sharing. Nor do I deny that in percentage terms, heterosexually acquired infections, especially those contracted by young American women, may now be growing at a faster rate than other types of HIV infection in this country. In fact, in those inner cities where injection-drug use is widespread, the second-wave heterosexual HIV epidemic is already in progress, with as many as one in fifty women of childbearing age currently HIV-infected.[5]

I am not minimizing the risks of other sexually transmitted infections. The same Americans who take their chances on HIV are concurrently risking syphilis, hepatitis B, gonorrhea, chlamydia, herpes, chancroid, genital warts, bacterial vaginosis, and trichomoniasis, to name a few. Those sexually transmitted diseases (STDs) are no picnic either. Advanced syphilis can cause brain damage; chronic hepatitis B infection can cause liver cancer; and pelvic inflammatory disease from gonorrhea or chlamydia can cause female sterility. But let's not get sidetracked. We lived with those STDs before the first AIDS cases were identified in 1981, before the discovery of HIV in 1983, before the HIV-antibody blood test was invented in 1985. Back then, before HIV, local school governing boards and PTAs all over America weren't debating whether schools should distribute condoms, or whether teachers should even mention condoms. Back then, people weren't convicted of attempted murder for intentionally transmitting HIV to their unknowing sex partners.[6] HIV framed the public dialogue. HIV made the difference because HIV infection ultimately leads to AIDS, and because AIDS, with few exceptions, is deadly.

I am not pronouncing the public health establishment, the surgeon general, the media, the opinion makers, or anyone else as misguided or obstinate. I don't begrudge them. As I shall explain later, there are good reasons why they need to say what they say. Nor am I espousing an entirely new point of view. In the past few years, the medical literature has contained sporadic protestations over "absolutism" and "perfectionism" and the "all-or-none approach" and two-faced messages that say one thing and mean another.[7] I am not lambasting the scientific community for failing to come up with useful findings on sex and HIV. Quite the contrary, washloads of valuable information are readily available in the public domain. The information is out there, but it's been bleached, decolorized, squeezed through perfectionist rollers, and wrung absolutely dry.

As American adults, we want to know how to *eliminate* risk but also how to *reduce* risk. We seek information that helps us to discriminate between higher-risk and lower-risk sexual encounters, so that we can decide ourselves how much precaution is warranted. We want information that permits us to tailor our choices to personal circumstances. What we get instead are sanitized dicta on abstinence, monogamy, and condoms, imposed upon us as if we were bad kids who didn't know any better, as if our every sexual encounter were tantamount to a death sentence. And the whole time, we're trying to determine whether we're at risk at all. The public dialogue is so narrowly framed that important facts fail to register. They slip by.

It is undoubtedly correct, as stated in my opening surgeon general's warning, that HIV *can* infect any human being. But is it possible that some humans might be *more* susceptible to HIV infection than others? If so, might there be some means, however imperfect, to assess a person's susceptibility? It is probably correct, as the warning states, that any HIV-infected person who is physically capable of sex *can* transmit the virus to his or her partner. But does that mean that *every* HIV-infected person is *equally* infectious? If not, might there be some method, however imperfect, to assess a sex partner's infectivity?

It is certainly true, as the warning states, that HIV-infected people *may* look perfectly normal. But are they *likely* to look normal? How about those who are most infectious to others? Do they look normal, too? *Perfectly* normal? It is entirely accurate, as the warning states, that HIV-infected people *may* not reveal the fact of their infection. But does that necessarily mean *all* of them will conceal it? If not, then what are the best ways of finding out? What are the right questions to ask?

The warning states that, failing abstinence, you should engage in sex with a one *permanent* partner. But exactly how long is *permanent*? Suppose that your boyfriend or husband slept with other women in the past but has been faithful since he met you. If he had been infected by another woman two years ago, then his chances of having AIDS by now would be less than one in twenty. If he'd been infected four years ago, his chances would be only one in eight. By nine or ten years, it would still be only one in two.[8] Do we therefore conclude that men who have been faithful to their partners for ten years still need to get tested for HIV? Or else use condoms? Is there no other information that would help one decide?

The warning states that a new latex condom is required for each and every sex act. This admonition is based on the entirely accurate proposition that HIV infection can occur during a single exposure to the virus. But does it necessarily mean that every sexual contact is equally dangerous? Is there absolutely no information out there, however imperfect, to help a man or woman decide when it is most or least important to insist on a condom? It is indeed accurate that one can contract HIV orally.[9] But does that necessitate the use of a latex condom during every instance of mouth-to-penis contact, or of a dental dam during every instance of mouth-to-vagina contact? Is there no alternative to a latex condom, even a *partially* effective alternative?

There are surely skeptics who believe the foregoing questions to be irrelevant. The emergence of HIV, they will contend, has transformed the American sex scene. People are heeding the warnings on abstinence, lifetime monogamy, and latex condoms. Behaviors have changed. The message has gotten through. Not so.

Sexual initiation before entrance into high school has become commonplace. Loss of virginity before graduation is the rule. In a 1990 nationwide survey of 11,600 high school students, one-third of the males and one-fifth of the females had had sexual intercourse before the age of fifteen, while almost two-thirds of the males and over half of the females had lost their virginity before age seventeen. By senior year, three-quarters of the males and two-thirds of the females had done it. And not as a one-time experiment. Forty-two percent of high school boys and 36 percent of high school girls had had sex during the preceding *three months*. By senior year, more than half of both men and women are sexually active. About one in four high school boys and one in eight high school girls has already slept with *more than three* different people. By senior year, the four-partner threshold was surpassed by three out of eight males and one in six females.[10] Other surveys show similar trends in early sexual initiation, continuing sexual activity, and multiple lifetime partners among white, black, and Hispanic teenagers, among high school students in different metropolitan and rural areas,[11] and among drug users and "good kids" alike.[12]

High school students use condoms in the minority of their sexual encounters. In the 1990 nationwide survey, 49 percent of sexually active males and 40 percent of females said they had used a condom the last time they had sex.[13] In nonschoolbased surveys, even lower rates of condom use have been reported.[14] There is little evidence that these low rates of condom use are caused by teenagers' somehow missing the message on sex and HIV.[15] In 1988, 93 percent of students in the San Francisco Unified School District knew that anyone infected with the AIDS virus can infect someone else during sexual intercourse. So did 90 percent of the teenagers incarcerated in a San Francisco adolescent detention center.[16] In 1989, the departments of education in ten major cities reported that 74 to 98 percent of students knew that sexual intercourse without a condom puts you at risk for HIV.[17] By 1991, five out of every six high school students nationwide had received classroom instruction on HIV.[18] Most teens say they have talked about HIV with their parents,[19] and most parents report discussing AIDS with their children, especially those parents who have seen public service messages on radio or TV.[20]

Studies of male and female college students show similar trends in sexuality.[21] Seven out of eight women who consulted gynecologists at one university student health service in 1989 were not virgins.[22] Nearly three in four had had sex with more than one man, and 21 percent had slept with *more than five* men in their lifetimes. Almost every nonvirgin had slept with a man during the past year, and one-quarter of them had slept with three or more men. The majority of women students admitted to being worried about HIV, and almost half thought their partners might even be at risk for HIV. Yet only 46 percent of the nonvirgins reported "always or almost always" using a condom during sexual intercourse. Condoms were more frequently used by college women in 1986 and 1989 than in 1975, during which time there had been a big drop in the use of birth control pills. The rising popularity of condoms seems to have resulted not so much from the students' concerns about HIV and other STDs as from widespread publicity about the dangers of the pill.

The explosion of teenage and college-age sex is not a passing fad, but part of a well-documented long-term national trend.[23] In fact, by every measure, sexual activity among all adult Americans has been on the rise for decades.[24] Three underlying forces are most responsible for this long-term trend: increased postponement of marriage; increased divorce and separation; and more reliable methods of contraception. These forces are now so ingrained and so powerful that it seems inconceivable that current trends could be significantly reversed, even by a continuous barrage of messages on abstinence and monogamy. After a decade of TV specials, public service announcements, magazine articles, and videos, the vast majority of the American population, even the most disadvantaged and least educated, has seen or heard the message on sex and HIV.[25] Yet there has been at best a minor dent in the seemingly impervious American sex machine.[26]

Survey upon survey belies the myth of the monogamous American. In the National AIDS Behavioral Surveys of 1990–91, which polled over 8,200 adults in twenty-three cities, 18 percent of heterosexual men and 7 percent of heterosexual women reported having had sex with more than one partner in the preceding year. Broken down by marital status, that's 28 percent of never-married adults; 17 percent of separated, widowed, or divorced adults; and 3 percent of married or cohabiting adults. Broken down by age, that's 22 percent of eighteen- to twenty-nine-year-olds; 12 percent of thirtysomethings; 7 percent of people in their forties; 4 percent of people in their fifties; and 3 percent of those aged sixty to seventy-five. While 12 percent of eighteen- to forty-nine-year-olds were non-monogamous during the preceding year, about 43 percent had had multiple partners within the past five years.[27]

A person with two or more sex partners did not necessarily sleep with them concurrently. Perhaps there was a series of successive relationships with one partner at a time, each of which was at least temporarily faithful. The problem with this "serial monogamy" interpretation is that many adults have multiple partners within a very short time interval. The 1988 National Survey of Family Growth, for example, found that over 4 percent of women aged fifteen to forty-four had had multiple sex partners during the past three months alone.[28] For divorced and separated women, the three-month multi-partner rate reached 9.5 percent. In the 1988 General Social Survey, 6 percent of men and 1.2 percent of women aged eighteen to forty-four reported sex with at least one casual date or pickup during the past year. What's more, 4.6 percent of never-married men under age thirty and 2.9 percent of never-married men aged thirty to forty-four years had had sex with *ten or more* women during the past year.[29] We cannot escape the conclusion that many heterosexually active American men and women have no serious relationship with their sex partners.

But do they use condoms? While drugstores have reported a recent boost in retail sales,[30] the answer still remains, at best, sporadically.[31] When the National AIDS Behavioral Surveys asked adults who had had multiple sex partners in the past year, 38 percent reported no condom use, and 17 percent said they always used condoms, while the rest used them sometimes. When the researchers polled adults whose main sex partner was non-monogamous, had injected drugs, or had a positive HIV blood test, they found that 70 percent never used condoms and only 13 percent always did.[32]

Similarly low rates of condom use have been found among heterosexual white, black, and Hispanic men and women,[33] among male and female injecting-drug users and their sex partners,[34] and among men and women who attend STD clinics.[35] A person with multiple partners is, in fact, less likely to use condoms with his or her "steady" partner than with other casual partners.[36] Prostitutes likewise use condoms much less often with private sex partners than with commercial partners.[37] Most of the five hundred million condoms purchased annually in the United States are probably used by married couples for contraception.[38] Many of these couples have switched to condoms because of the widely publicized side effects of the birth control pill and IUD. More than a few condoms are no doubt being purchased by millions of homosexual American men.

To create an intelligible, realistic framework that helps us to make our sexual choices, we need a context, a set of relevant facts, an example. To that end, I ask you to consider the unique choices faced by a hypothetical person named Dinah. You might imagine that you have just rented a newly released video entitled *Dinah's Choice.* You rewind the tape to the start, and begin to play. At critical junctures, you hit the PAUSE button, and we discuss what's transpired. Then you hit PLAY again, and we repeat the process. We can even speculate what might transpire before the tape resumes. The fact that you're viewing a videotape, however, should not alter your perspective. Dinah's story is fictitious, but her problem is real.

It is, of course, impossible to construct a meaningful story about sex and HIV that is devoid of moral overtones. Accordingly, lest you reject Dinah's predicament out of hand, I make a preliminary request: Withhold judgment. Agreed? Rewind the tape and press PLAY:

Dinah is a thirty-two-year-old, recently divorced woman with two young children. One weekday evening after work, at the WestSide Fit-Club, while her mother is still watching the two kids, Dinah gets into an extended conversation with thirty-eight-year-old Caleb.

This isn't Dinah's first encounter with Caleb. Once or twice, he helped her rack some dumbbells. Occasionally they made small talk, and they always smiled and said hello at the water cooler. Caleb, she now learns, has been divorced a lot longer than she. He is of the same race and religion. He does not look kinky or weird. While Caleb doesn't say it outright, he sends unmistakable signals that he's tired of all the dates he's had since his separation, that he wants to settle down.

Dinah, for her own reasons, decides that Caleb's the one for her. Still wearing her leotard and aerobics sneakers, she says to herself: "Come on, Dinah, just do it. Play hard. Go for it." Were it not for the deadly risk of HIV, she would entertain the idea of sleeping with him. After an hour or so, Dinah actually finds herself sitting in Caleb's car. "Where to?" he asks.

PAUSE: The list of potential objections to this story is virtually endless. You may argue that Dinah ought to be spending her free time with her kids; or that she, as a recent divorcée, ought to be staying away from romance right now, concentrating instead on getting her act together, acquiring more marketable skills and, ultimately, a better job. Without denying the merit of such objections, I ask you to accept Dinah's predicament, to try to decide what you would do in her position. Resume PLAY:

Dinah was just a kid during her premarital courtship, but she's all grown up now. And her mother isn't there to wave a finger at her; she's back at her own house giving her two grandchildren a bath. Dinah knows all about birth control. She used the pill before she had the kids, and a diaphragm with spermicidal jelly after the youngest was born. She still has her diaphragm at home, but hasn't used it since her separation. Dinah has read and heard all about sex and HIV in newspa-

*pers and magazines and on television. Yet this evening, none of that
seems to be terribly helpful. She did watch one TV program where somebody in a white coat pinched the little receptacle at the tip of a latex
condom, then unrolled it onto a banana. But Dinah herself has never
touched a condom in her life.*

PAUSE: Having had sex with other women before he met
Dinah, Caleb has already broken the rule on abstinence or
permanent mutual monogamy. For that matter, so has Dinah.
Dinah and Caleb aren't teens anymore, so nobody can admon-
ish them to abstain until adulthood. They cannot be revirginalized.[39] Having been through at least one courtship and marriage, neither Dinah nor Caleb is completely naive. Nor are
they so intoxicated or so horny that they cannot exercise judgment. Both are divorced. Adultery is not an issue. Now resume
PLAY:

*Dinah directs Caleb to her place. She asks him in for a drink. He
accepts. The kids, she thinks to herself, can sleep at Grandma's; it
won't be the first time. Dinah and Caleb are sitting together on a sofa
in her living room, beers in hand. She is trying to remember whether
her old tube of spermicidal jelly has passed its expiration date. They
talk. Then, a kiss. Caleb excuses himself to go the bathroom. As he gets
up from the sofa, Dinah can see him unbuttoning his shirt.*

PAUSE: Dinah's ultimate objective is to establish a long-term
monogamous relationship with Caleb. She may be taking a
chance—a very big chance—but the best time to start that
relationship may be tonight. Within the next fifteen minutes,
Dinah will decide whether to have sex with Caleb. If she
chooses to have sex now, then she will also need to decide
about contraception, as well as protection against HIV and
other STDs. But those aren't Dinah's only choices. There's a
lot more for her to think about tonight.

Whatever Dinah chooses tonight, it will not be the last of
her decisions. If she defers sex now, and if she and Caleb continue to see each other, then she will surely face the same decision somewhere down the road, maybe this weekend, maybe
next month. If she has sex with Caleb and employs a condom
tonight, then she will need to decide whether to use a condom
on each subsequent sexual contact and, eventually, when not

to use one. Whatever she decides tonight, Dinah will have to decide anew tomorrow and tomorrow.

Dinah wants to know whether Caleb is HIV-infected. More precisely, she wants to know how likely it is that Caleb might be HIV-infected. Even more precisely, Dinah weighs her degree of suspicion that Caleb is HIV-infected against many other factors in deciding whether, when, and how to have sex with him. I have framed Dinah's decision in probabilistic terms because there is no practical way that Dinah can monitor Caleb's present and future HIV status with absolute certitude. Even if he had a negative HIV-antibody blood test just last week, it is still entirely possible that he might have contracted HIV within the last few months, but hasn't had the infection long enough for his body to produce the antibodies necessary for a positive blood test.[40] Even if he kept notarized copies of his medical records in the glove compartment of his car, Dinah would still need to rely upon his promise that he had no recent sexual contacts and had not shared needles or other drug-injection equipment with an illicit drug user. The uncertainty is intrinsic to Dinah's decision-making problem. It is not simply a limitation of current technology. Even if Caleb had an affordable, reliable, and rapid HIV blood test tonight, Dinah has no guarantee that Caleb won't contract HIV tomorrow, next week, or next month. In theory, we may contemplate Caleb's getting a gold-standard HIV blood test in advance of each sex act. But in practice, Dinah will at some point need to assess the credibility of Caleb's promises of continued faithfulness. There is really no way around it.

Dinah and Caleb could try to play strictly by the rules. They could defer all sexual intercourse until they got tested for HIV antibodies. If they were both HIV-negative on the first go-around, then they could both promise to remain abstinent for six months, when a second set of blood tests would be performed. If these tests were also negative and if the pair continued to remain faithful, then they might have unprotected sex thereafter. Alternatively, Dinah and Caleb might engage in protected sex, possibly tonight or on some future date, and continue to use latex condoms during every sex act until they got the results of their first round of HIV-antibody blood tests. If the blood tests came back negative, then Dinah might decide that Caleb's fidelity is unquestionable and that a sec-

ond test is unnecessary. She might even decide thereafter to
stop using condoms. But these aren't the important cases. We
want to know what happens if Dinah breaks the rules tonight,
if she commits even a minor infraction, if she and Caleb conduct their lives as real, fallible American adults.

I now want to play out four possible scenarios. In no way have I
tried to exhaust all potential outcomes. Nor have I arbitrarily
manufactured these scenarios. My goal is to make Dinah's
choices concrete, to create a context. We are still on PAUSE.
We're merely contemplating what might transpire, not what
actually happens:

*SCENARIO #1: Dinah asks Caleb about his sexual history, as well as
HIV testing. Caleb says that he tested negative "about six months ago,"
that he's had sex with only one unnamed woman since he took his
blood test, and that this unnamed woman told him that she had a negative test, too. Attaching significance to the fact that Caleb doesn't
appear weird or kinky, Dinah does not press him about other partners
or sources of HIV exposure in the months immediately preceding or following his negative HIV test. Nor does she inquire about exactly when
his nameless other partner took her HIV test. She decides to engage in
mouth-to-penis sex tonight, without a condom, bringing Caleb to
orgasm but paying careful attention not to permit his semen to pass her
lips. She defers any future decision about penis-into-vagina intercourse. She will see what develops in their relationship. If any suspicious information on Caleb should later come to light, Dinah thinks,
she can broach the subjects of condoms and testing at that point.*

*SCENARIO #2: Dinah specifically asks Caleb whether he ever injected
drugs, ever had an HIV blood test, ever had sex with another man, or
ever had sex with a prostitute. Caleb says no, no, no, and yes but just
once, in connection with a bachelor party. Dinah excuses herself to
find her diaphragm in the medicine cabinet, whereupon she returns to
the sofa to ask Caleb how many women he's slept with since his separation. Caleb doesn't remember, but regardless of the exact number, he
says they were "all nice girls," just like her, except for the call girl that
one time. Dinah returns to the bathroom, checks again that her
diaphragm is intact and fits snugly, and that her spermicide hasn't
passed its expiration date. For good measure, she applies extra spermicide directly into her vagina. At least she has contraception, Dinah*

thinks. She knows that her diaphragm, which is up against her cervix at the back of her vagina, cannot shield the rest of her vagina or her external genitalia from HIV. But she recalls reading that spermicidal jelly contains a detergent (nonoxynol-9) with at least some HIV-killing effect, at least outside the body. Returning again from the bathroom, she asks one final question about Caleb's willingness to make a long-term commitment. He answers in the affirmative, whereupon Dinah accepts Caleb's potentially deadly penis, uncloaked by a condom, just this once.

SCENARIO #3: Dinah asks him about protection, and Caleb says he has it. Somewhat surprised, Dinah asks him whether he was planning to seduce her. Caleb says that he uses condoms because "I care about myself. As a matter of fact, I care about us both." He fetches his three-condom packet from the glove compartment of his car. Only two condoms are left. The first one looks dried, brittle, and unusable, so they discard it. Unfortunately, Caleb loses his erection after the last remaining condom is already in place on his penis. When Dinah tries to arouse him again, the condom tears on her ring. Dinah takes Caleb's willingness to use a condom as a sign of his commitment and caring. Making no further demands or inquiries, she decides to have condomless sex, at least tonight. She'll get some fresh condoms tomorrow.

SCENARIO #4: Caleb returns shirtless from the bathroom. Dinah offers to give him a back rub, thinking that she'll go all the way. She notices a red bumpy rash over most of Caleb's back. Caleb says that he's seen two dermatologists, who both told him it was some kind of oily skin condition. Suddenly frightened, Dinah explains that she's got to get her children from her mother's place. She walks him back to his car.

Each of these scenarios appears quite different, yet they all share a common feature. Dinah has to rely upon imperfect information about Caleb. She also has had to consider how she might acquire better information about him. In scenario #1, Dinah considers it informative that Caleb doesn't appear weird or kinky. She finds his description of his sexual past sufficiently informative to engage in oral sex but not vaginal intercourse. In scenario #2, Caleb's disclosures alone are insufficient, and Dinah remains unsure until she finally receives his assurance of a long-term commitment. In #3, Dinah takes

Caleb's willingness to use a condom, and his statement of caring "about us," as favorable signs. In #4, she sees his rash as a telling sign. There is, of course, considerable room for disagreement about Dinah's interpretation of these assurances, acts, and signs. But they constitute information, just the same.

Before she decides whether, when, and how to have sex, Dinah collects information. Can she possibly acquire the information she needs in the next fifteen minutes? What additional information on Caleb might be forthcoming over the next few days and weeks that she could not acquire tonight? How might the prospect of additional information affect her decision about sex tonight, or tomorrow?

Dinah's problem is fundamentally one of timing. She wants to advance her relationship with Caleb, to move from a transient smile and hello at the health-club water cooler to a lasting intimacy. But she also needs time to learn about her partner. Should Dinah adopt a holding strategy? Should she temporize until she gets more information on Caleb? Was Dinah's decision to have only penis-into-mouth sex (scenario #1) a reasonable, low-risk temporizing strategy? Was her decision to have penis-into-vagina sex with a diaphragm and spermicide (scenario #2) pushing her luck? At some point, Dinah may believe that she has learned enough about Caleb to engage in unprotected sex. It is conceivable that she already knows enough. But did Dinah go just a bit too far in trusting Caleb when the last condom broke (scenario #3)? She planned to have unprotected sex just once. Is that such an unreasonable risk? Dinah could conceivably learn something about Caleb in the next fifteen minutes. In fact, as we will soon find out, there's a lot she could learn about him. But was Caleb's rash (scenario #4) really a telling sign? Did Dinah overreact when she walked him out?

If Dinah ever intends to have a relationship with Caleb, she needs to ask questions and he must answer them. Even more crucially, Dinah needs to evaluate the credibility of Caleb's answers. Asking the right questions is a difficult task. It requires skill and no little bravery. In each scenario, one might argue that Dinah doesn't ask enough questions, that she believes Caleb too soon, or that she doesn't trust him enough. One way or another, asking questions and assessing the credibility of the answers is a central part of Dinah's choice. Word-less sex is not an option.

My prefatory surgeon general's warning, however, doesn't suggest a single question that Dinah might ask Caleb. Nor does it offer any hints about to how she might react to the answers. In fact, Dinah isn't advised to ask any questions. Instead, she is warned to abstain from sex or to use latex con-doms every time, while Caleb gets tested twice for HIV. Why? Under the standard American paradigm on sex and HIV, Caleb's oral testimony is to be discounted, because Dinah can-not tell for certain whether Caleb has been truthful, and even if he passed a polygraph test, Caleb himself may not know that he's infected by HIV. As *Cosmopolitan* put it: "Most of us can't be absolutely sure about someone else's behavior. . . . Don't rely on someone else's promise to protect your health."[41] Any means of "knowing your partner," aside from serial HIV test-ing, is per se unreliable. The logic of this proposition is so faulty that it destroys the credibility of the paradigm itself.

The American paradigm has a hidden message: If the answer is to be discounted, then the question isn't worth ask-ing in the first place. Accordingly, it's not worth asking whether Caleb has ever been tested for HIV and, if so, when each test was performed and what the results were. It's point-less to inquire whether he's ever had man-to-man sex and, if so, whether another man ejaculated into his rectum. It's a waste of time to ask Caleb whether he's ever visited Africa, whether he's had sex with a person from Haiti, Nigeria, Rwanda, Uganda, or Zaire. It's useless to ask whether Caleb had sex with a person who was sick or who had a positive test, or whether anyone with whom he had sex ultimately devel-oped AIDS, even if that person appeared well at the time. It's pointless, so the message implies, to ask Caleb whether he ever had gonorrhea, syphilis, herpes, hepatitis, or chlamydia; to ask him in nontechnical terms about "bad blood," or the "clap," or "leak," or "drainage," or "coolant," or "bore"; or whether he ever took antibiotics because of a discharge from the tip of his penis; or whether he ever had sores on his penis or his groin that didn't go away.[42]

It's a total waste, according to the paradigm, to ask Caleb whether he ever injected heroin, smack, crack cocaine, speed, or any other street drugs; or whether he ever shared needles or drug-injecting paraphernalia with anyone, including spoons or bottlecaps for heating crystalline heroin and dissolving it in water. Dinah shouldn't even bother, the message implies, to ask Caleb whether he ever traded sex for heroin or cocaine or angel dust or hallucinogenic mushrooms; or whether he ever had sex with somebody in a crack house; or whether he ever gave or received mouth-to-penis sex in return for crack cocaine; or whether he ever had sex with transvestites, street-walkers, or teenage runaways; or whether he has been tattooed recently. Dinah will get nowhere, the message implies, if she asks Caleb whether he's a hemophiliac and received a transfusion of blood-clotting factor; or whether he received a transfusion of whole blood or any blood product from the beginning of the HIV epidemic around 1977, to the point where the American blood supply began to be screened in March 1985.

According to the standard American paradigm, the only interpersonal skills worth acquiring are how to say no to sex, how to ask for an HIV blood test, and how to request and use a condom. But just as a prosecuting attorney asks a defendant his whereabouts on the night of the crime, and just as juries assess the credibility of the witness's answers in reaching a verdict, Dinah must learn to ask questions and assess Caleb's credibility. She must develop the interrogatory skills to ask the right questions. The fact that these skills entail imperfect information-gathering methods does not invalidate them. Nor is the difficulty of learning to ask questions a legitimate excuse not to try.

The magazine features, the AIDS education pamphlets, and the celebrity videos all attempt to teach Americans the required skills to buy, to ask for, to talk your partner about, to put on, and to take off a condom. Caleb's statement (scenario #3) that "I care about us both" is a standard line in many pamphlets that attempt to teach such condom-using skills.[43] I'll have more to say about condoms later. For readers who were unaware that condoms shouldn't be stored in the hot glove compartment of a car, let me say that condom-using skills are not a trivial matter either to teach or to learn. Anyone who has been unable to find an expiration date on a condom without spermicide already knows better.[44] Anyone who's had a semen-filled condom left inside her after her partner's postorgasmic penis got soft already knows better. Anyone who has learned the hard way that too much saliva prevents the condom from gripping the penis firmly and staying on tight while the man moves back and forth inside her already knows better. Anyone who has found out the hard way that an uncircumcised penis with an especially redundant foreskin isn't exactly the same as the banana that Dinah saw on a TV demonstration already knows better. If you happen not to be one of these people, then consider the proposition that condom use entails technical *and* social skills, and that the required social skills are not necessarily less complex or more teachable than the interrogatory skills and credibility-assessing skills that Dinah really needs tonight, tomorrow, and in her every sexual encounter.

Consider the first question Dinah might ask Caleb: "Have you ever been tested for HIV and, if so, when was each HIV blood test performed and what were the test results?" She asks him that in scenarios #1 and #2. That's not a stupid question. Obviously, Caleb might know he's HIV-positive and lie about it, or he might be unaware that he's infected. But one thing is certain. If Caleb tested HIV-negative, he's not going to tell Dinah that he's HIV-positive. In other words, it cannot hurt, and can only help, to ask.

If Caleb knew he was HIV-infected, wouldn't he always withhold this information from Dinah? Not necessarily. In formal research studies, between one-half and seven-eighths of the people who know they're HIV-positive will inform their sex partners, especially their steady as opposed to casual partners.[45] The implication is clear. Dinah is more likely to get a straight answer from Caleb if they're in the midst of an ongoing relationship, and not just a one-night stand. Dinah may still decide that having sex tonight is a prerequisite to a long-term relationship. One way or another, if she can keep going out with Caleb, she will actually "get to know" her partner. And the longer she stays with him, the more she will learn.

But if Caleb were HIV-infected, wouldn't he surely be unaware of it? Again, not necessarily. HIV blood testing is now widespread in this country. In a 1990 nationwide survey, about one-quarter of all American adults reported having had an HIV blood test.[46] While most people were coincidentally tested while donating blood, millions of adults have voluntarily taken an antibody blood test to find out their HIV status.[47] By 1991, about five million Americans had undergone voluntary HIV testing in publicly funded programs alone, of whom 240,000 were HIV-positive.[48] Publicly funded testing appears to identify slightly less than half of all positive HIV blood specimens.[49] Accordingly, by 1991, somewhere between a quarter-million and a half-million Americans actually knew they were HIV-positive. That's nearly a quarter to a half of all HIV-infected Americans.[50] Sure, many people who know they're at risk for HIV infection have refused to be tested.[51] But the inescapable conclusion is that a substantial fraction of HIV-infected people already know their diagnosis.[52] To be sure, many people who know they're HIV-infected have AIDS or advanced HIV disease. But, as I will explain shortly, these are the people most likely to infect their sex partners.

Asking questions and probing answers is not going to identify every HIV-infected person. Still, in research studies, where people fill out anonymous questionnaires and don't have to answer questions face to face, as many as one in three or even one in two of HIV-infected people can be identified.[53] Is one in three really so small? Let's say that Caleb's chances of being HIV-infected are 0.3 percent. Dinah asks him questions, and he says no across the board. She just reduced Caleb's chances of being HIV-infected by one-third, to 0.2 percent. Dinah didn't eliminate the risk. She reduced the risk.

Researchers are currently working on computer programs to screen potential blood donors for HIV infection. These computer programs ask people not only whether they've had an HIV blood test, but many of the same questions I have enumerated. They also ask the potential donor whether he's been sweating so much at night that his pillow and sheets are drenched by morning; whether he's had white spots or unusual sores in his mouth that don't go away; whether he's lost at least ten pounds without explanation; whether he's been constantly running fevers that weren't merely symptoms of a cold or flu; whether he continually has diarrhea; whether he's had lumps in his neck, armpits, and groin for at least a month; whether he's had purplish, discolored areas in or under his skin that were not bruises; whether he's had pneumonia, trouble breathing, or a persistent cough; and whether he's had sex with anyone who had these symptoms.[54]

With so many things to ask, are there any organizing principles that govern the choice of questions? Actually, yes—there are four main categories of questions. One category directly addresses Caleb's past history of HIV testing. A second, related set of questions addresses Caleb's risk of being HIV-infected, including his past sexual contacts, past exposure to blood products, and experience with drugs and injection equipment. The third category probes Caleb's history of sexually transmitted diseases other than HIV. The fourth focuses on the possibility that Caleb not only is HIV-infected, but has advancing HIV disease. (That's why the computer asks potential blood donors about sweats, mouth sores, weight loss, and fevers.) The last two categories are especially important to Dinah tonight, because they speak directly to an issue of immediate concern: Is Caleb a superinfecter?

Let's get back to the problem of holding strategies. In scenario #1, Dinah decides to have oral sex, at least tonight. After that, she'll see how the relationship evolves. In #2, equipped with diaphragm and spermicide, Dinah accepts Caleb's uncloaked penis "just this once." In #3, after the last condom tears, Dinah has unprotected sex, at least tonight. Tomorrow, she'll get more. Although each scenario may entail a different level of risk, Dinah is basically thinking the same way: If she can get through tonight, she'll have more options later.

Just this once. Is there a modicum of soundness to the logic of these words? After all, if Caleb were HIV-infected, what are the chances that he'd give the virus to Dinah in a single act of penis-to-vagina sexual intercourse? Isn't the one-time risk supposed to be very low? Granted, Dinah could fall into the classic trap in which every time is just this one time. Still, doesn't she need to have sex many times with Caleb to build up a significant risk of HIV transmission?

The answer depends not merely upon whether Caleb is infected, but whether he's *infectious* as well. Not every HIV-infected person has the same degree of infectivity. In fact, Dinah's choice of holding strategy tonight hinges critically on whether Caleb might be a *superinfecter.* It also depends on Dinah's degree of susceptibility, for not every uninfected person is equally susceptible to sexual HIV transmission. In fact, some may be more resistant, while others are *supersusceptible.* That means Dinah's got some hard questions to ask herself, too.

You may have read that the chances of male-to-female transmission of HIV in a single heterosexual encounter are well
below one in a hundred, probably closer to one or two in a
thousand. In interviews with the press, and in my own writings,
I have been one of the perpetrators of this wholly misleading
statistic.[55] If the chances were really 0.002 per individual act of
coitus, then mathematically motivated readers could calculate
that Dinah's chances of becoming infected wouldn't pass 50
percent until they'd done it 347 times. But counting numbers
of sex acts is the wrong way of looking at HIV transmission. If
Caleb is a superinfecter and Dinah is supersusceptible, then
they can get the job done in just one shot.

Where did the two-in-a-thousand statistic come from? It's a
misleading average. For some couples—namely, the superinfecters and the supersusceptibles—the chances of transmission
in a single sex act are more like one in five. For other couples,
the chances must be much lower than one or two in a thousand. In fact, they must be minuscule. If Caleb turned out to
be a superinfecter, repeated sex with him would be a death
sentence. It wouldn't matter whether Caleb and Dinah practiced mutual monogamy.[56] In fact, if she didn't get HIV from
him tonight, Dinah would be better off never seeing him
again. What really matters is not how many times you have sex,
but with whom you have sex.

Scientists have studied male-to-female transmission of HIV
by tracking "discordant" couples, in which the male partner
was known to have been infected outside the relationship and
the female partner was known to be uninfected, at least initially.[57] In almost all these studies, only 10 to 30 percent of the
women became infected, despite repeated acts of unprotected
sex.[58] In general, these studies show no connection between
the risk of HIV transmission and the duration of the couples'
relationship or the number of times they had sex.[59] Some
women get infected in one or just a few contacts; others
remain uninfected after hundreds of acts of unprotected sex.[60]
In one study of fifty-five men infected by blood transfusion,
only ten of their wives (18 percent) contracted HIV.[61] One of
the infected wives slept with her husband *just once;* another
had eight contacts since he became infected; and another just
sixteen. The thirty-seven women who didn't contract HIV had
had unprotected sex an average of 156 times. In fact, none of

the women who had unprotected sex over 200 times became infected.[62] The only reasonable interpretation of these studies is that some male-female liaisons are much more prone to HIV transmission than others: The infected man is highly infectious, the uninfected woman is highly susceptible, or the man and woman, acting together, facilitate passage of the virus.

What might make a man a superinfecter? Or a woman supersusceptible? Many possibilities have been explored, but the near-unanimous consensus from the discordant-couple research is that the more advanced the man's HIV disease (that is, the closer he is toward full-blown AIDS), the more likely he is to infect the woman.[63] Moreover, men with a history of STD, and especially those with current STDs, are even more likely to be superinfecters. Likewise, women who have an active vaginal infection or vaginal bleeding are more susceptible to HIV infection.

Many lines of scientific evidence bolster the conclusion that men with advanced HIV disease are much more likely to be superinfecters. Individual histories of known superinfecters are a case in point. In 1985, several HIV-infected Belgian women identified the same man as their sex partner, a civil engineer whom I'll call Augustus. Five years earlier, Augustus had had sex with several prostitutes during a trip to central Africa. At the end of his trip, he ran an unexplained fever (his "primary HIV infection," as I'll explain shortly). When doctors contacted Augustus, he admitted to having genital herpes. On examination, they found swollen lymph glands throughout Augustus's body. His CD4 count, a blood test that tracks the progressive deterioration of the immune system, was way down. Augustus could identify nineteen recent female sex partners, of whom eighteen submitted to HIV testing, and of those eleven were HIV-infected. Four of these infected women had had penis-into-vagina sex with Augustus just two to five times, and two women had slept with him just *once*. Six months later, Augustus developed full-blown AIDS. He was dead in a year.[64]

Clearly, HIV transmission does not necessarily take place every time an infected man inserts his penis and ejaculates into the vagina of an uninfected woman. For transmission to occur, there must be HIV in the infected man's semen, or possibly in an open sore on his genitals. Semen is not the same thing as sperm. The semen is a fluid, manufactured by the man's prostate gland and other reproductive organs, in which sperm cells swim. (The prostate gland is inside a man, situated under the root of a man's penis, its bottom side almost touching the wall of the rectum.) If there is HIV in a man's semen, it will not be inside the sperm themselves. Instead, the virus will either circulate freely in the fluid, or it will be contained in white cells (called "mononuclear cells") that have migrated from the blood to the man's reproductive organs in response to an infection or inflammation.[65] Thus, the semen of a vasectomized man may have no sperm, but it could still contain HIV.[66]

While the field of HIV-semen analysis is still evolving, it has become clear that not every HIV-infected man has HIV in his semen. Among those who do have HIV in their semen, not every man has the same amount of virus. Although the evidence is not airtight,[67] two main identifiable factors appear to influence the amount of HIV in semen: how advanced the man's HIV disease is; and whether he has had a sexually transmitted disease.[68] That's exactly what one would expect from the discordant-couple research and the case histories of super-infecters.

Once a man ejaculates HIV-laden semen into a woman, the virus must then pass through the lining along the sides of her vagina, or possibly through the cervical opening at the back of her vagina, and then get into her body.[69] HIV transmission from man to woman is enhanced by virtually anything that inflames the woman's vagina or cervix, but especially if the woman has a concurrent sexually transmitted infection. These infections cause microscopic tears, which become openings for the virus to enter. STDs also stimulate the flow of blood to the inflamed organs, which in turn increases the chances that HIV will be transported from its entrance point directly into the woman's body. Infections and bleeding disrupt the vagina's natural acidity, which tends to protect against HIV.[70] A woman with an abnormal Pap smear is also more susceptible, because the associated lesions in her cervix create an opening for the virus.[71] A woman who inserts foreign objects or irritating substances into her vagina can also cause tears and bleeding that may help the virus to enter her body.[72]

These facts send a clear message to Dinah. If she has or

thinks she has an abnormal Pap smear, sexually transmitted disease, or vaginal infection or inflammation, she may be a supersusceptible woman, and she'd better think twice about the most appropriate holding strategy for tonight.

There is a widely held perception that HIV-infected people are basically well until AIDS strikes suddenly. One reason for this view is that most people don't publicly disclose their disease until they are very sick. Another reason is the popular scientific explanation of AIDS—the idea that AIDS precipitously occurs when the body's immune defenses have been so damaged that the gates are laid wide open to pneumonia, tuberculosis, toxoplasmosis, herpes, and numerous other infections by bacteria, fungi, and viruses. This catastrophic model of AIDS, however, is incomplete, misleading, and entirely outmoded. In fact, it is so outmoded that scientists are on the verge of abandoning the term *AIDS* altogether, and speaking instead of various stages along the entire spectrum of *HIV disease*.

Once HIV is transmitted to a susceptible person, that person has acquired a *primary HIV infection*. Within about two weeks, but possibly up to twelve weeks, most newly infected people develop an acute, temporary illness that resembles the flu.[73] They have fevers, headaches, diarrhea, sore throats, and rashes; they lose their appetites and feel tired. The illness usually lasts a week or two, but can persist for months. In many cases, the symptoms are so mild that they go unnoticed,[74] but some people are sick enough to be hospitalized.[75] This is the very first illness caused by the AIDS virus,[76] but it is not the same thing as AIDS, which comes much later.

During a primary HIV infection, the virus actually circulates in the afflicted person's blood, a phenomenon called *viremia*. As he recovers from the primary HIV infection, the viremia subsides, and his immune system begins to make antibodies against the virus.[77] Once these antibodies are detectable in the blood, he will have a positive HIV-antibody test. This can happen in a few weeks or a few months. By one estimate, half of the HIV-infected people will still test negatively nine weeks after their primary infection. At six months, one in twenty will still be negative.[78]

Once the primary infection has subsided, HIV doesn't go away. The virus seeds throughout the afflicted person's body, mostly in the lymph nodes and certain white blood cells (mononuclear cells), which serve as the main reservoir from which the virus will spread. From that point onward, it is a chronic, progressive illness called *HIV disease.* During the course of this chronic disease, a sequence of events, spread out over at least two years and often more than ten years, will ultimately lead to the development of AIDS.[79] In particular, the virus progressively infects and destroys a particular set of mononuclear white blood cells (the CD4 cells) that are critical to a person's immunity.[80] As HIV disease advances, the CD4 count in the blood falls.[81] Uninfected people have a CD4 count of about 1,000 to 1,200.[82] By the time a person has one of the serious infections or cancers that characterize AIDS, it has usually fallen below 200.[83] In fact, the Centers for Disease Control now defines a person as having AIDS if his or her CD4 count falls below 200.[84] (When doctors examined Augustus, his CD4 count was down to 108.) As death approaches, the count plummets to below 50 and can reach single digits or zero.[85]

During the course of HIV disease, the virus is periodically released into the blood from infected mononuclear cells.[86] These episodes of viremia become ever more frequent, and with each one the amount of freely circulating virus progressively increases.[87] HIV then spreads to other tissues, including the kidneys, muscles, brain, and other parts of the nervous system. What's more, both free virus and virus-laden mononuclear cells increasingly find their way into the afflicted person's sex organs, including the prostate and urethra.[88] (The urethra is the tube that runs down the underside of a man's penis, connecting to the slit at the very tip, through which urine and semen pass.) Once the virus has seeded the reproductive tract, it gets into the semen. In principle, the virus could seed a man's reproductive tract at any time during the course of HIV disease, and theoretically HIV could appear in the semen of a man with a newly acquired primary HIV infection. Still, the pattern is clear. The more advanced a person's HIV disease, the more frequent the episodes of viral seeding, the more likely it is that HIV will be found in his semen.

As HIV disease advances, HIV-infected people—men and women alike—gradually become ill.[89] They suffer persistent fatigue, fever, night sweats, sore throats, coughs, diarrhea, and

new or unusual bruises, rashes, or skin discolorations.[90] They
have swollen glands, not just in the front and back of the neck,
but also in the armpits and groin. They become short of breath
on exertion, first as a result of anemia and later from respiratory infections. They have headaches, sleeplessness,[91] memory
loss, apathy, inability to concentrate, and depressive symptoms,
all probably a direct effect of HIV on the brain.[92] They get tin-
gling and numbness from nerve damage.[93] Their muscles ache.
They lose ten pounds or more. They have bleeding problems.
As their immune systems begin to deteriorate, they get more
respiratory infections, including bronchitis and pneumonia.
They get viral infections of the eyes. They come down with
increasingly serious yeast infections. The most common, called
thrush, appears in the mouth and is present even in many HIV-
infected people who say they feel well.[94] It often presages more
serious immune breakdown.[95] Women with HIV get chronic,
often severe vaginal yeast infections that do not respond to
medication.[96] They also have abnormal Pap smears.[97]

People with HIV disease can develop these pathological
changes with increasing frequency five years before AIDS
arrives, before their CD4 counts drop below 200, before many
of them even know that they're HIV-infected.[98] By one estimate, a third of HIV-infected people have persistent fatigue,
rash, fever, or thrush as early as two and a half to three years
before they come down with AIDS, when their CD4 counts still
average 500.[99] For every person with AIDS, two additional HIV-
infected people seek medical care, and among those thrush is
present in one-ninth with CD4 counts over 500, one-fifth with
CD4 counts between 200 and 499, and over half with CD4
counts below 200.[100]

In short, not every HIV-infected person looks and feels perfectly normal. This proposition does not contradict my opening warnings. It goes beyond them. It tells Dinah that there are
yet other ways to discriminate between higher-risk and lower-
risk encounters, if only she knows what to look for.

In scenario #4, Caleb returns shirtless from the bathroom, and
Dinah offers to give him a back rub, thinking they'll have sex.
Suppose—just suppose—that Caleb is lying face down on the
sofa, and Dinah is straddled atop his brief-covered buttocks. As
she runs her palms back and forth from the small of his back

to his shoulders, she notices some swellings under his armpits. Caleb turns face up, his head resting on a sofa pillow. Dinah, now facing him, astride his hips and groin, runs her fingers slowly up his chest all the way to his temples. Caleb sighs. Along the way, she feels what seem to be swollen glands in his neck, too. She reaches for a new can of beer from the coffee table. It's still cold. She rubs it over his nipples. Caleb fidgets and laughs. He asks her for a swig. She pops the can open. He opens his mouth, eyes closed, shirtless, waiting. Now suppose—just suppose—that as Dinah is about to pour cold beer into Caleb's open mouth, she notices that his tongue is covered with creamy, white, curdlike patches.

You may now be protesting that Dinah would be incapable of detecting swollen glands in a person's armpits. Or she would be incapable of spotting a yeast infection in a strange man's mouth while straddling his crotch and pouring brew down his gullet. How would she know that the white stuff wasn't left over from something Caleb ate? The answer is that the beer would wash away meringue topping or frozen yogurt, while the patches of yeast would cling to his tongue and the inside of his mouth. What's more, his mouth might look inflamed and his lips may be crusty. If you were a medically sophisticated reader, you might further protest that Caleb's thrush could be caused by something other than HIV disease. He might be taking steroid inhalants for asthma, or he might have been on high-dose antibiotics for some innocent infection unrelated to HIV, or maybe his immune defenses were hampered by diabetes, severe burns, or leukemia.[101] Those are possibilities, but for a thirty-eight-year-old man such as Caleb, HIV disease is the odds-on favorite.

Now suppose—just suppose—that Dinah is waiting on the sofa, but Caleb doesn't return from the bathroom so fast. Five minutes go by, ten minutes, and Caleb's still occupied. Finally, after fifteen minutes, Caleb emerges, ready to receive his back rub. But it's too late. The beers have disappeared. The sofa is empty. Dinah is standing, Caleb's car keys in hand, ready to escort him straight from the bathroom door to the exit.

What happened? Did Dinah see needle tracks on Caleb's forearm when he got up from the sofa? No, it can't be that. She would have seen them long before then, while Caleb was racking the dumbbells in his tank top at the WestSide FitClub.

Was he coughing and short-winded going up the stairs to her place, a tipoff that he had some sort of HIV-related respiratory infection? No, Dinah would also have noticed his breathlessness at WestSide.

What was he doing in the bathroom? Perhaps he had a protracted case of diarrhea. That could be a sign of either primary HIV infection or advancing HIV disease. Or it could be a sign that Caleb is bisexual and has a bowel infection from anal sex. Perhaps Caleb took so long because he had difficulty urinating. That's it. Maybe it was painful to urinate. Maybe a discharge emanated from the tip of his penis whenever he tried to urinate. Maybe he had gonorrhea or chlamydia or something like that. Should Dinah have waited until they got into bed to see if he had a discharge, or open sores on his penis or his groin, or warts or fissures around his anus? No way.

Of course, Dinah wouldn't know for certain whether Caleb had swollen lymph nodes or thrush, and even if he had these conditions, she couldn't be totally sure that they were signs of HIV. And she didn't know for certain why Caleb spent so much time in the bathroom. But we're not going after certainties. We're exploring ways that Dinah can use information about Caleb's physical appearance and comportment to determine whether he might be a superinfecter. Yes, I know that Dinah might not want to hear or see anything bad about this thirty-eight-year-old eligible guy. But let's not go out of our way to insult her. She is entitled to develop the skills necessary to evaluate her sex partner's body and his actions, just as she is entitled to learn how to ask him questions and assess his credibility, just as she is entitled to learn how to use a condom or, for that matter, a diaphragm.

Even if Dinah adopts a completely different holding strategy, even if they have a frank discussion about slow dating and don't touch each other tonight, she's eventually going to look at his body. Even if Dinah plays 100 percent by the surgeon general's rules, she's still got to look. Suppose they decide to sleep together, but only after they both have negative antibody blood tests. Suppose they get married. Two years later, Dinah finds a new ulceration at the tip of his penis. He's coming down with chills and fevers and losing weight. Dinah still needs to learn what these physical signs mean. She cannot ignore them.

Perhaps Dinah's reaction to Caleb's rash, in scenario #4, was not so hasty after all. But what about the bachelor party that Caleb described in scenario #2? Should Dinah make much of the fact that Caleb had sex with a prostitute? After all, it was just once.

In essence, we're asking whether an infected woman can serve as an HIV superinfecter and whether an uninfected man can be supersusceptible. Much less is known about female-to-male transmission of HIV in the United States. Although discordant-couple studies suggest that a man has a much lower *average* chance of becoming infected this way,[102] it could mean merely that there were fewer female superinfecters in the couples under study. A second-wave heterosexual HIV epidemic among women is now under way in the major urban centers. As this female HIV epidemic becomes older, more women will enter the advanced stages of their HIV infections, and more will likely become superinfecters. If so, then researchers will soon find that the female-to-male heterosexual transmission rate isn't as low as we first thought.[103]

In the United States today, some but not all groups of prostitutes have high rates of HIV infection.[104] If Caleb had had sex with a call girl, as in scenario #2, I would have found it disturbing that he did not later have an HIV-antibody test. If I were going to give him the benefit of the doubt, I would press his memory on four points. First, did he or any of his friends develop any STD after the bachelor party? If anyone developed chlamydia, gonorrhea, herpes, or anything else, that would be an indicator that the call girl, too, had an STD. If so, given our current state of knowledge, we have to assume that a woman with an STD is a potential superinfecter.

Second, I would ask Caleb whether cocaine was used at the party, or whether the call girl offered anyone a line of coke. A new wave of syphilis in the United States has been propagated by the spread of cocaine, particularly by the practice of giving mouth-to-penis sex in return for crack. This crack-fellatio-syphilis nexus may also be responsible for the spread of HIV.[105] Third, I would ask whether the call girl had anal sex with anyone at the party, since this might be a clue that she regularly engaged in such a high-risk sexual practice. Finally, I would ask whether any of Caleb's friends may have been a bisexual man, or might for any reason have been HIV infected. If someone like Augustus had been at the party, then the call girl's vagina may have served to expose Caleb to another man's HIV-laden semen.[106]

This is not the place for a lecture on the proper techniques for purchasing, storing, putting on, and taking off latex condoms. Still, I cannot but emphasize that arguments about condoms not filtering every single particle of virus are irrelevant. What matters is not the technical capacity of latex condoms but their success rates in actual use. The fact that a certain percentage of American men and women report using condoms does not mean that they are using them correctly, either for contraception or for the prevention of HIV or any STD.

My own experience in medical practice is that many adults routinely made mistakes when they use condoms. They do not ensure that there is no air bubble at the tip of the condom, so that there will be room for the man's semen when he ejaculates. They don't always unravel the condom with the correct side out. Women don't use two hands when unraveling a condom on an uncircumcised penis, and they fail to start tucking the man's pulled-back foreskin under the rubber after it's been unraveled about a third of the way down. Men and women do not know what size condom to buy, only to find that it does not reach the base of the man's penis. Women use their mouths to stimulate their partners' erections, only to find that too much saliva isn't a good precondom lubricant.

Men and women don't know that the man must withdraw immediately after his orgasm, lest the walls of the woman's vagina start collapsing around his softening penis, thus allowing his semen to leak out the sides. They don't know the correct way to withdraw the penis after the man's orgasm, so that the rim of the condom is gripped together with the penis at its base. Women do not know to keep their legs wide open after the man ejaculates, with their heels remaining atop the man's buttocks, so that either partner can reach under to grasp the rim of the condom. Instead, some women immediately rest their legs flat on the bed after the man stops moving, changing the angle of the vagina and making it more difficult to remove the detumescing penis and condom in tandem. They don't realize that a postorgasmic man may not be able to feel a con-

dom slipping off his penis. They don't realize that if the condom is too short, then its rim can catch on the woman's
fourchette (the little piece of skin connecting the two inner
labia at the bottom of the vaginal vestibule).

One woman who developed gonorrhea in the throat was
unaware that proper prevention technique bars any contact
between a mouth and an unsheathed penis. Strictly speaking,
the woman shouldn't permit a condomless penis to touch her
unprotected labia, clitoris, or any part of the vaginal vestibule,
especially if the man ejaculates while they rub their genitals
together. About the only thing that my patients seem to know
consistently is that salad oil, cooking oil, baby oil, mineral oil,
Vaseline, butter, and margarine are totally inappropriate lubri-
cants to use with a condom.

There is still considerable debate about the degree of protection against HIV and other STDs afforded by other barrier
methods, particularly the diaphragm with spermicide. In theory, these other barrier methods should not be as effective
against these diseases as condoms. But in practice, they may
actually be superior preventive devices, possibly because their
proper use entails only one person's skill and not the cooper-
ation of two people.[107] While the risk of HIV transmission via
mouth-to-penis and mouth-to-vagina sex is probably quite
low, the same can hardly be said about the risk of other STDs
from oral sex, particularly syphilis and gonorrhea. In scenario #1, Dinah attempted not to let Caleb's semen pass her
lips, but we do not know whether it touched her lips or any
other part of her body. We are, accordingly, faced with the
possibility that Dinah's use of a barrier contraceptive with
extra spermicide (scenario #2) may actually have been a
superior STD-preventive measure than oral sex alone. Moreover, as soon as we cross the line from the artificial domain of
absolute certainty into the real world of probabilities, we must
face the fact that Dinah's use of both oral sex (scenario #1)
and diaphragm-with-spermicide sex (scenario #2) as temporizing strategies were far superior to her best intentions to use a
condom (scenario #3).

How did we get into this logjam anyway? Why does the public
dialogue on sex and HIV seem so irrelevant to Dinah's
predicament?

Many analysts see Dinah's problem as rooted in politics. The AIDS information campaigns of the past decade, they argue, were hamstrung by narrow-minded ideologues whose foremost concern was the propriety of uttering the word *condom* in public.[108] This view is, at best, only partly right. Neither the government nor the public health establishment has ever been a monolith. Squadrons of stuck-in-sand zealots have not been the main obstacles standing between Dinah and the facts. There are fundamental constraints on what the surgeon general, or any government official responsible for the public's health, can and cannot say.

From the surgeon general's standpoint, advice on sex and HIV must be extremely conservative. The surgeon general cannot suggest that a small risk of HIV transmission is acceptable, because even very small risks, when multiplied by hundreds of millions of sex acts, could lead to hundreds or thousands of AIDS deaths. This built-in conservatism is enhanced by the one-sided nature of the surgeon general's mission. The public health is advanced whenever the risk of HIV transmission is reduced. But the surgeon general scores zero points if Dinah, Caleb, or anyone else has a meaningful sexual experience.

The surgeon general's inherent conservatism is further bolstered by the communicable nature of HIV. When people decide whether to take their chances with unprotected sex, they're watching out mostly for themselves. To be sure, Dinah may realize that if she should contract HIV now, then she might later harm other innocent persons, especially a future spouse and children. But she's not likely to consider whether a newly acquired HIV infection would perpetuate the epidemic and thus harm the public's health in general. The overall public health, however, is exactly what the surgeon general is supposed to worry about.

There are even more basic reasons why Dinah doesn't find the standard American message on sex and HIV terribly helpful. Public health authorities have strong incentives to target their messages to people at the highest risk of HIV infection. Communication, after all, is expensive. Dollar for dollar, a public service message aimed at sexually active teenagers, or injecting-drug users and their sex partners, or Hispanic and black young women in inner cities is, at least in theory, more likely to reduce HIV incidence than a message tailored to Dinah's or Caleb's personal needs. This inherent bias to communicate with high-risk audiences is hardly lost on Dinah, who discounts the standard messages as being meant for others. The irony, of course, is that teenage runaways, crack-addicted prostitutes, and young gay streetwalkers may follow the same logic—*everyone else* should wear latex condoms every time.

The surgeon general must tell a crystal-clear story. An ambiguous plot may sell movie tickets and novels, but it just doesn't cut it as public health policy. To communicate lucidly, the surgeon general must issue messages that are short, simple, closed-ended, and unqualified. This creates a strong bias toward absolute prescriptions. Never drink and drive; always buckle up. No sex at all; sex forever with one unscathed partner; latex condoms every time.

To tell the public that some condom use is better than none is to declare the self-evident. But that would implicitly condone partial compliance, in other words, unprotected sex. The proper level of condom compliance would then remain open-ended, unresolved, and susceptible to misinterpretation. There would be an implicit message that some degree of risk is acceptable, but the message itself wouldn't give a formula for evaluating the risk. The same goes for the obvious admonition that one should have sex with low-risk partners. The communication is open-ended; it doesn't have an appendix on partner evaluation. To heed the warning, one needs more information that is to be found somewhere else.

The public health establishment does not always follow these rules of communication. A public service advertisement to the effect that "HIV kills" is, by itself, unquestionably simple and unqualified. But the message is instantly transformed when the TV screen flashes the toll-free telephone number for the viewer to get more information. Now the message says: "HIV kills, but there's more to it." But my intent here is not to tell anybody how to do his job. I'm saying that important principles of communication govern the surgeon general's utterances. Purging the politics from public health might be a good idea, but it will not change these principles.

That's why I haven't pronounced the media, the opinion makers, or anyone else as misguided or obstinate. That's why I don't begrudge the surgeon general. My goal is solely to bridge the gap between two sides, to open the channel between the senders of the message and the receivers, the people like you, me, and Dinah, who go home, sit on the sofa, and choose. Now resume PLAY:

Caleb returns from the bathroom. His shirt is buttoned. He is laughing.

"You know, Dinah, you're not gonna believe this."

"Believe what?" *Dinah asks nervously.*

"Well, it's sort of a reproductive issue with me. It's a man's issue."

"What sort of a reproductive issue?"

"Well," *Caleb continues,* "Mary and I thought we'd never be able to have kids. I never understood it, but they said my sperm and her body fluids didn't match. Anyway, just when our marriage was starting to fall apart, Mary got you-know-what."

"No, I don't know what."

"Pregnant. For nine months, she carried Simeon around in her belly. And for nine months, I carried a stone around in my own belly, worrying there'd be something wrong with him, worrying he'd be deformed, or have a fatal disease, or that I'd given Mary something that he'd catch."

"Given him what? Is he alive?"

"Simeon? Of course he's alive. I wish I had custody, damn."

"He's not sick or anything, is he? You didn't give him anything, did you?"

"Oh, no way." *Caleb is still chuckling to himself.*

"What's so funny? Let me in on it."

"Well, you see, I didn't speak a word until I was almost five years old. They thought my mother had 'bad blood.' They thought I'd gotten it from her."

"What's 'bad blood'?" *Dinah asks.*

"Syphilis," *answers Caleb.*

"You have syphilis?"

"No way. Actually, my mother didn't have it either. They call it a 'false positive,' but I guess they didn't know about false positives in those days. Anyway, I just had this terrible fear that Simeon would be deaf and dumb."

"And he's okay? He doesn't have syphilis or anything?"

"No. He's three years old, and guess what: He's a championship talker. But you know what else? He can't say hamburger. He calls it handgerber." *Caleb's laughter is almost uncontrollable.* "You should *hear him say it. You'd double up. And he opened the refrigerator last weekend, and he said, 'Daddy, you have blumberries?'"* Caleb sits on the sofa, guffawing. *"You've got two kids, don't you?"* he asks.

"Uh-huh. . . ."

"I'll bet they'd really like Simeon's company, especially if they're a little bit older."

"Caleb. . . ." Dinah is looking at him.

"Well, anyway, thanks for the beers. I am totally pooped from that workout at WestSide tonight." Caleb gets up to leave.

"Caleb, I haven't had sex in two years."

"You know something, Dinah. We all ought to get together. Next weekend Simeon's staying with me. Anyway, I want to get back and call him before his bedtime."

3

Spring Training
Exercise

Stephen is a forty-six-year-old married professional. For two decades, by his own admission, Stephen's most strenuous regular physical activity has been taking the elevator. Now things are different. Stephen has joined WestSide FitClub. It is 12:11 P.M. on a weekday in early January, and Stephen is exactly eleven minutes into his very first bench-stepping aerobics class. He is wearing his new heart-rate monitor, a holiday present from his wife.

Tamar, the twenty-three-year-old aerobics instructor, can shout and exercise simultaneously. Having taken the class through a ten-minute warm-up and stretching routine, Tamar begins the first in a series of rhythmic, choreographed bench-stepping movements, timed to loud contemporary music, that will continue for the next thirty-nine minutes. Stephen, being a step virgin, has set his adjustable-height stepping bench at six inches.

"Basic sequence, ten repetitions!" shouts Tamar. "Step up right foot, step up left foot! Step down right foot, step down left foot!" The energetic woman directly in front of Stephen knows the moves. "You got it! Now add the arms!" Tamar rhythmically closes and opens her arms, first at the elbows, then at the shoulders. "Up, up! Down, down! Circle right! Circle left! Seven more!" Tamar's arms swoosh in huge arcs.

Stephen is breathless. His arms are fatigued. His thighs burn. He is uncomfortable. He cannot go on much longer.

Imagine that you have been viewing an issues-and-commentary program on network television. The foregoing video vignette was the lead-in segment to a feature story entitled "Stephen's Choice." After the commercial break, we switch locales from WestSide FitClub to the network studios, where a moderator introduces two panelists who, having watched the same segment as the TV audience, are prepared to offer their best advice to Stephen at this juncture. PANELIST ONE is experienced in step aerobics, while PANELIST TWO is plainly not a fitness aficionado.

MODERATOR: *Should Stephen try to finish the class?*

PANELIST ONE: *If the combination of upper-body and lower-body exercise is too taxing for you, Stephen, then stop the arms altogether and just continue with the footwork.*

MODERATOR: *You're saying that Stephen should continue?*

PANELIST ONE: *Use your pulse meter, Stephen. As a beginning exerciser, you want to keep your heart rate between 60 and 70 percent of the maximum for someone your age. Subtracting your age from 220, you'd get a predicted maximum pulse of 174. So your target range is 104 to 122 beats per minute. If your pulse exceeds the 122-beat limit or you feel uncomfortable, then reduce your bench height to four inches. Don't be daunted if Tamar performs advanced movements, such as sideways plyometric lunges. Just keep time with basic, up-down steps. Take breaks to catch your breath. Get some water. Even if you're pooped, come back for the situps and warm-down stretch at the end of the class. Stephen, you're not the first person to go through this. After a while, it gets easier, really. And remember, no one is looking at you.*

PANELIST TWO: *What is a forty-six-year-old professional man doing in a step-aerobics class with two dozen women half his age? Reclaiming his lost youth? He'll burn out in two weeks, maximum three.*

PANELIST ONE: *Step aerobics may not be the optimal choice for Stephen. He might prefer to work his upper body with resistant-tubing aerobics. If WestSide has a pool, he might try aquatic aerobics.*

PANELIST TWO: *Stephen has fallen victim to an aerobics fad. Whatever happened to plain golf? Or plain bowling? Why can't he go out in his yard and rake some leaves? Or shovel some snow? Anybody remember dancing? My co-panelist, the fitness expert over there, would want to know only whether the fox-trot burns more calories per minute than badminton does, or whether the cha-cha works the muscles in your buttocks. Why does ordinary physical activity have to be remade into a butt-busting, body-sculpting, fat-burning, cardio-aerobicized workout?*

ONE: *Stephen doesn't have to take any aerobics class. He could take a brisk walk on the treadmill instead. The important thing is that he exercise sufficiently to get his heart rate into the target aerobic-training range for at least twenty minutes three times per week. As his fitness improves and he tries to raise his pulse to 75 or even 80 percent of maximum, he might work up to jogging. If he still wants to work his buttocks and thighs, he might try a computerized stair-climbing machine. He could program it for high-intensity intervals.*

TWO: *Stephen is breathless and uncomfortable. Can we be confident he isn't having chest pain, too? Do heart problems run in Stephen's family, especially heart attacks before age sixty? Does Stephen have diabetes? Does he smoke cigarettes? If Stephen had undetected coronary heart disease, he could conceivably drop dead at the age of forty-six, right in the middle of his first aerobics class.*

ONE: *If Stephen has been sedentary for so long, he probably needs some strength work, too. On Mondays, he could do horizontal barbell bench presses and supplementary dumbbell flyes. That would work his pectorals, his back, and his triceps, too. On Wednesdays, he'd do biceps curls and maybe military presses for his shoulders. On Fridays, he could do leg extensions and work his way up to barbell squats. He could do aerobics on the alternate days and take Sundays off.*

TWO: *Even if he doesn't drop dead, Stephen could still hurt himself seriously. He could blow out his pectorals on the bench press, tear his rotator cuff in the military press, or strain his lower back on the squats, trying to lift too much weight.*

ONE: *Stephen should learn proper weight-lifting techniques. He should increase the weight to be lifted by 5 percent only after he can perform two sets of ten repetitions unassisted. A regular spotter wouldn't hurt, either. Stephen's a professional, so maybe he can afford a personal trainer.*

TWO: *Just imagine poor Stephen magnificently attired in a panoply of overuse injuries, inflamed tendons, bone spurs, and stress fractures.*

ONE: *You're exaggerating.*

TWO: *Exaggerating? Why are sports medicine and physical therapy booming businesses? Ever seen people drudging through these aerobics classes with orthotics and knee braces? Is that what Stephen wants from his twenty minutes three times a week, from his com-*

puter-programmed high-intensity intervals, from his sideways plyo-
metric lunges? Bad knees?
MODERATOR: *Heart attack or no heart attack, bad knees or good knees,*
why is Stephen exercising at all? What are his goals?
ONE: *Maybe he wants to improve his cardiovascular endurance.*
Maybe he wants to add bulk to his major muscle groups, thereby bol-
stering his self-esteem. Perhaps he's trying to strengthen a weak
lower back. Perhaps he wants to burn off his accumulated abdomi-
nal fat. Maybe he's trying to keep his blood pressure down.
TWO: *Maybe he doesn't have a clue why he's exercising.*
MODERATOR: *What form of exercise is right for Stephen? How many*
times per week should he exercise? How hard and for how long
should he exercise each time? Should Stephen continue the aerobics
class? How much exercise is enough? We'll tackle these and other
critical questions—and find out what actually happened to Stephen
in Tamar's class at WestSide FitClub—when we come back.

Fadeout to local stations.

You may have already taken sides. Or you may have a different
view of Stephen's predicament than either of the panelists.
Whatever position you adopt, you would undoubtedly prefer,
as a TV viewer, to see an entirely new and authoritative person
intrude upon the scene after the station break and politely set
ONE and TWO straight. After that, the producers could put
Tamar on camera at WestSide FitClub for her commentary,
and then segue to breathless Stephen for the wrap-up. Thesis,
antithesis, and synthesis. What a show. Except for one thing:
What does this new character say?

If I could book myself a guest appearance on "Stephen's
Choice," here's what I would say:

ME: *Neither panelist looked at Stephen's choice from the proper angle.*
The whole argument was wrongly framed.
MODERATOR: *What is the proper angle? Should Stephen try to finish*
Tamar's class?
ME: *Stephen, you need a long-term perspective. Don't focus myopically*
on the next five minutes of aerobics. Don't worry whether your pulse
is always in range or you're burning enough calories. Don't get
hung up on this week's or next week's exercise schedule. Don't get
frazzled if you miss your regular workout, or if you can't lift the

*same weight as last time. Don't overanalyze whether the treadmill is
inferior or superior to the stair-climbing machine.*

*You're forty-six years old, Stephen. Keep moving. Stay active. But
do not confuse activity with athleticism. Remind yourself that there is
a vast middle ground between supreme fitness and total immobility.
Take precautions, Stephen, yet try to progress, to get better, to attain
competence. But do not confuse physical competence with physical
prowess. And be sure to take rests, for that will make you a true athlete. Don't seek a magic formula for the intensity and frequency of
your physical activities. Instead, seek variety in their intensity and
frequency. As your body progressively ages—and it will—adapt to
your new physical limits. Don't be afraid to change. Above all, think
in terms of years. Think five years, ten years, twenty years.*

*In twenty years, when you're sixty-six years old, when Tamar is
forty-three, who will remember whether you finished this or the next
fifty step-aerobics classes? In twenty years, it would matter little that
you were a serious aerobicizer or even a marathoner for one or two
years if you went back to elevator-only mode for the remaining eighteen years. It would matter little that you had an injury at age fifty-
three if you made a comeback at age fifty-four. What will ultimately
matter, what you'll feel, is the cumulative effect of your entire
twenty-year career of physical activity.*

*How much exercise is enough? It's an interesting question, and
it's certainly not a trivial matter, especially if one's focus is the next
five minutes or the next six weeks. But the answer is secondary.
What matters, Stephen, is how long you persist.*

MODERATOR: *That's all we have time for.*

ME: *But there's a lot more to say, especially about persistence—*

MODERATOR: *Thanks to all of our panelists. We'll return to Stephen
and Tamar at WestSide FitClub right after this short break.*

Exercising my prerogative as author, I shall now divulge everything that I was about to say on the air before the moderator
cut me off. Then we can find out what happened to Stephen.

PANELIST TWO threw a lot of different punches. One set of
attacks was aimed directly at Stephen, at his allegedly unrealis-
tic goals, at his supposed lack of insight. Stephen was the victim of a fad, said TWO, trapped in a youth-regeneration fantasy,
thrashing his arms and straining his thighs without a clear
notion as to why.

This criticism is unfair. It is certainly possible that Stephen has joined WestSide without the slightest fore-thought; that he has hooked up his pulse meter without know-ing how to use it; that he has ventured randomly into his first aerobics class without any notion that it could be so difficult; and that he is now absolutely paralyzed as to what to do next. Even if that were true of Stephen, it would hardly be a fair crit-icism of the millions of other Americans who, like Stephen, have tried or contemplated resuming physical activity at some time in mid-life. Most people in Stephen's shoes would have some idea why they're exercising. They would have some type of exercise plan, even if merely a short-term one. And they would have some reasonable expectations about the benefits and risks of such a plan.

A second set of attacks was aimed not at Stephen but at exercise itself. Even if Stephen does not die from a heart attack, said PANELIST TWO, he'll incur all sorts of pulls, sprains, tears, fractures, and whatnot. Implicitly, the dangers of exer-cise outweigh the benefits.

This attack is overbroad. It is conceivable that Stephen does have a significant family history of premature heart attacks; and that he has bounded into Tamar's class, intending to push himself to the limit, without so much as discussing the possibil-ity of an exercise stress test with his doctor. But, again, that's not a fair characterization of the typical forty-six-year-old per-son who has just joined a health club. Regular physical activity can have important benefits, which I shall discuss shortly. It would be unreasonable to claim that, for every person engag-ing in such physical activity, the attendant risks of sudden death, heart attacks, and overuse injuries generically outweigh the benefits.

The third set of attacks, aimed at PANELIST ONE, was the most subtle and yet the most potent. TWO accused ONE of sci-entizing ordinary physical activity, of wanting to know how many calories the fox-trot burns. PANELIST ONE's technical-sounding recommendations were echoed mockingly: "Is that what Stephen wants from his twenty minutes three times a week, from his computer-programmed high-intensity intervals, from his sideways plyometric lunges? Bad knees?" PANELIST ONE was sardonically labeled "the fitness expert over there."

PANELIST ONE is a pseudo-scientifico, a pseudo-athletico, and, by innuendo, a fraud.

Is this third criticism so far-fetched? It's not that PANELIST ONE said anything off the wall. Still, there is an artificial rigidity in ONE's approach, a false precision that strains credibility. Would Stephen gain no benefit if he exercised only nineteen minutes three times per week? Would all be lost if Stephen's heart rate fell outside the target range? Must Stephen strengthen every major muscle group in his body? Would it be so terrible if he increased his dumbbell weight by 6 percent, instead of 5 percent, and after he had completed only one set of nine repetitions instead of two sets of ten?

Why must PANELIST ONE translate the exerciser's subjective sensations into objectively defined end points? Why must Stephen "improve his cardiovascular endurance" or "add bulk to his major muscle groups"? Why can't he merely "feel better" from exercise? Even the MODERATOR has been co-opted, asking the panelists and the television audience about the recommended frequency, duration, intensity, and modality of exercise. It's as if physical activity were a subdiscipline of subatomic physics: decomposed and quantized into calories, heartbeats, repetitions, intervals, and muscle fibers.

Something lies hidden between the lines of the thousands of messages about getting in shape and working out that are transmitted day after day to Stephen and his fellow Americans. What lies hidden, what goes unstated, is a specific scientific model of physical activity, which I shall call the *training paradigm*. The problem is not that the training paradigm is scientifically invalid, or even that it's scientific. The problem is the translation from scientific model into popular discourse.

Properly and fully stated, the training paradigm has three components: the *training effect;* the *overtraining effect;* and the *detraining effect*. In our culture, the first of these components has been vastly overplayed; the second has been misunderstood; and the third has been all but ignored. The end result is a framework for our popular discussions of exercise that is scientifically rooted but painfully misleading.

Hundreds of scientific studies have shown that people who exercise can achieve measurable physical and psychological benefits after a relatively short period of time, usually within a few weeks. These short-term improvements are known collectively as *training effects*. In most studies, little or no improvement is observed unless the person exercises a specific number of times per week at a specific level of intensity and for a specific amount of time, and unless he or she continues the specified exercise regimen for a sufficient number of weeks. The basic idea is that the human body adapts favorably to specific types of salutary physical stresses, provided that these stresses are sufficiently large and are repeated sufficiently often. These stresses (or *training stimuli*) actually produce minor but reversible injuries, and the favorable adaptations are part of a repair process that shields the body from further similar insult. The aphorism "no pain, no gain" is an oversimplified description of training adaptation. More accurate is: "If the stress is inadequate or too transient, then the body won't adapt to it."

Some scientists narrowly apply the term *training effect* to a specific bodily adaptation to regular aerobic exercise, which I shall discuss later on. Here, I use the term broadly. If Stephen found it progressively less taxing to perform step aerobics, to the point where he could use both his arms and his legs or increase the bench height, then that would count as a training effect. If Tamar progressively gained upper-body strength and endurance from lifting free weights, or from rowing or swimming, then those, too, would count as training effects. So might improvements in Stephen and Tamar's balance and coordination, or changes in the distribution of their body fat, or increases in the density of their bones.

In *overtraining*, by contrast, the physical stress is too intense or too frequent, or it is applied for too long. As a consequence, the body maladapts. In simplistic terms, "too much pain, no gain." For every training effect, there is a corresponding overtraining effect. If Stephen has a heart attack from going whole hog in an aerobics class, that would be an overtraining effect. If Tamar develops a stress fracture in her ankle from teaching too many high-impact aerobics classes, that would be an overtraining effect. If Stephen performs barbell squats so frequently that his thigh and buttock muscles have no time to recover, to the point where his strength actually deteriorates, then that would be an overtraining effect. In the first example, the physical stress is so intense that Stephen's circulatory system breaks down. In the second, Tamar's ankle-bone is stressed so frequently that it does not have time to repair itself. In the last example, the stress is applied so often that Stephen's muscles do not have sufficient time to dispose of metabolic waste products, to load up new energy stores, and to grow bigger fibers.

In *detraining effects,* the body's favorable adaptations go away when the salutary physical stresses are removed. In simplistic terms, "stop the pain, lose the gain." For every training effect, there is also a corresponding detraining effect. Just as training effects can develop in a few weeks, so detraining effects can occur within a matter of weeks. Detraining, however, is not exactly the reverse of training.

Remember the energetic woman directly in front of Stephen? Let's say her name is Rachel. She knew the arm-and-leg combinations so well that she didn't have to think about them. She could easily get through the class with an eight-inch bench. That includes even Tamar's lateral plyometric lunges—alternating sideways leaps, where one foot lands atop the bench and the other foot lands on the floor. Rachel has been trained in step aerobics. Now suppose that Rachel volunteers to participate in a scientific study, in which she is put on complete bed rest for a whole month, after which she would be allowed to get up and return to Tamar's regular noontime bench-stepping class. What would happen?

Rachel would still remember virtually all the choreographed bench-stepping movements, because they have been hard-wired into the nerves that connect her muscles to her brain. These neuromuscular learning effects, which develop after hundreds and thousands of repetitions, can take a fairly long time to go away. On the other hand, Rachel would be far more breathless and uncomfortable than before. Her body would have lost much of its previously acquired ability to absorb oxygen from the air, to pump it through her blood-stream to her muscles, and to use it as an ignition spark for leg stepping and arm waving. Rachel would not be in the same shoes as Stephen, but she would have lost most if not all of her aerobic fitness.

This is obviously an extreme case that I have manufactured to make a point. If Rachel had forgone step aerobics but was allowed to maintain a sedentary life-style for a month, the deterioration of her aerobic fitness would be less extreme. If she had been permitted to take regular brisk walks on a treadmill during that time, the detraining would still occur, though it would be even less extensive. And if she went jogging for a month, she may still have had difficulty with Tamar's lateral plyometric lunges, because such sideways movements require certain muscles that are not used during straight-ahead jogging and because Rachel's lateral-movement muscles would have been detrained.

The short-term nature of training effects contributes to the misperception—better still, the illusion—that "getting in shape," "firming up," and "becoming fit" are achievable in the here and now. But the overtraining phenomenon reminds us that these gains in well-being and performance cannot be achieved so quickly, because the training stimulus can't be applied too hard or too fast. What's more, the detraining effect tells us that such short-term gains can just as rapidly evaporate when one removes the training stimulus and stops exercising. To "stay in shape," "stay firm" and "stay fit," one must continue the training stimulus, in measured quantities, over the longer term. Pulse meters, dumbbells, and computerized stair-climbers alone won't do it. You need *persistence*.

Back to Rachel. Two months after her return to regular aerobics classes, Rachel had still not lost the five pounds she gained during her layoff. Nor did she feel as energetic, strong, and flexible as she used to. On Tamar's suggestion, Rachel increased her step-aerobics frequency from four to seven days per week. After two months of daily classes, Rachel was chronically tired, slept poorly, and had actually gained five more pounds. This was a very difficult period for Rachel, who, unlike Stephen, had never been a sedentary person. After two years of trial and error, Rachel finally found the right combination of jazz dance, martial arts, and outdoor bicycling. She took only an occasional aerobics class. Rachel's sequel is not about short-term training but about a wholly different phenomenon: long-term *progression*.

At the same time that Stephen joined WestSide FitClub, his old college classmate Raphael decided to run the local marathon, an event held annually in the fall. It being early January, Raphael started a regular walk-jog routine on an indoor track, going twenty minutes three times per week. By late January, he could walk-jog thirty minutes at a time. By mid-February, he was up to four sessions weekly. At that point, Raphael could jog continuously for thirty minutes with no need for intervening walks. Raphael had achieved a short-term training effect. Now he was ready for the marathon, right? Obviously not.

I shall omit Raphael's checkered transition from indoor track to outdoor running, with its uphills and downhills, wind and puddles, dogs and cars. By early fall, Raphael was actually jogging on the road for fifty continuous minutes five days per week. Then, on a brisk Sunday, as planned, Raphael went for his first ultradistance run. Two hours later, he returned with severe tendinitis and horrible blisters. After a two-week rest, he tried again, but felt inexplicably tired and unmotivated. Thoroughly disheartened, Raphael stopped running altogether. A month later, he agreed to coach intramural soccer, running behind the kids on the field. At the end of the soccer season, after a good rest, Raphael resumed jogging. He vowed never again to prepare for a marathon.

As both Raphael's and Rachel's stories suggest, long-term progress is not necessarily achieved by a steady, monotonous increase in the training stimulus. It is not merely the accumulation of lots of smaller short-term training effects. There are long-term cycles of overtraining, detraining, and retraining. There are plateaus, valleys, and peaks.

As soon as we start talking about long-term progression, our parlance becomes far less scientific. This is to be expected. Scientists can study people over days, weeks, months, and seasons, but careful tracking of human subjects over years and even decades is much more complicated and expensive. There are mountains of books to help Raphael prepare for the marathon, cross-country skiing, and every other endurance sport. There are detailed manuals, some with computer spreadsheet programs, on how to train for everything from powerlifting to speedskating. Volumes have been written about off-season training, peaking, and tapering. Collectively, these sources offer at best an unsystematic and incomplete picture of medium-term progress. They say little about the long-term successful careers of serious athletes. They say even less about the long-term active careers of ordinary people who, like Stephen, seek physical competence rather than physical prowess.

While it is nearly impossible to generalize across all physical activities, long-term progression appears to have certain common features. First, it is *long-term*. As obvious as this may sound, it needs explicit stating, especially for adults like Rachel, Raphael, and Stephen. It takes an infant thousands of repetitions to learn to walk without consciously trying. It can take adults tens of thousands of repetitions to master complex movements. It takes years of experience not only to master jazz dance or karate or marathoning or speedskating but simply to learn, by trial and error, how much exercise is enough. Without a long-term perspective, with only a myopic focus on short-term training results, Rachel and Raphael may have dropped out for good.

Second, progression entails *variety*. The same training stimulus, applied over and over, becomes increasingly ineffective. Progress is often made only when novel training stimuli are substituted. That's exactly what happened to Rachel, who burned out on bench-stepping and prospered with other activities. Third, progression entails extended intervals of *rest*. Multiple overtraining effects accumulate over time. I'm talking not just about sprains, strains, and bursitis, or about incomplete recovery from an intense workout, but about extended periods of fatigue and demotivation, which, however poorly understood, can be even more crippling. Cessation of training stimuli is necessary to overcome these overtraining cycles. Raphael was fortunate in that regard. It took him only a season of coaching soccer before he could go back to jogging.

Finally, progression entails *adaptation*. No two people respond the same way to the same training stimulus. Progress is empirical. There are challenges and backslides. When one form of exercise doesn't work, when one schedule is too taxing, when one plan doesn't work, then change it. As obvious as this may seem to you now as you read it, it was not so obvious to Rachel during her two months of daily step aerobics. It was not so obvious to Raphael until well into the soccer season.

I'll have more to say about persistence, progression, variety, rest, and adaptation. But I want to reemphasize here that these ideas apply as much to adults in mid-life contemplating the resumption of physical activity as they do to serious athletes. In fact, it is the myopic overemphasis on short-term training results that brings out the worst performance not only in the average adult but also in the competitive athlete. It is ironic that our culture, having misidentified physical activity with athleticism, has offered us the kind of coaching that no athlete deserves.

There is widespread scientific agreement that a lack of exercise contributes to the long-run development of coronary heart disease in both men and women. One of the most widely cited research studies in support of a long-term cardio-protective effect of exercise is the Harvard Alumni Study.[1] It is no coincidence that this study is also the most widely misinterpreted.

In back-to-back mailings in 1962 and 1966, the Harvard alumni office sent a one-page, self-administered questionnaire to 31,700 known living men who had entered Harvard College between 1916 and 1950. The questionnaire asked each alumnus about his recent physical activity and also about smoking habits, personal medical history, and parents' illnesses. The alumni responses, most of which came from the 1966 mailing, formed the basis of a research study by Ralph Paffenbarger and his colleagues.

Dr. Paffenbarger's research team kept track of the Harvard men. They obtained the death certificates of virtually all deceased men reported to the alumni office, in order to find out the official causes of death. In 1972, they sent out a second one-page questionnaire, inquiring whether a doctor had diagnosed a heart attack or other diseases. Excluding unusable and missing questionnaires, as well as alumni who reported a past heart attack, the researchers ended up with a study population of 16,936 men who were thought to be free of heart disease at the time of the original 1960s questionnaire and whose medical status was known as of 1972. Based on the questionnaire responses and collected death certificates, they found that men reporting higher levels of physical activity in 1966 (or 1962) had lower risks of fatal and nonfatal heart attack in the ensuing six (or ten) years.

Dr. Paffenbarger's team did not, and could not, continuously track the physical activity of nearly 17,000 Harvard alumni throughout their lifetimes. They did go back to college records to see who had participated in varsity or intramural sports. Beyond that, all they had was a single self-administered snapshot of the recent physical activities of each Harvard man at some point in his mid-life. That was the sole datum upon which to relate physical activity to the subsequent risk of heart attack over the next six (or ten) years.

Suppose that Thomas, who was born in 1920 and entered Harvard in 1938, was a participant in the alumni study. In 1966, when Thomas was forty-six years old (the same age as Stephen now), he was sent a questionnaire inquiring: How many flights of stairs do you go up each day? How many city blocks (or their equivalent) do you walk each day? Do you engage in sports play or other spare-time activities such as yard work? If Thomas answered the last question affirmatively, he was then asked to specify the types of sports and the hours played per week.

What would Thomas say? Forget step aerobics—this was 1966. But the post–World War II recreation boom was well under way. Dwight Eisenhower had already established the President's Council on Physical Fitness. Television was already covering professional and college sports. Thomas and his fellow Americans had already heard the heartbeats of men in outer space. But they would have to wait four more years to read Kenneth Cooper's *Aerobics;* twelve more years to read James Fixx's *Complete Book of Running;* sixteen years to see Joan Benoit win Olympic Gold in the women's marathon; twenty-one years to watch *Kathy Smith's Winning Workout* video; and twenty-four years to experience stair-climbing machines.

Most Harvard alumni, such as Thomas, were professional people with sedentary occupations. Many older respondents were already retired. To the extent that these men were physically active at all, they participated in leisure-time sports. To gauge each alumnus's level of physical activity, the research team divided these sports into two groups: "light" sports, such as bowling, baseball, biking, golf, or yard work; and "strenuous" sports, such as basketball, running, skiing, swimming, and tennis. Assuming that light sports consumed five calories per minute and strenuous sports consumed ten calories per minute, they computed the total number of calories each alumnus expended in sports play per week. Further assigning four calories for each flight of stairs ascended and for each city block walked, they added up the total calories per week to create a "physical activity index."

Thus, if Thomas climbed six flights of stairs daily, that's 24 calories per day, or 168 calories per week. If he also walked four city blocks daily, that's 16 calories daily, or 112 per week. The stair-climbing and walking combined would thus yield 280 calories per week. If he also played golf two hours (or 120 minutes) every week, that would add 600 calories, and we're up to 880. Another two hours of tennis would bring it to a grand total of 2,080 calories per week.

But didn't Thomas also burn calories while he was just standing around, even while he was sleeping? Does tennis burn exactly ten calories per hour? Suppose it was doubles. For that matter, did Thomas carry his own golf clubs? Is all yard work properly placed in the "light" category? How about digging or shoveling? Dr. Paffenbarger's team never intended their physical activity index to measure exhaustively and precisely every calorie burned by Thomas and his classmates. Still, they figured that they were getting a pretty good indicator of the level of physical activity among a group of white-collar and retired men who were, by and large, not carrying bales of hay or laying down railroad tracks. Overall, their physical activity index ranged from under 500 to over 5,000 calories per week, with two-thirds of the alumni falling under the 2,000-calorie mark.

In figure 3.1, I have graphed the alumni physical activity index against the alumni heart attack rate.[2] For each of six categories of the activity index, the solid circle shows the observed heart attack rate, while the accompanying dashed line displays the statistical error range. Thus, for men whose physical activity index was less than 500 calories per week, the observed risk of a fatal or nonfatal heart attack was 7.4 per 1,000 per year, or 0.74 percent annually. The margin of error was from about 6 to 9 per 1,000, or 0.6 to 0.9 percent annually. The heart attack rate gradually falls as the physical activity index increases, at least until the 2,000–2,999 calorie range. After that point, there appears to be no further improvement in heart attack risk. While the numbers seem to rise from 3.2 to 3.8 per 1,000 men per year as we go past 2,000–2,999 calories, there is too much statistical uncertainty to conclude that they are actually reversing.

The research results shown in the chart, along with other similar findings from the Harvard Alumni Study,[3] have been widely misinterpreted to mean that Thomas—as well as Stephen, Rachel, Raphael, and Tamar—need to expend 2,000

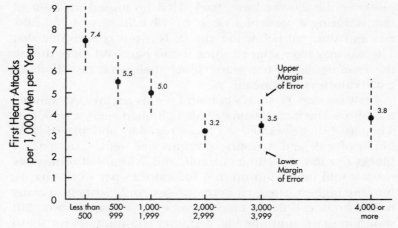

FIGURE 3.1
Heart Attack Rates in Relation to Physical Activity
Study of 16,936 Harvard Alumni, Aged 35–74, During 1962–72

Physical Activity Index, Measured in Calories per Week
Based upon Responses to Questionnaires in 1962 or 1966

SOURCE: Adapted from Ralph Paffenbarger et al., "Physical Activity as an Index of Heart Attack Risk in College Alumi," *American Journal of Epidemiology* 108 (1976):166.

calories per week to get the full benefit of exercise. As a major statement on exercise standards by the American Heart Association put it, "There is no evidence of a health benefit at more than 2,000 calories per week."[4] In many popular translations of the Harvard Study, the 2,000-calorie cutoff has been transformed into a requisite minimum below which no benefits accrue. "Walking a brisk 20 miles every week is the simplest way to use up the requisite 2,000," noted one newspaper editorialist.[5]

But the chart tells us only the relation between Thomas's reported *short-term* exercise level in 1966 and his risk of heart attack for the next six years. It doesn't say anything about his physical activity from 1966 to 1972. It tells nothing about his *long-term* progression over that period. It doesn't say whether he varied his physical activities, whether he learned and progressed, whether and when he took extended periods of rest, whether and when he became injured, whether he adapted or recovered, or whether he backslid or persisted.

In the foregoing numerical example, Thomas's two hours of golf and two hours of tennis, combined with his walking and stairclimbing, managed to put him at 2,080 calories per week, just over the 2,000-calorie mark. Had he missed an hour of tennis during a particular week, he'd backslide to 1,480 calories and thus fall below the cutoff. Is it not conceivable that Thomas may have skipped some tennis here and there during the ensuing six to ten years? If so, then what do Thomas's 2,080 calories really mean?

Let's say that Thomas's golf and tennis partner, Alexander, was also a Harvard classmate. Alex climbed stairs as much as Thomas, but he walked 8 blocks per day, and played 4 ½ hours of golf and 4 hours of tennis per week. The extra 4 blocks per day, 2 ½ hours of golf, and 2 hours of tennis per week would move him up to 4,142 calories per week, that is, into the highest category. Perhaps Alex could sustain so many hours for a couple of months, or even a year or two. But would he have continued at that level continuously for six to ten years? Some Harvard alumni, such as Alexander, may indeed have burned 4,142 calories per week at the time they answered the 1966 (or 1962) questionnaire. Others, such as Thomas, may have expended only 2,080 calories per week. That doesn't mean the Alexanders consistently maintained twice the level of leisure-time physical activity as the Thomases for years at a time.

My interpretation of the Harvard Alumni Study is completely different. Even a small amount of physical activity, the slightest increment beyond a totally sedentary life-style, appears to reduce substantially the risk of coronary heart disease. The exact amount of risk reduction and the required minimum level of physical activity cannot be determined from the Harvard Alumni Study alone, because the study merely took a one-week snapshot of exercise habits. What the study did not measure, and what we need to measure, is physical activity over the long term, that is, *progression*. The Harvard Alumni Study provides absolutely no support for a magic 2,000-calorie cutoff. The chart could just as well mean that the benefits of exercise continue to accrue at higher levels of activity, but that many people, even many Harvard men, cannot consistently sustain such activity levels over six or ten years.

Years after the public and the experts decided what the Harvard Alumni Study meant, Dr. Paffenbarger and his colleagues published a new wave of findings. The research team had sent out a second set of physical activity questionnaires to surviving Harvard alumni in 1977 and had kept track of death certificates until 1985.[6] This time around, the researchers had not asked alumni whether their doctors diagnosed heart attacks, so their new, second-wave study had to focus on death rates rather than heart attack rates. Nevertheless, as in the first wave, alumni with even minimal physical activity had mortality rates that were significantly lower than those of the most sedentary alumni.

There was, however, one important difference in the second-wave results. Those alumni with the very highest physical activity scores in 1977, in the range over 3,500 calories, had lower death rates than men with intermediate scores, in the range of 2,000 to 3,499 calories. This new finding demolished the accepted story line that an alumnus received the full benefit of exercise when he reached the 2,000-calorie cutoff, or even the 3,500-calorie level. My reading of these second-wave results is that in 1977, some Harvard alumni had *progressed* to 3,500 calories on the physical index, and had managed to *persist* at or near such a high level of activity for several more years. These men reaped the payoff from their persistence.

The researchers matched up the alumni's second-wave questionnaire responses in 1977 with their first-wave responses in 1966 (or 1962). What they found should be no surprise. The typical alumnus couldn't maintain the same level of physical activity for years at a time. In fact, the correlation between an alumnus's reported activity in the 1960s and his activity level in 1977 was remarkably weak.[7] In each wave, the researchers classified alumni who fell below the 2,000-calorie cutoff as "less active" and those above the 2,000-calorie cutoff as "more active." Thirty percent of alumni who were *less* active in the 1960s had become *more* active by 1977. Conversely, 40 percent of alumni who were *more* active in the first wave had become *less* active by the second wave.[8] Two counteracting trends were taking place. On the one hand, the Harvard men had gotten eleven to fifteen years older between the two waves. As they aged, one would expect some of them to become less active. On the other hand, the late 1960s and early 1970s were a time when jogging, biking, skiing, swimming, racquet sports, and home exercise equipment soared in popularity. By 1977, a great many alumni, especially older men, had newly taken up these pursuits.

When they looked at mortality during 1977–85, the researchers found that alumni who were *persistently* more active in the 1960s and the 1970s had the lowest death rates. Those alumni who *progressed* from lower to higher levels of activity likewise showed improved longevity, while those who backslid had the highest death rates. Alumni who took up moderate and vigorous sports in 1977, including men in their sixties, seventies, and eighties, had much lower rates of death from all causes, and especially from coronary heart disease, than those who did not.

The Harvard Alumni Study has now embarked on third and fourth waves. A questionnaire on physical activity was sent to the alumni in 1988 and 1993. As in the second wave, the researchers found that an alumnus's activity index in 1977 was poorly correlated with his index in 1988. Nevertheless, some men had managed to maintain high levels of physical activity far into their seventies. When the mortality results of the third wave are compiled, it will be interesting to see how much long-term benefit these persistently active older men have reaped.

The Harvard Alumni Study is far from perfect. More than a few alumni did not return questionnaires, especially in 1972, and these nonresponders had curiously higher death rates. During the 1960s and 1970s, many alumni quit smoking, watched their weight, and controlled their blood pressure. While these preventive measures did not alone explain the improved longevity of the active men, the researchers did not measure changes in alumni dietary practices. Still, the Harvard Alumni Study makes it absolutely clear that people don't automatically stay active for years on end. They have to work at it, to persist, and to progress. Those who do are likely to reap the benefits of their efforts.

It is unfortunate that Dr. Paffenbarger and his colleagues explicitly recorded their physical activity index in calories per week. Such an accounting practice has only reinforced the illusion that physical activity can be broken down into calorie-sized quanta, to be burned up Mondays, Wednesdays, and Fridays. It has obscured the fact that these men, who passed through middle age and reached old age in the 1960s and 1970s, probably

never took a step-aerobics class, never did a stint on a computerized stair-climbing machine, never retained personal trainers,
and never wore pulse meters. They did what people did in
those days. Indeed, they burned calories. But the single most
important unit for measuring physical activity is not the calorie
but the year.

PANELIST ONE recommended that Stephen take up weight
training in addition to aerobic exercise. On Mondays, said
ONE, Stephen could do bench presses and cross-chest dumbbell flyes for his pectoral, triceps, and back muscles. On
Wednesday, he'd switch to biceps curls for his arms and military presses for his shoulders. On Fridays, he could do leg
extensions and eventually work his way up to the queen bee of
weight-lifting exercises, the barbell squat. Proper technique,
however, was required. Stephen should have a regular spotter,
even a personal trainer. What is more, said ONE, Stephen
should increase the weight to be lifted by 5 percent only after
he can successfully perform two sets of ten repetitions without
assistance. PANELIST TWO attacked these recommendations, saying that Stephen would end up a tangle of torn muscles, dislo-
cated joints, and slipped discs.

The risks of recreational weight lifting are a controversial
area. Some people are going to get hurt, especially if they
don't warm up in advance and if they attempt to lift too much
weight with improper technique and no assistance. Those with
coronary heart disease have to be especially careful about
straining and breath holding. On the other hand, some
researchers have suggested that medically stable heart patients
can safely perform bench presses, military presses, standing
biceps curls and leg extensions at weights equal to 80 percent
of maximum.[9] Moreover, there is a strong case that assistance
devices such as weight belts can reduce the risks of injury.[10]
Many sports specialists and researchers have argued that
weight training strengthens joints and actually prevents injury
from other physical activities.[11]

If we put PANELIST TWO's objections in perspective, isn't
there an important gain to be made from strength training? Is
PANELIST ONE such an extremist? Stephen may take my advice
and adopt a long-term perspective, but doesn't he still need to
decide whether to lift weights, or possibly combine strength

work with other forms of exercise? Isn't there any short-term guidance we can offer him?

There is widespread consensus that men and women lose muscle mass and strength as they get older, especially in nonagrarian societies such as ours. The age-related deterioration in strength tends to be much greater in the lower body (the feet, legs, thighs, hips, and lower back) than in the upper body. In fact, the muscles least affected by aging are those involved in hand gripping.[12] In the population as a whole, strength tends to increase during puberty through one's mid-twenties. After that, there is a plateau, followed by a slow-decline phase during one's thirties and forties. Once a person gets into his fifties, the drop in strength accelerates with each passing decade.[13]

Specialists in physiology have long debated whether the decline in strength is an intrinsic part of the aging experience. Some scientists believe that people inevitably lose certain "fast-twitch" (or "type IIb") muscle fibers as they get older. These muscle fibers cannot be recovered because the nerves that once connected to them have died out. These scientists point to the fact that "explosive" muscular activity, such as sprinting and jumping, deteriorates markedly with advanced age. Others suggest that type IIb fibers can be preserved or perhaps regenerated with physical activity. Even if some loss of strength is inevitable, they argue that most of the age-related decline is a reversible consequence of disuse. People who don't use their muscles will lose their strength. If they use their muscles again, they'll get stronger again.[14]

The debate about the retrainability of muscles is extremely important for older people, who fall down with increasing regularity as they enter their sixties, seventies, and eighties. These falls are serious business. A precipitous tumble in an octogenarian can be a disaster, even a terminal event, especially if it results in a hip fracture. While there is an entire field of research about why older people fall and how their falls can be prevented, a loss of strength in the lower body is unquestionably a key factor. The muscle that is most important in the prevention of falls seems to be the quadriceps muscle (or "quads") in the front of the thigh, the one that straightens the leg at the knee joint. Some researchers have observed that older people who continue to walk and climb stairs have the greatest quadriceps muscle strength, and that their quads retain the most fast-twitch fibers. What's more, older people tend to lose their leg strength in the winter, when they cannot walk outside. This is exactly the season in which dangerous falls are more likely to happen.[15]

Stephen, unfortunately, has been taking the elevator for all these years, not the stairs. His quadriceps muscles undoubtedly need strengthening. He could retrain his quads by riding a bicycle (indoors or outdoors), working an electronic stair-climbing machine or a stationary skiing machine, or taking a step-aerobics class. Snow skiing, water skiing, ice hockey, mountaineering, in-line roller skating, or even ice speedskating would do the trick, if only Stephen could break into these sports. Some training specialists would argue that these activities do not specifically focus on improving quadriceps strength, and that Stephen will need to sit on a leg-extension machine and perhaps do other weight-lifting exercises to get his leg strength back. Others will argue that activities such as stair climbing, step aerobics, and skating simultaneously increase the strength of many leg and hip muscles while improving balance and coordination. One way or another, the inescapable conclusion is that Stephen needs to take step aerobics even more than Tamar, Rachel, or any of his other two dozen younger female aerobics classmates do. Stephen may be thoroughly daunted by the younger men and women at WestSide who grunt their way through leg extensions, leg curls, leg presses, squats, and whatnot. If so, he has to realize that his parents need to strengthen their legs even more than he does.

Specialists in rehabilitation medicine are seriously studying the effects of strength training for people in their sixties and beyond. Most research studies involve the use of a leg-extension machine to retrain the quadriceps muscles. In virtually every case, the researchers have come to the same conclusion. Elderly people can be made stronger. They get stronger not merely because they learn to use the muscles they already have but also because they get bigger muscles. But you can't train older people's quads with itty-bitty weights. You've got to push their muscles near their limits, to stress them sufficiently to achieve a strength-training effect.[16]

Perhaps the most widely publicized of these weight-training studies is a short-term trial of quadriceps strengthening in ten frail, institutionalized nonagenarians. The eight-week training program involved leg extensions three times per week. The research subjects attempted to perform three sets of eight repetitions at a weight equal to 80 percent of the maximum they could move even once. That's hardly a light load. While one eighty-six-year-old man was advised to stop in mid-course because he felt a groin pull, three other men and six women completed the full training program. At the end of eight weeks, these nine people could move weights that were 174 percent greater than at baseline—almost a tripling in strength.[17]

You may have read how these ninety-year-olds were able to walk faster than their children, how some no longer needed a cane, and how a few actually managed to get out of a chair without using their arms. Much less publicized is what happened when the training period ended. When seven of the nine subjects were retested, their quadriceps strength gains fell from 136 percent at eight weeks, to 115 percent at ten weeks, to 92 percent at twelve weeks. Before the start of the study, the typical nonagenarian could barely manage to straighten one leg against a seventeen-pound resistance. After strength training, she could move forty pounds. But two weeks later, she could move only thirty-seven pounds, and four weeks later only thirty-three pounds. If we could get her to walk regularly, take the stairs, and use her legs, then her posttraining strength loss might level off. But at that rate of *detraining,* if she resumed her cane and the wheelchair, she would be back to square one in another eight weeks. From what we know about detraining in general, Stephen would experience a comparable strength loss if he, too, stopped leg extensions and all other quadriceps-training exercises for several months.[18] What is more, the nonagenarians were still getting stronger at the end of the eight-week training period. They hadn't reached a strength plateau. Had they continued with two sets of eight repetitions at 80 percent of maximum, they would likely have broken through the fifty-pound ceiling for a one-leg extension. That's no baby weight. Again, from what we know about weight training, Stephen would also continue to *progress,* provided he stuck with it.

PANELIST ONE recommended that Stephen keep his pulse rate in the "training zone," initially at 60 to 70 percent of the maximum for his age, for at least twenty minutes three times per week. Where did this training-zone idea come from? Where did the twenty minutes three times per week come from?

PANELIST ONE did not invent these exercise standards. The American College of Sports Medicine recommends that healthy adults perform twenty to sixty minutes of continuous aerobic activity, at 60 to 90 percent of maximum heart rate, for three to five days per week.[19] The Scientific Council of the American Heart Association recommends "large muscle dynamic exercise for extended periods of time (30–60 minutes, 3–4 times weekly)."[20] When the U.S. Centers for Disease Control reports that 63 percent of high school students are not physically active, they're employing a standard of "at least 20 minutes of hard exercise that makes them breathe heavily and their hearts beat fast 3 or more days per week."[21] When the CDC likewise reports that 58 percent of Americans have a sedentary life-style, they mean that Americans report either no physical activity or exercise "fewer than three times per week and/or less than 20 minutes per session."[22]

These recommendations are based upon research studies, conducted mostly in the 1970s, that tried to determine the minimum amount of aerobic exercise necessary to achieve a short-term training effect.[23] Such training effects were gauged by a specific measure of fitness called the "maximal oxygen consumption," or "V-Dot-O_2-Max." The basic idea is to put someone like Stephen on a treadmill or a stationary bicycle and have him breathe into a mouthpiece-and-tubing system that measures the amount of oxygen he's using. The researcher then makes Stephen exercise harder and harder to the point of exhaustion, until Stephen can't take in or use any more oxygen. The V-Dot-O_2-Max is the gold standard by which to measure fitness in the world of exercise science and sports medicine.

So far, Stephen has been in step-aerobics class for eleven minutes. During the first ten minutes, Tamar took the class through a warm-up and stretching routine. That means Stephen has been doing step-up, step-down on his six-inch bench for only one minute. It usually takes three to five minutes after the start of aerobic exercise before a person's heart, lungs, muscles, and circulation get completely going.[24] So, unless Stephen is feeling faint or in pain, he probably ought to follow PANELIST ONE's advice and hang in there a little longer, even if it means forgoing the arm movements.

Of course, PANELIST ONE and the experts are telling Stephen more than just to hang in there for five more minutes. Even if he finishes the entire aerobics class, his V-Dot-O$_2$-Max is quite unlikely to budge.[25] Stephen's got to continue to do step aerobics with some minimum regularity before his aerobic capacity improves measurably. If he keeps dropping out after the warm-up, if he misses a lot of classes, if he doesn't push himself at all, he's not going to get anywhere. If he sticks with it, however, then after a while it will get easier, just as ONE promised.

Beyond that, Stephen ought not to take PANELIST ONE's advice too literally. If he travels as part of his work, Stephen's literal adherence to ONE's advice will mean bags of sneakers and sweats tucked into airplane overhead compartments and evenings of stair climbing in strange hotels, rather than an opportunity to give his body a rest. If he has an important lunch meeting, he'll have to make it to WestSide at night, but if his wife wants to go ballroom dancing instead, he'll have to insist on the swing dance or, better still, the quickstep, provided that they dance for at least twenty minutes and that Stephen can free his outstretched left hand from his wife's grasp long enough to check his neck pulse. If his children want to go "plain bowling," he'll have to decline on the grounds that it may not produce an aerobic-training effect. If his dutiful wife spends her days picking up laundry and carrying hampers to the basement washer, hand-mowing the lawn, raking leaves, and playing erratic doubles tennis and social badminton, he might very well complain that she's not getting enough exercise. And when Stephen comes down with tendinitis or a minor sprain and has to lay off temporarily, he'll sink into the deepest misery because his V-Dot-O$_2$-Max is, day by day, going down the drain.

In fact, a good case can be made that Stephen ought to throw out the experts' advice entirely. There is an ever-growing body of evidence that people vary widely in the amount of exercise necessary to produce aerobic-training effects, much more widely than previously thought. Some middle-aged, previously sedentary people like Stephen may take six months to get used to exercising. These people can achieve aerobic-training effects at lower levels of exercise, but it might take longer. The 1970s short-term research studies that lasted for only fifteen or twenty weeks would miss these training effects. Newer research studies suggest that middle-aged men can boost their V-Dot-O_2-Maxes with repeated bouts of exercise that last much less than twenty minutes or a half hour, even possibly as short as ten minutes.[26] Many newer research studies show that older people can be aerobically trained, often at much lower intensities than middle-aged or young people.[27]

The purist devotion to aerobic training is increasingly seen as misplaced. The old-school view was that training-induced gains in V-Dot-O_2-Max were caused by major improvements in heart-pumping and circulatory efficiency. The new view is that once someone has reached middle age, aerobic training is more a form of leg muscle conditioning than heart strengthening.[28] For people like Stephen, those forms of exercise that were always called "aerobic" are actually mixtures of cardiovascular and strength training. What's more, researchers are finding that the amounts and types of exercise necessary to strengthen one's bones,[29] prevent diabetes,[30] lower one's blood pressure,[31] redistribute one's body fat,[32] improve one's cholesterol,[33] gain mental agility,[34] or improve one's self-esteem[35] may be quite different from those necessary to boost one's V-Dot-O_2-Max. Even serious athletes are coming to understand that aerobic training isn't everything, that two bicyclists with the same V-Dot-O_2-Max don't necessarily have the same endurance.[36] Eric Heiden, who took five gold medals in Lake Placid in 1980, had a V-Dot-O_2-Max of 63.8 in October 1979, well above the typical value of 40 for an active twenty-year-old, but way below the 70 and 80 values of many champion marathoners, cyclists, cross-country skiers, and triathletes.[37]

The Harvard Alumni Study inquired whether *active* men had fewer heart attacks. New research studies have asked whether aerobically *fit* people have lower disease rates. The new studies have consistently found that the least fit men and women have higher cardiovascular mortality, but that people with the highest V-Dot-O_2-Maxes don't seem to fare that much better than people with medium aerobic conditioning.[38] These findings have been widely misinterpreted to mean that the full benefits of exercise are attainable by regular brisk walks, or by some other physical activity that gets you out of the totally sedentary category. What these studies are really showing is that fitness counts, but *aerobic* fitness isn't everything. Other dimensions of exercise matter, too. The Harvard alumni who stayed active in later life didn't live longer just because they had higher V-Dot-O_2-Maxes. They were stronger, more coordinated, and more mentally agile. Their bones were more resilient. They didn't get diabetes as much. They didn't suffer catastrophic falls.

PANELIST TWO asked, Whatever happened to plain golf, or plain bowling? Was that question so far off the mark? As soon as we escape from the target-heart-rate-twenty-minutes-three-times-per-week mentality, we can start thinking about the benefits of a much wider range of human physical activity. To be sure, most readers would agree that bowling probably burns fewer calories than step aerobics. But we can't be too rigid about ranking different types of activities. For the person who won't do step aerobics, a pronouncement that bowling doesn't rate is an invitation to do nothing. What's more, the level of energy expenditure in these activities depends a great deal on who is doing them and how hard he is trying.

To begin with, the number of calories you burn per minute in stair climbing, walking, bowling, or step aerobics depends crucially on your weight or, more precisely, your muscle mass. If you have viewed TV advertisements that claim you'll burn "up to 800 calories per hour" on such-and-such an exercise machine, you should be aware that 800 calories per hour would be decent exercise if you were a 170-pound man, but if you're a 115-pound woman, you probably ought to try running a 2:45 marathon instead.

To take a person's weight into account, researchers have relied increasingly on a unit of energy expenditure called the MET, which is an abbreviation for *met*abolic equivalent. A person who is working at 1 MET is burning 1 calorie per hour per kilogram of body weight. That's about as much energy as you would expend reading this book, provided you were quietly sitting down and hadn't used it to practice hook shots into the trash can. The new MET system is slowly working its way into medical textbooks and personal-trainer manuals. Some of the latest electronic stationary bicycles will tell you your effort level in METs.

Since we live in a country of pounds and not kilograms, I

find it easier to express energy expenditure in CHPs (pro-nounced "chips"), which stands for *c*alories per *h*our per *p*ound of body weight. Working at 2.2 METs is the same as 1 CHP, which is about as much work as clearing dishes from the table after dinner or putting away clean laundry. It's a little more work than playing the cello while seated, but a little less than playing the violin standing, at least for the average player.

Everything from fishing and hunting to sexual activity to driving a car has now been rated for energy expenditure.[39] The problem with these ratings is that they're only an average. Dancing the fox-trot would be about 1.4 CHPs, provided you didn't up the tempo into a quickstep. The waltz would also be about 1.4 CHPs, provided it wasn't the Viennese, and a fast cha-cha might get you up to 2.5 CHPs. If you ran a nine-minute mile, you'd be up to 5 CHPs, but the exact amount depends critically on your running efficiency. The same goes for swimming a fast crawl or a butterfly stroke, which are also rated in the 5-CHP range. Playing golf runs at about 0.9 CHPs, provided you don't pull or carry your clubs. Walking on the level at about a fourteen-minute-mile pace would burn about 2 calories per hour per pound, but again it depends on your stride and rhythm. Plain bowling weighs in at 1.4 CHPs, while raking the lawn burns 1.8 CHPs. Shoveling snow burns 2.7 CHPs or more, depending on the speed of shoveling and the weight of the snow. Social badminton is 2.0 CHPs, but compet-itive badminton is up to 3.2 CHPs. Competitive speedskating, to put things in perspective, runs at about 7 CHPs, which would be the same as running a 6:23-mile pace. Cross-country skiing on hard snow uphill at maximum effort would be 7.5 calories per hour per pound.

It cannot be overemphasized that these calorie rankings depend crucially on the level of effort. For Stephen's female classmates in step aerobics, working out with a six-inch bench seems to burn about 3.7 CHPs. At an eight-inch bench, it's up to 4.1 CHPs, and at a ten-inch bench, it's up to 4.5 CHPs.[40] Nor do the MET or CHP ranking systems really tell Stephen the required level of effort. Walking fourteen-minute miles may expend 2 CHPs. For Eric Heiden, whose pre-Olympic maximum was 8.7 CHPs, that's less than a 25 percent effort, but for someone whose maximum is 4 CHPs, that's a 50 per-cent effort.[41]

The expert reports and blue-ribbon panel recommendations almost always contain a qualification that the most desirable physical activity depends upon the exerciser's age and sex, and that exercise programs should be tailored to individual needs. They caution that more research needs to be performed on the health benefits of "light" exercise, such as housekeeping, golf, and pleasure walking. But they need to go one step further, to extricate themselves from the narrow focus on this week's exercise schedule and next month's training results. The experts, like Stephen, need a long-term perspective.

I have lost count of the number of hours I have spent talking to my patients about exercise. Many have come to tell me how much they enjoyed aerobics classes, yet a year or two later, they have stopped. They're too busy, they say. Their membership expired. Others have insisted that they'll start walking outdoors as soon as the weather improves. Yet winter seems to linger through spring and beyond. Some have bought stationary bicycles and resistance machines, only to donate them to the school auction the following year. Others have stacks of free weights in the basement—dumbbells, bars, plates, and all—which have grown dusty after they hurt their backs pushing themselves a little too hard. Many have told me how much they wish they could join a gym and work out. But they are embarrassed. Some have video exercise programs, with their own stepping benches, ankle and hand weights, and elastic bands. But they're hungry after work and eat too much to exercise afterward, and anyway, it's almost bedtime. Still others say they're too old to exercise. But they say it with body language that reveals they know differently.

For all these people, I do not have a perfect answer. Still, I have come to the conclusion that my patients should be treated, in a sense, as if they were all competitive athletes, all Olympic material. No, I don't mean that Stephen should quit work and train full-time. I mean that Stephen has to worry not about the next thirty-nine minutes of aerobics but about his own personal equivalent of the 1994 Games and beyond. Instead of telling Stephen that it's perfectly all right to take a rest, I would tell him he has to taper. Instead of telling him that he needs variety in his physical activities, I would tell him he needs to cross-train. Instead of telling Stephen that he's too preoccupied with his aerobics schedule, I would tell him he's overtraining. Above all, I would emphasize the attainment of competence. Just as the athlete wants to win, Stephen, Tamar, Rachel, Raphael, Thomas, Alexander, and everyone else want to do well. By the time Tamar gets to be Stephen's age, she will not have the same maximum heart rate or V-Dot-O_2-Max, but she might be a Masters Women aerobics champion. By then, Rachel may have her fourth-degree black belt in karate.

I am serious. Walking and climbing stairs in the wintertime is so manifestly beneficial for older people, especially older women, that I tell them that they actually have it in them to be championship walkers. To someone who thought she could only lift an ice cream cone, I have said: "Did it ever occur to you that you could be a powerlifter?" To one elderly man I said: "You look like you could dance Latin." To another I said: "You have the balance and agility to learn speedskating." As trite as it sounds, to all of them I said: You can do it.

It is 4:25 P.M. The bench-stepping aerobics class has long ended. Tamar and Stephen are on a bicycle path in a park not too far from WestSide FitClub.

"Tamar, you didn't let go the right way!"

"Okay, Stephen, I'll try to let go the right way next time."

"No more next time. I can't do it. I never learned to ride a bicycle when I was a child. I can't learn now. Period."

"Look, Stephen, do you know what patience is?"

"Yeah, like when someone else is in the bathroom first."

"Come on, Stephen, you managed to stay on the bike for ten whole seconds. So what if you fell in the grass? You got up."

"The seat is too high."

"No it isn't, Stephen. Rest a little and try again."

"You didn't tell me when you were going to give me a push. Tamar, you let go before I was ready. You were talking while you were pushing, and it broke my concentration."

Stephen mounts Tamar's bike again. She runs alongside, holding the seat as he pedals. She lets go. Stephen manages to wobble for about twenty seconds and then collides with a tree.

"You got it, Stephen! That was the tree's fault, right?"

Stephen is perspiring and uncomfortable. He pedals once again, sustaining his balance this time: ten seconds, twenty seconds, thirty seconds. Tamar tries to run alongside, breathless. At the end of the path is a large, immovable cast-iron fence, toward which Stephen is directly headed.

"Turn, Stephen. Turn around!"

Stephen back-pedals to a perfect, split-second stop in front of the fence. "Wow, Tamar. That was my world record."

4

Body Mass Index
Weight Control

At age thirty, Eve is chief resident in psychiatry at a university-affiliated hospital. Standing 5'5" tall and weighing 162 pounds, she is neither flashy nor homely.

Eve has just completed a regular clinic session with her patient Leah, a twenty-one-year-old student who is as tall as Eve but who weighs only 114 pounds. After months of concealment and denial, Leah has finally admitted to Eve that she never stopped her binge-eating and vomiting.

Still in her office, Eve overhears Leah pleading with the receptionist in the hallway: "Can I possibly have an appointment with a different psychiatrist? Do you have any specialists in bulimia who aren't so fat?"

Eve is the protagonist in this chapter. Leah is merely a foil, an expository device, an excuse to pose questions. This is Eve's choice.

Leah has an eating disorder. She gorges and disgorges. Like many people with bulimia, Leah is so mortified by her binging and purging that she has concealed it even from her doctor. Now that her secret is out, she may be relieved and even grateful to Eve. But she is also angry and even more embarrassed for having lied and been caught. Preoccupied with thinness and bodily dimensions, Leah may actually believe that her own thighs or tummy are too heavy. Feeling inferior to Eve in every other respect, Leah attacks her doctor the only way she can. She calls Eve a fatso behind her back.

Obviously, Leah's bad-mouthing doesn't automatically make Eve a fat person. But her attack brings up a tough question: What actually makes a person "fat"?

Is it enough for somebody else to think that Eve is fat? Does it matter who that somebody else is: her parents, her colleagues, her patient? Is Eve fat because our culture (that is, everyone else, taken collectively) says she's fat? Is fatness merely a label, a matter of name calling? Would Eve be fat if she herself thought she was fat, even if no one else thought she was fat? If so, then is Leah fat merely because she herself thinks she's fat? Does Leah's bulimia disqualify her from assessing her own fatness or Eve's fatness? Does Eve's education and professional status, on the other hand, qualify her to assess her own fatness? Is it conceivable that Eve, too, has an eating disorder and is therefore similarly disqualified? Are there objective criteria for fatness, or is it entirely subjective?

Leah, I hope we agree, may be thin but still has a normal weight. What makes Leah abnormal is her behavior, not her weight. Had Eve weighed 192, we would surely concur that she was overweight. But Eve is a 162-pound, accomplished, well-trained, empathic physician who wants to help Leah. From what we know so far, Eve's conduct is normal. It's her weight that is problematic.

When Eve graduated from high school, she weighed 132 pounds. She gained 6 pounds during college; 6 pounds in medical school; 12 pounds during her internship; and has so far acquired another 6 pounds during her psychiatry residency. Eve's internship was especially stressful. With no leisure time and little exercise, she virtually subsisted on coffee, chocolate-chip ice cream, and miniature doughnuts.

Eve has never attempted to lose weight. She has never even contemplated a diet. As a well-informed physician and a specialist in eating disorders, Eve knows the scientific literature that says diets don't work. She knows that many authorities have voiced skepticism about the long-term success rates of commercial weight-reduction programs.

On Eve's desk is one of the hundreds of unsolicited brochures that she receives and discards monthly. This one advertises a structured, balanced-deficit plan: 1,200 calories daily, with specially formulated foods, group sessions on relapse prevention, and optional individual counseling. Another unproved gimmick, Eve thinks to herself.

Leah has gone. The receptionist gave her another appointment with Eve, who now picks up her phone and dials the 800 number.

Should Eve stay on the line or put the receiver down? If she hangs up, is there anything else she can do about her weight, or should she just forget the whole thing? Eve has gained thirty pounds in twelve years. Even if she isn't overweight, shouldn't Eve be taking some sort of action now to prevent further weight gain?

We can read Eve's mind, as she holds the receiver to her ear, as she envisions all those women in all those before-and-after testimonials, in all those print ads and television commercials, on behalf of all those weight-control programs, all those diet pills and replacement meals, all those sweating and bouncing exercise routines and body-squeezing and spot-reducing machines, all those women who gained thirty pounds in a dozen years, but who all shed those very same thirty pounds within a dozen weeks. And for every woman in every testimonial, Eve can now see three others who abandoned the group sessions or the pills, who gave up on the meals or the machines. And of all those women who stuck to their program, Eve can see as many as two-thirds regaining the weight within one year and nearly all within five years. She sees thousands of them now, trapped by their diets in shackles of undernutrition, psychologically trampled by their failures to maintain weight loss, physically abused by repeated cycles of weight loss and regain. She sees a thousand Leahs, a thousand receptionists, a thousand new appointments, a thousand fat psychiatrists.

To speak with a courteous sales associate, press "1" now.

I am no fan of fashion models. I think they're too skinny. Nor am I a worshiper at our culture's altar of the slim. I have no financial ties to any commercial weight-control program or product. I try not to discriminate against overweight people. So much for apologies. Eve has a weight problem.

That does not automatically mean that she should register

for the weight-loss program advertised in the brochure, or that she needs to lose thirty pounds or even twenty pounds, or that she is capable of controlling her weight, or that her current weight presents a serious medical or psychological risk. But the plain fact is that Eve can no longer ignore her weight problem. It is not a figment of anybody's imagination. It won't go away even if Eve's parents think she looks terrific.

So, do I agree with Leah that Eve is a fat psychiatrist? I said only that Eve had a "weight problem," not that she was "fat." The difficulty with the word *fat* is that it has too many different connotations, encompasses too much. Actually, we wouldn't do much better if we called Eve an "obese" psychiatrist, and only slightly better if we called her an "overweight" psychiatrist. There are many different types of weight problems. Some may have no solution or at best a half-solution. Others may have a distinctly best approach. Still others may be amenable to many weight-control strategies. Not all obese people are the same. They shouldn't be treated the same. To call Eve "fat" is to put her in the same ballpark with many other so-called fat people who, in reality, aren't even in the same league.

I need not bore you with the reams of surveys that reveal how just about everybody from Leah to Eve to Eve's aunts and uncles has tried, is trying, or is contemplating trying to lose weight. All these Americans in all these surveys are not psychiatrists specializing in eating disorders. They cannot tell you the percentage of people who default on such-and-such a diet, or who relapse within one year or five years. Yet, even without advanced education, they instinctively know that the television and magazine testimonials are merely personal anecdotes, that they prove little. They know what it means when the fine print says "individual weight loss may vary." They know that if there really were a single, distinctly superior method of long-term weight control, then everyone would already be using it. They already know that weight control is not merely a matter of self-discipline and willpower. They already know that many people later regain the weight they have lost. They already know that some but not all people are stuck at a certain weight. They don't need a new wave of skeptics to tell them how diets don't work. Still, like Eve the specialist, they pick up the phone and dial the number anyway.

All these Americans are trying to lose weight because they

believe that they are each different, that there must be some strategy of weight control that works for them if not for everyone else. They view the assertion that "diets don't work" as meaning that the average diet doesn't work for the average person, but that the right diet could still work for them. To ask whether unsupervised dieting works, whether commercial programs work, whether exercise machines or specially formulated foods work, is to misstate the issue. The problem, properly framed, is one of matching up people with solutions. Eve, holding the phone to her ear, is no hypocrite. She is not acting in bad faith. She may envision a thousand fat psychiatrists. But a full census would yield a count of one thousand and one.

I do have some ideas about matching people to weight-control solutions. But I have no magic algorithm that says Eve is such-and-such type overweight and therefore needs so-and-so weight-control strategy. It may take Eve a long time to find out what solution, if any, is right for her. The task is not painless. There is a legitimate question about whether Eve should try to control her weight at all. But we can still get Eve started in the right direction. We can still ask the questions she needs to ask.

Indeed, most weight-control strategies haven't been adequately evaluated. Indeed, many programs that have been systematically tested appear to have poor long-term track records. Indeed, repeated attempts and failures at weight control, especially when they entail so-called weight cycling, may have adverse consequences.[1] But these are mitigating facts. They don't automatically mean that Eve should give up and do nothing about her weight.

Maybe Leah's soft-spoken request for a not-so-fat psychiatrist will be the sonic boom that finally scares Eve out from behind the curtains of rationalization and denial.

Standing 5'5" and weighing 162 pounds, Eve has a *Body Mass Index* of 27. To compute her Body Mass Index (abbreviated "BMI"), I divided Eve's weight in pounds by a factor of 6. To compute your own BMI, divide your weight by the conversion factor corresponding to your height in figure 4.1.

The BMI is an important measure of body weight that takes a person's stature into account. That's why the conversion factors in the chart vary with height. The taller one is, the larger the

FIGURE 4.1
Body Mass Index (BMI)

If your height (in feet and inches) is:	Then divide your weight (in pounds) by:
4'9"	4.91
4'10"	4.77
4'11"	4.94
5'0"	5.11
5'1"	5.28
5'2"	5.46
5'3"	5.63
5'4"	5.81
5'5"	6.00
5'6"	6.18
5'7"	6.37
5'8"	6.56
5'9"	6.76
5'10"	6.95
5'11"	7.15
6'0"	7.36
6'1"	7.56
6'2"	7.77
6'3"	7.98
6'4"	8.20

Example: Reuben stands 6'0" tall and weighs 184 pounds.
To compute his BMI, Reuben divides 184 by 7.36, which
equals 25.

factor. Consider a sixty-year-old grandfather named Reuben,
who stands 6' tall and weighs 184 pounds. From the chart,
Reuben's BMI would be 184 divided by 7.36, which equals 25.
Reuben thus weighs more than Eve, but when we correct for his
taller stature, Reuben's BMI is less than Eve's. By contrast, Leah
stands 5'5" and weighs 114 pounds. From the chart, her BMI
equals 114 divided by 6.00, which gives 19. As these examples
show, the formula for calculating BMI depends only upon
weight and height, and not upon age, gender, or any other per-

sonal characteristic.[2] In the past ten years, the vast majority of researchers and medical specialists have adopted the BMI as the standard index for assessing a person's weight in relation to his or her body size.

There is no unanimity on the exact BMI at which a person becomes overweight. But there is general agreement that for young people such as Eve and Leah, a BMI from 19 to 25 is healthy. BMI values from 25 to 29 fall into a gray zone of overweight, where a person is beyond the healthy range but not necessarily in medical trouble. BMI values from 29 and up would usually be considered medically significant obesity, although some authorities might set the cutoff at a BMI of 30. A person with a BMI of 35 has entered the medically dangerous zone, and a BMI of 40 would usually be considered medically severe (or "morbid") obesity. That puts Eve, with her current BMI of 27, right in the gray zone of overweight. For a 5'5" tall person such as Eve, this gray zone corresponds to a weight range of 150 to 174 pounds.[3]

When she graduated from high school at age eighteen, Eve weighed 132. At presumably the same height, she had a BMI of 22. By college graduation four years later, Eve's BMI had risen to 23 points. By the end of medical school at age twenty-six, her BMI was up to 24. During her one-year internship, Eve's BMI jumped two more points to 26; and during her three-year psychiatry residency, it has so far risen another point to its current value of 27. That's an overall gain of five BMI points in a dozen years, with three out of the five points amassed since Eve graduated from medical school four years ago. If Eve continued to add three BMI points every four years, then by age thirty-four she'd reach a BMI of 30, which for her is equivalent to a weight of 180 pounds.

For American women aged eighteen to twenty-four, the median BMI is 21.6 (that is, half the women have a BMI below 21.6, and half have a BMI above that level).[4] So, when Eve graduated high school, her BMI of 22 placed her pretty close to the average for her age group. But that was twelve years ago. Now Eve's BMI of 27 puts her in the eightieth percentile of twenty-five- to thirty-four-year-old American women, whose median BMI is 22.6. That statistic does not by itself make Eve a rare bird. After all, 20 percent of the women have a BMI above Eve's. What is far more exceptional about Eve is that she gained five BMI points during a time when the typical American woman gains only one point.

Nobody can legitimately squeeze Eve's entire life into a single statistic. To say that Eve's BMI is 27 is to say nothing about those long, doughnut-laden nights of her internship, not to mention the chocolate-chip ice cream. Still, by tracking the path of Eve's BMI over the past twelve years, we can begin to see her problem more clearly. It is not so much where Eve stands now as which direction Eve is heading and how fast she is headed there.

Leah's life history can be no better summarized by a number than can Eve's. To say that Leah's current BMI of 19 puts her at the fifteenth percentile of eighteen- to twenty-four-year-old women is to leave out her vomiting, her perfectionist obsession with thinness and body parts, and, for all we know, far more doughnuts than Eve ever consumed. Still, the same principle applies. If Leah's BMI were headed downward from the twenties, then she would likely be entering a restrictive, anorexic phase of her illness. If her BMI fell below 16, which would correspond to a weight of 96 pounds, she would be getting into the danger zone of malnutrition, fragile bones, disrupted menstruation, heart rhythm problems, and worse.[5] On the other hand, if Leah's BMI were headed upward from the teens, it could signal a new chapter in her life, where her rigid, primitive eating strategies have collapsed, and where experimentation with food is no longer forbidden.

I already said that the median BMI for American women aged eighteen to twenty-four was 21.6, and that it was 22.6 among women aged twenty-five to thirty-four. For women aged thirty-five to forty-four, the median BMI is 23.8; and for women aged forty-five to fifty-four, it's up to 24.8. In the subsequent two decades, it rises further to 25.3 and then to 25.9. Accordingly, the typical adult American woman who has just graduated high school or college can expect to gain 4.3 BMI points over the next five decades, with the rate of BMI increase being greatest during her thirties and forties. For a 5'5" tall woman like Eve, a 4.3-point BMI gain would correspond to a twenty-six-pound weight gain.

As they pass through middle age, increasing numbers of American women enter the gray overweight zone of BMIs from 25 to 29, as well as the medically obese range of BMIs from 29 and up. At twenty-five to thirty-four years of age, about 15 percent of women have a BMI in the gray zone and another 15 percent are in the medically obese range. Ten years later, about 20 percent will fall in the gray zone, while another 20 percent will have a medically obese BMI. As American women reach their seventh and eighth decades of life, the proportions are 25 percent in the gray zone and 25 percent medically obese.

For American men, the pattern of lifetime weight gain is somewhat different. At ages eighteen to twenty-four, the median BMI is 23.0, and by ages twenty-five to thirty-four, it's already up to 24.7. In the next two decades, the median BMI rises to 25.6 and then 25.9, after which it levels off and drops slightly. So the typical American man who has just graduated high school or college can expect to add about 2.9 units of BMI over the next three decades, with the greatest velocity of weight gain in his twenties and early thirties.[6] By ages forty-five to fifty-four, about 35 percent of American men have a BMI in the gray zone, from 25 to 29, while another 23 percent are medically obese.

Some authorities believe that the healthy range of BMI should be allowed to rise with age. They point out that older people with BMIs of 19 or 20 have higher rates of certain diseases such as cancer. But that's because their cancer made them lean, not the other way around. In the U.S. government's recent guidelines, the healthy range for BMI was set at 21 to 27 points for people over thirty-five years old.[7] Basically, you're allowed two points once you get into middle age, whether you're male or female. The rationale for this recommendation is not crystal-clear.[8] American women tend to gain weight with successive pregnancies. In our modern culture, we can't expect women to shed all their pregnancy-acquired pounds by breast-feeding children until age three or four. Once menopause arrives, the argument is that the change in a woman's sex hormones tends to add more fat to her upper body, including her chest and arms, as opposed to her abdomen, hips, and thighs. Even if we accept these judgments about healthy weights in middle age, it's only a 2-point BMI gain, which is a lot less than the 4.3-point gain experienced by the average woman. And it certainly won't do thirty-year-old Eve very much good. As for men, I don't have a clue why they should get a 2-point BMI credit, and shall not speculate as to the influence of middle-aged and older men on blue-ribbon scientific panels.

Let's pretend that we got Eve to go to the doctor for a checkup. Which doctor do I recommend? Let's make you the doctor.

If you happen to have actually gone to medical school, please restrain yourself from exhaustively listing every known medical cause or complication of weight gain. Don't expect to run up a big bill, either. Eve will not receive an ultrasound test of her gallbladder. You won't perform a laparascopy of her ovaries. And she's not going to have an injection of radioactive iodine to scan her thyroid gland. You're just going to pose a question or two, then take her blood pressure and get a fasting blood-sugar level.

You ask Eve how she's been feeling lately. She answers, "Doctor, I've had so much trouble getting to sleep. I just can't concentrate. I have to force myself to do things. It seems as if I'm always coming down with another cold or stomachache. Even when I'm not sick, I feel run down. Sometimes I feel like crying." Well, doctor, what do you make of it?

You may be hearing the symptoms of severe stress. It turns out that Eve, in her final year of medical training, has been applying for permanent positions. She has just received a rejection notice from another university-affiliated hospital. As a female professional, Eve has undoubtedly been held to a higher standard than her male counterparts. That goes not just for her psychiatric skills but also for her personal appearance. It is ironic, you muse to yourself, that Leah wants unrealistically to be perfect. Yet it is Eve who, realistically, has to be perfect. Fair or unfair, Eve is alerting you that her weight has already become a significant medical problem. Quite apart from the psychic stresses of professional and social rejection, the plain fact is that Eve's long-run professional career prospects will be significantly hampered by her obesity, especially if it gets worse.

Eve says, "Doctor, I have pains under my kneecaps whenever I run down the hall. I have this gnawing ache in my butt when I sit in the bucket seat of my car. And I still haven't gotten over those back spasms from digging my car out of the snowdrift."

Eve's 162 pounds may have already begun to overload her major weight-bearing joints, especially the back, hips, and knees.[9] The overload might be compounded by a loss of flexibility from being inactive. As you listen to her complaints, you say to yourself: If Eve had gained only eighteen or even twenty-four pounds since high school, instead of thirty, she might not have had these orthopedic troubles. Eve may not know it, but it could have been the last six or twelve pounds of weight gain that really overloaded her joints.

You take Eve's blood pressure, and it's 130 over 90. That's barely into the range of mild hypertension. You will probably want to get a few more readings before taking action, and you may decide not to give her any antihypertensive drugs, at least for now. But that's not the point. You ask Eve about her blood pressure in the past. She says, "I definitely remember it was 110 over 70 during my pre-internship physical, and I can't remember any other blood pressure measurements since then." Eve, you realize, may be one of those people whose blood pressure is weight-sensitive. It was twenty points lower when her BMI was three points lower. Actually, you don't know exactly when Eve's blood pressure went up. It's possible that it rose the full twenty points only with the last six or twelve pounds of weight gain.

Eve's fasting blood-glucose level turns out to be 120. You're not going to prescribe antidiabetes pills or insulin injections for a blood sugar that is barely beyond the range of normal. Again, that's not the point. You ask Eve about her blood sugar a few years ago. She doesn't remember having a test. But now you're thinking that Eve's blood sugar might be also weight-responsive, just like her blood pressure.

As Eve's doctor, you know that weight sensitivity of blood pressure and weight sensitivity of blood sugar tend to go together in the same person. Most such people, you know, have a blood triglyceride level that also goes up with weight gain.[10] When these people put on extra weight and acquire more body fat, the excess fat disturbs the body's internal control systems for blood pressure, blood sugar, triglyceride, and cholesterol. These weight-sensitive people have higher blood sugars, as do diabetic patients, but they don't run out of insulin hormone, as some diabetics do. Actually, their bodies make extra insulin, but their extra body fat keeps their insulin from working effectively. Some specialists, in fact, would check Eve's fasting insulin level, to see if it's higher than normal.

But you don't want to get fancy. You just want Eve to get better. So, as her doctor, you advise her, "Eve, your blood pressure is only at the borderline of hypertension. Your fasting blood sugar is only slightly beyond the normal range. Still, these are signals that your current weight of 162 pounds is already giving you medical problems, and that further weight gain could produce genuine hypertension and diabetes, as well as high triglyceride and cholesterol. I'm not saying you're going to keel over tonight. But these conditions will place you at much higher risk for heart attack, stroke, and other circulatory problems in the future."

Eve interrupts, "I know I've got to lose the 30 pounds that I've gained since high school. At least I should lose 24 pounds and get down to 138."

"Not necessarily," you say.

"Isn't that the way you're supposed to do it? Aren't you supposed to set a weight goal?" Eve asks.

"Fair enough, Eve. But why should 132 or even 138 be your goal?"

"Because the life insurance tables in my office say that a medium-framed 5'5" tall woman should ideally weigh 127 to 141 pounds, with 3 pounds of clothes on."[11]

"Don't use those so-called ideal weights to set your goal. That's not the best approach to your weight problem, Eve. It's entirely possible that your blood pressure and blood sugar will come down with only a twelve-pound, or possibly even a six-pound weight loss."

"You mean it might help me just to get down to 150 or even 156?"

"Look, Eve, you've gained five BMI points in a dozen years, but the last one or two BMI points were very likely the most dangerous to you. And if you keep gaining weight, the next one or two BMI points may be even more dangerous."

"I'm going to feel great with just a small weight loss?" Eve asks.

"Since you didn't feel the extra blood pressure or the extra blood sugar on the way up, you may not feel it on the way down. But that's not crucial. What's important is that your BMI of 27 puts you in a gray zone of overweight. And the results of your checkup suggest that you're in the dark gray region of the gray zone. You've got to get out of dark gray and into light gray. That's the crucial first step."

"If I were large-framed, my ideal weight would be 137 to 155 with clothes, so that would be okay. Doctor, do you think maybe I'm large-framed? Aren't you supposed to measure my elbow?"

"You're still worrying about the 'ideal' weights from those life insurance charts. Eve, you can't go by those numbers. When they first worked out those life insurance statistics in the 1950s and 1960s, how many women had life insurance policies?"

"Not very many, I suppose."

"Eve," you continue, "the first step in gauging your weight problem was to calculate your BMI. The second step was to determine how rapidly your BMI has been increasing. The third step was to see whether your weight gain is already giving you medical problems. The fourth step was to set a reasonable weight-loss goal that is based on a simple principle: The last few points of BMI were the most dangerous, and the next few will be even more dangerous."

"Is there a fifth part, doctor?"

"Yes, indeed. That's where we start matching you up with an appropriate weight-control strategy. But the checkup's not over. I still have one more question."

"Uh-huh."

"Eve, do you smoke cigarettes?"

Figure 4.2 shows how a woman's risk of coronary heart disease depends upon her Body Mass Index. There are three curves: one for current cigarette smokers (triangles); another for past smokers (circles); and another for women who have never smoked (squares). The curves were derived from a study of 115,000 American nurses between 1976 and 1984.[12] The design of this Nurses' Health Study was very similar to that of the Harvard Alumni Study described in chapter 3. Nurses aged thirty to fifty-five answered a mailed questionnaire in 1976. From each nurse's reported height and weight, the researchers computed a BMI. The researchers then related the nurses' BMIs to their risks of coronary heart disease over the next eight years.

I have grouped the nurses' BMIs along the horizontal axis

FIGURE 4.2

Risk of Coronary Heart Disease Among 115,886 Nurses from 1976 to 1984 in Relation to Their Body Mass Index and Cigarette Smoking Status in 1976

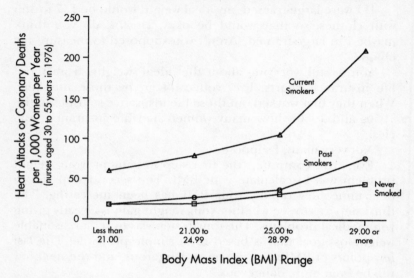

SOURCE: Adapted from JoAnn Manson et al., "A Prospective Study of Obesity and Risk of Coronary Heart Disease," *New England Journal of Medicine* 322 (1990): 886.

into four ascending ranges. The figure shows that the risk of coronary heart disease goes up with a woman's Body Mass Index, and that the risks associated with overweight are greatly enhanced by her cigarette smoking.[13] For each smoking category, but especially for the current smokers, the risk curve gets steeper as the BMI passes 25 points into the gray zone and then enters the medically significant range from 29 and up. The Nurses' Health Study did not separately report on women with very high BMIs. But the scientific evidence, taken as a whole, indicates that the curve relating BMI to the risks of disease rises ever more steeply as the BMI increases beyond 35 and 40.[14] That is, the last few units of BMI were the most dangerous, and the next few units will be even more dangerous. While Eve may have been concerned about getting her weight well below 150 (that is, a BMI of 25), the figure suggests that she would have attained little if any further reduction in her risk of heart disease, provided that she was a nonsmoker.

Just as in the Harvard Alumni Study, the figure is based on the BMIs of the nurses only at the time they filled out a questionnaire. If a nurse had a BMI of 27 in 1976, the chart alone doesn't say whether her weight had been increasing in the recent past or whether she'd been at 27 her whole adult life. To be sure, most people's weights don't vary nearly as much as does their level of physical activity.[15] Still, separate analyses of the Nurses' Health Study showed that a nurse's recent weight gain, and not her weight upon graduation from high school, determined her risk of heart disease and diabetes.[16] In other words, the rate of increase of BMI matters.

Similarly, the nurses' smoking practices could have changed during the eight-year tracking period. A nurse who currently smoked cigarettes in 1976 could have quit at some time from 1976 to 1984. Therefore, the curve of "current smokers" that connects the triangles in the chart actually measures the risks of a mixed group of continuing smokers and quitters. If anything, the actual risks of the continuing smokers would be even greater. But the curves tell us more than the fact that cigarette smoking and obesity are a bad combination. They tell us that, as least so far as coronary risk is concerned, it pays to quit smoking, even if you gain a lot of weight after quitting.

The figure shows the curve for past smokers (circles) to be well below the curve for current smokers (triangles). Only the most overweight quitters, with BMIs exceeding 29, had coronary risks that were comparable to those of the leanest current smokers, with BMIs under 21. To put it more concretely, consider Daphne, a 5'4" woman who weighs 122 pounds and smokes cigarettes. From figure 4.1, her conversion factor is 5.81, so her BMI is 122 ÷ 5.81, which equals 21. If Daphne kicked the habit, she'd have to gain at least 8 BMI points in order to cancel out the improvement in her coronary risk from smoking cessation. But 8 BMI points is equivalent to $8 \times 5.81 = 46.5$ pounds. In other words, it would pay Daphne to quit smoking unless she gained 46.5 or more pounds after quitting. Most people who quit smoking gain much less weight than that. In the decade after they quit, women gain an average of 1.5 BMI points over continuing smokers. One in eight such quitters gains 5 or more BMI points. Men who quit smoking gain an average of 0.8 BMI points over the long term, and one in ten male quitters gains 4 or more BMI points.[17]

The chart is only about coronary risks. It doesn't tell us how much Daphne could cut her risks of cancer or emphysema, or her risk of having a sick newborn, by quitting smoking. Nor does it say anything about the psychic stresses and orthopedic consequences of any resulting weight gain. But now I'm going too far afield. I'll get back to quitting smoking in chapter 6. In the final analysis, the overall equation for quitting smoking is very unlikely to change, even for the one in eight women who gains more than 5 BMI points after quitting. What we can say now is that if Eve smokes, then she's got to be treated as a special case, whether she quits or not. If she continues to smoke, her weight is going to be especially dangerous to her. If she quits, we'll need to be on guard for an acceleration in her weight gain.

For that matter, the figure tells only about the coronary risks of middle-aged women. Nothing is said about older women, or about men of any age, or about overall mortality. If we put together all the long-term follow-up studies of weight and health, we'd pretty much get the same relationship for both sexes, for older and younger people, and for overall mortality as well as coronary disease.[18] In the Harvard Alumni Study, in fact, both the initial questionnaire (in 1966 or 1962) and the second-wave questionnaire (in 1977) asked men about their weight and height. At the time of the first wave, the vast majority of Harvard men had a BMI below 26. More than a decade later, 11 percent of these men had gained enough weight to pass the 26-point mark. These gainers had about a 35 percent higher chance of dying per year than those men whose BMIs stayed below 26.[19] Parenthetically, some researchers have suggested that the weight-mortality relationship may be different for blacks, and that there is little if any connection between weight and mortality in black women.[20] If the scientific community ever manages to amass data bases on black Americans as large and detailed as the Harvard Alumni Study and the Nurses' Health Study, I believe that these speculations will turn out to be wrong.

When she came to see you for a checkup, Eve brought up the height-weight tables from the life insurance industry, which are often used to establish so-called ideal weights. You criticized the tables because they were based on the experience of a small number of selected women. Still, is there a so-called ideal weight at which one's risk of disease is lowest? Are height-weight tables such as those from the insurance industry of any use in establishing weight-reduction goals?

In theory, every person has her own "ideal" weight. Eve's ideal is not necessarily the same as Leah's or Daphne's. The best we can say at this point is that most ideal BMIs, if they do exist, are in the range of 19 to 25. To give you some sense of the individual variability in ideal weights, the BMIs of thirteen women on the 1992 U.S. Olympic speedskating team in Albertville ranged from 20.9 to 26.6. (The women at the extremes, by the way, won medals.) The BMIs of thirteen male Olympian speedskaters ranged from 22.0 to 26.6. (None won medals.) The speedskaters' BMIs varied, in part, because they had different amounts of "lean mass" (muscle and bone), and the same goes for the rest of us non-Olympians.

When the life insurance industry studied the mortality of policyholders of different weights, they drew artificial distinctions between small-, medium-, and large-framed people. A person's frame was supposed to be gauged by the breadth of his or her elbow. But elbow breadth isn't an accurate indicator of a person's lean mass, especially muscle mass. Anyway, when the industry first collected information on policyholders' body frames, the examining doctors didn't measure elbows. They just eyeballed the examinees' body frames, and that's basically what's done today. Such body-frame distinctions probably do more harm than good. They convey a false sense of precision about "ideal" weights. In practice, many people are likely to be misclassified.

What's worse, the industry didn't distinguish between smokers and nonsmokers. They just lumped them together. Since smokers tend to be leaner, the policyholders with the lowest weights were overrepresented by smokers, who in turn had higher death rates. That made the lowest weights appear riskier than they actually were. The failure to distinguish smokers from nonsmokers, coupled with an artificial distinction by body frame, created a statistical illusion that there was a narrow range of "ideal" weight at which mortality is lowest, when in fact the minimum-mortality range may be much broader.

But who cares? We're not interested in Eve's "ideal" weight. And if we knew what it was, we wouldn't use it to establish a weight-reduction goal. We want Eve to lose one or two BMI points, or at the very least to stop gaining any more weight. That's a reasonable and realistic goal. The question is: How can Eve do it?

You have probably read somewhere that obesity is an unsolved puzzle, "a complex disorder," as they say. People who gain weight must somehow be taking in more calories than they burn up. Beyond that, nobody's entirely sure whether overweight people eat more, whether they have slower metabolisms, or whether they tend to retain excess fat. Some writers make a big deal of the fact that obesity is inherited, at least partly, because identical twins tend to have the same BMIs.[21] That's no help. They're just saying that they can't explain obesity either, and so whatever it is, you might have gotten it from your parents. Here's a clue to the puzzle. Any time the scientific community says that the cause of a "complex disorder" is unknown, it's a good bet that the so-called disorder is really ten disorders, maybe twenty, artificially rolled into one.

Actually, I think it's impolitic to call obesity a "disorder." We already have genuine "eating disorders," such as anorexia nervosa and bulimia nervosa. The American psychiatric community has been toying with the idea of a new "binge-eating disorder," but that would basically be a form of bulimia without the vomiting or the laxatives.[22] People with these eating disorders are disturbed. It's not just their weight, or for that matter their eating, that's the problem.

Take Leah. Even at 114 pounds, she obsesses over her thighs. She tries rigidly to control her diet, counting her breadsticks, doing ten situps for each stalk of celery. But then, on the way to her appointment with Eve, ridden with self-hate, she binges at the doughnut shop. And then, as if to spew forth doughnut poison, she vomits it all back into the bathroom toilet at the gas station. Every day, sometimes several times a day, this binge-purge cycle is repeated.

Eve may be overweight, but she's no Leah. Perhaps Eve doesn't like her shape, but that's not the same as a delusion that one's thighs are too fat. Eve ate doughnuts during her internship, but not several dozen in a half-hour. Eve doesn't make herself vomit, and even if she admitted to purging a few times in high school or college, that doesn't make her bulimic. Leah, by contrast, upchucks like clockwork.

You have probably read that our culture is driving young women to eating disorders. I am not about to deny that our social preoccupation with thinness plays a role in the development of anorexia and bulimia. But don't think for a minute that every young woman who has downed a quart of chocolate-chip ice cream, cried about her cellulite, gone on a starvation diet, or tried to vomit should automatically be classified as "disordered." Millions of American women and men, young and old, are legitimately concerned about their weight and shape. They're not psychiatric material, like Leah. Eve has enough excuses. To tell her to ignore her weight problem because our culture overemphasizes thinness is just another rationalization. It's baloney.

Language matters. Branding obesity a "disease" would be no less impolitic than calling it a "disorder," and labeling it an "eating disease" would be even worse, especially since we don't know whether eating is the cause. Perhaps we could call it a "condition," as in the phrase "skin condition" or better still, a "process," as in "the aging process." The latter term suggests that overweight is internally programmed, sort of computerized. In effect, Eve's central weight-processor chip has been set in overweight mode. She can't simply replace it with a new chip because, sadly, it's soldered to the main motherboard. Unlike computers, however, Eve can't replace her motherboard. Overweight is hard-wired, cybernetic, almost robotic.

You have probably read about the so-called setpoint theory of weight regulation. It is the ultimate in body-weight determinism. According to setpoint, overweight people are programmed to be overweight, just as lean people are programmed to be lean. Their weights are set. If Eve succeeded temporarily in losing weight, her internal weight-control system would swing into action, forcing her ultimately to regain the weight she had lost. Eve's weight, according to the theory, is stuck in a set range around her 162-pound setpoint.

The setpoint theory is another lame excuse for Eve to do nothing. Eve weighed 132 after graduation from high school. Was 132 pounds her setpoint at that time? If so, then why did she gain 6 pounds in college and 6 more pounds in medical school? Setpoint proponents will respond that Eve's setpoint was "reset" at 144 pounds. But Eve then gained 12 pounds during her one-year internship. How come her internal weight-control program didn't zap those 12 pounds off when her internship was over? Reuben, the six-foot-tall grandfather, has weighed about 184 pounds his entire adult life. How come his setpoint was never "reset" upward, as was Eve's? Setpoint theory doesn't really have a setpoint; it has a ratchet. It's a ratchet theory. Actually, it's a ratchet tautology. Reuben's weight hasn't gone up because something keeps it from going up. Eve's weight has gone up because nothing keeps it from going up, but something keeps it from going down. Sauerkraut.

So then, what do we call overweight? One way out is to make up a new word. Overweight people, we might say, are *dysponderal*. ("Pondus" means "weight" in Latin.) After all, we've already got dyslexia and muscular dystrophy, not to mention dyspepsia, dysphagia, dyskinesia, and dysentery. To label Eve "dysponderal" is to impart legitimacy to her condition. Imagine Leah asking the receptionist, "Do you have any specialists in bulimia who aren't so dysponderal?" Anyway, here's the point. Dysponderal people are a motley crew.

Not every dysponderal person overeats, but some do. Not every dysponderal person binges, or eats at night, or eats from depression, or eats a high-fat diet, but some do. Not every dysponderal person has a slow metabolism, or underexercises, but some do. Not every dysponderal person has cellulite, or a pot belly, or a spare tire around the waist, but some do. Not every dysponderal person is chronically dieting, or has cycles of weight loss and weight regain, but some do. Not every dysponderal person has dysponderal parents, but some do. Not all dysponderal people are the same, and they shouldn't be treated the same.

Some weight-control problems may have no solution, or at best a partial fix. Others may have a singularly best approach. Still others may be amenable to many approaches. But how do we classify people into different types of overweight? How do we match each type of overweight with a suitable weight-control strategy?

Under currently recommended medical practice, overweight people are basically sorted according to the severity of their weight problems, with the most obese people receiving the most intensive measures.[23] As the degree of overweight increases, the dietary caloric restriction gets more severe; the program entails more medical supervision; the weight-control curriculum is more structured and less discretionary; the counseling becomes individualized rather than group-oriented; and there is greater reliance on specially formulated foods and supplements.

While there are no universally accepted rules, people in the gray overweight zone with BMIs over 25, such as Eve, are usually offered low-calorie diets (called "LCDs") in the range of 1,200 to 1,500 calories per day. These diets are typically self-administered, with periodic help from a nutritionist, and often entail so-called food exchanges. People with medically significant obesity, with BMIs over 29 or 30, also receive LCDs, sometimes as low as 1,000 calories per day. There is greater reliance on prepackaged foods to replace self-cooked meals, and the weight-control programs are more organized. There are exercise classes; group therapy to teach people to identify their weaknesses, build their problem-solving skills, and reward themselves for good behavior; and special maintenance sessions to prevent relapse.

For people with medically dangerous obesity, with BMIs over 35, and especially for people with severe or morbid obesity, with BMIs over 40, we're into very low calorie diets ("VLCDs"), typically in the range of 800 calories per day or lower.[24] (Eve's BMI would reach 40 points when she weighed 240 pounds, at which point she'd be in the top 2 percent of all women in her age group.) Basically, VLCDs are medically supervised starvation. Because serious complications can develop, VLCDs are not for everyone. People on VLCDs need to get enough protein (and the right kinds of protein), as well as supplements of vitamins and minerals. In some VLCDs, the protein is administered as a powder to be mixed with water. In others, such as the protein-sparing modified fast, the protein comes in the form of carefully apportioned servings of lean meat, fish, or poultry. VLCDs are major productions, entailing regular blood tests and checkups. They can't last more than three or four months, because it would be too dangerous to stay below 800 calories per day for longer than that. At some point, the dieter has got to make a transition back to an LCD and regular food. Finally, at the point of morbid obesity, at BMIs over 40, when all else fails, we're into various surgical methods of turning one's normally expandable stomach into a small pouch.[25]

The greater the degree of overweight, the more severe the measures undertaken. The more extreme the intervention, the greater the need for medical supervision. The greater the degree of medical oversight, the greater the opportunities for systematic evaluation. We are thus led to the paradox that the most overweight people, the top 2 to 5 percent of the adult population, are actually in a position to make the clearest, most informed choices. At this end of the spectrum, it is hardly the case that no weight-loss programs have been evaluated.[26] True, a great many people can't get through these programs. For those who stick it out, weight regain is commonplace afterward. Still, the degree of weight regain may be only partial, and the long-term net weight loss may be significant.

Of course, there aren't any fixed rules. Some overweight people attend worksite programs; others attend commercial programs; others go away to residential programs, where their entire lives are restructured. Some people have private counselors. Although subject to controversy, some practitioners use the new generation of appetite-suppressant drugs.[27] Still, the matching algorithm underlying these programs is basically the same. The higher your BMI, the more weight you have to lose, and therefore the more extreme the intervention. These matching systems are actually quite primitive. There's no genuine classification of people into different styles or types of obesity. It boils down to who's who on the pecking order of extra pounds.

For someone like Eve, way back at a BMI of 27 points, these manifold weight-reduction technologies must seem overwhelming. There she sits, receiver in hand, contemplating the "1"-button on her phone, perusing a brochure about a structured, balanced-deficit plan, 1,200 calories daily, with specially formulated foods, group sessions on relapse prevention, and optional individual counseling. There she sits, smack in the middle of the gray zone of overweight, trying to lose only six or twelve, or maybe eighteen pounds.

No wonder Eve rejects these state-of-the-art offerings as gimmicks. No wonder Eve lumps them together with the thousands of too-good-to-be-true ten-day meal plans; and the too-gorgeous-to-be-real people on those exercise devices, whose percentage body fat drops lickety-split before your eyes; and the refrigerator magnets and diet journals and the innumerable entertaining self-control tidbits that she reads and hears about daily. Would you blame Eve for her rationalizations, her cynicism, her denial?

Eve doesn't smoke cigarettes. But that alone doesn't take the heat off, because now you've got her worried about her blood pressure, her blood sugar, her stress level, and her back spasms. She knows that no matter what her current degree of overweight is, her rate of recent weight gain is especially high. Eve sees herself as different from other 162-pound, 5'5" tall women. Yet at the same time, she's right in the center of the same gray zone that is occupied by half of the overweight women in America and nearly two-thirds of the overweight men. Eve is unique unto herself. Yet she is Everywoman.

People who have gained weight must have taken in more calories than they burned up. It is standard to equate each pound gained with 3,500 excess calories. Eve has gained thirty pounds in a dozen years, so she accumulated 105,000 excess calories. Twelve years is 4,383 days. So, on average, Eve has consumed about 24 excess calories per day since high school. That's as many calories as in a cup of cauliflower florets. A sedentary young woman of her size probably burned up around 2,000 calories per day. So, over a twelve-year period, Eve consumed about 1.2 percent more calories every day than her body burned up. But that's the long-term average. Eve gained twelve pounds during her internship alone. By the same sort of calculation, her daily caloric excess during her year of peak weight gain would equal about 115 calories. That's the equivalent of one banana plus a whole prune per day. Put differently, it's an excess of 5.7 percent daily.

This type of calculation suggests that Eve could lose twelve pounds in a year if she could cut back on her average caloric intake by about 115 calories per day. But it could just as well be interpreted to mean that she's got to burn an extra 115 calories per day. At this point, we could make a bunch of pseudoscientific computations about the number of cookies Eve would have to forgo or the number of miles she'd have to walk per week. (If walking at a fourteen-minute-mile pace has an intensity of about 2 CHPs, then a 162-pound person would burn about 324 calories per hour, at least at her initial weight. That means 115 extra calories would be expended in 0.35493 hours of walking, which over seven days would come to 2.48451 hours or, equivalently, 10 miles, 1,140 yards, and 10 $^{15}/_{16}$ inches of walking per week.) But that would be pretty much a waste of time. You just can't be that scientific about it. Eve isn't going to know whether caloric restriction works until she tries it for a sustained period, at least a month or two but probably longer. The same goes for physical activity. The superior method of finding out whether her weight responds to dieting, exercise, or both is the empirical method. Eve has to do the experiment to know the answer.

To solve the matching problem, Eve should be classified not by the degree of her obesity, or even its underlying cause, but by what interventions work for her. She needs to test her responses to specific weight-control challenges. She needs to figure out whether she's a *diet-responder* or an *exercise-responder.* If she's a diet-responder, then she needs to see whether she's a *calorie-restricter* or a *fat-restricter.* If she's an exercise-responder, she needs to see whether she's a *high-intensity* exerciser or *high-volume* exerciser. Maybe she's a combination. Maybe she's none of the above. Time will tell.

There are so many dietary variables that Eve's task of finding out what works seems daunting, almost hopeless. Eve could try avoiding all doughnuts and ice cream, or, for that matter, all desserts. Or she could stay away from the fast-food restaurant next to the hospital. Or she could try a "nibbling" strategy under the supposition that large, infrequent meals, especially "gorging," predispose to weight gain.[28] Or she could stock rice cakes and celery for especially vulnerable moments. Of course, Eve can't live on rice cakes and celery alone. She's got to get adequate protein, vitamins, and minerals. But when it comes to Eve's testing the hypothesis that she's a diet-responder, only two variables really matter: her total calories consumed, and the proportion of her calories that is consumed in the form of fat.

The human body relies upon two main sources of fuel: *carbo-fuels* and *fat-fuels.* Protein is a secondary source of fuel, and for people who drink a lot, alcohol can be a significant component in the overall fuel equation.[29] These fuels are used to perform work. They make Eve's muscles contract, her heart pump, and her intestines rumble. They keep her warm-blooded. They support the building and repair of her skin, bones, muscles, and other tissues. If Eve were pregnant, she'd use fuels to help feed the fetus growing inside her. If she were nursing, the fuels would be called upon to make her baby's milk.

When a person eats, she takes in fuel. The *ingested fuels* are broken down in the intestines and absorbed into the bloodstream, where they circulate through the tissues. These *circulating fuels* can be used directly by the body's organs, or they can be saved as *stored fuels* for later use. Carbohydates and fats assume different chemical forms as ingested fuel, as circulating fuel, and as stored fuel. For example, ingested carbo-fuels come as simple sugars, such as nondiet sodas, table sugar, corn syrup, and honey; or as complex carbohydrates, such as the starches in pasta and baked potatoes. The main circulating carbo-fuel is a simple sugar called glucose, which was measured in Eve's blood glucose test. Carbo-fuel is stored mainly as a starch called *glycogen* in the liver and muscles.

Ingested fats also assume many chemical forms, depending on whether they come from animal or vegetable sources. Most ingested fat-fuel comes in the form of *triglycerides*. (We'll worry about cholesterol in chapter 5. It's usually less than 1 percent of your dietary fat.) Once ingested and absorbed into the bloodstream, triglycerides can be broken down into *fatty acids,* which serve as the main circulating fat-fuels. The circulating fatty acids can be repackaged (three at a time) into *tri*glyceride, which is then stowed away in specialized fat cells. These fat cells are in turn clumped together as fatty tissues throughout the body: under the skin, layered between the muscles, and surrounding various internal organs, especially within the abdominal cavity.

Once ingested, the human body can convert carbo-fuels into fat-fuels, and vice versa. But that doesn't mean that the body treats carbos and fats interchangeably. For one thing, carbo-fuel stores are limited, while fat-fuel stores can expand almost without limit. We usually associate the complete exhaustion of a person's carbo-fuel stores with extreme endurance sports, such as "hitting the wall" in the marathon. In fact, it is possible to deplete the body's entire carbo-fuel storage system with twenty minutes of superintense exercise. Even when a person's carbo-fuel stores are totally emptied, however, it takes only a day of normal eating to fill them up again.[30] By comparison, all but the very leanest people have weeks worth of fat-fuel, stored as triglycerides within their body fat.

Imagine Eve eating some mixture of carbo-fuels and fat-fuels. If she consumes more fuel than her body currently needs, then the excess fuel will be stored someplace. If the carbo-fuel stores in her muscles and liver are already filled up, then the excess fuel will go into body fat. It won't matter whether the extra fuel was ingested as carbo-fuel or fat-fuel. But suppose that the total amount of fuel that Eve consumes is not more than her body needs. Or suppose that Eve's carbo-fuel stores are not completely filled. Then it can matter how the calories are consumed. Eve may be one of those people who tend to convert ingested fat-fuels into circulating fatty acids and send them directly into fat storage as triglycerides.[31] These people preferentially fill up their fat stores, even when they need the circulating fat-fuels to perform work and even when carbo-fuel stores are unfilled.

There is a huge, nearly endless controversy over whether overweight people actually eat more than other people.[32] They don't seem to record more calories in their food journals, but some don't document everything they eat.[33] When spied upon by research sleuths, some overweight people are found to overeat, but others undereat. The undereaters, of course, may be dieting because they are overweight. There is just as much controversy over whether overweight people eat more fat than others do. For those people who actually eat more calories than they burn, it's not going to matter whether it's fat-fuel or any other fuel. The extra calories will end up as body fat. But for those people who aren't overeaters but who are prone to convert dietary fat into body fat, the fuel mix can matter.[34]

We get no more agreement when we ask whether overweight people have slower metabolisms than others.[35] While Eve is thirty pounds heavier than she was at age eighteen, her resting metabolic rate may actually be higher than it was when she graduated high school. As I'll explain shortly, Eve has not only more fat than before, but also more muscles, and those muscles are burning extra calories all the time, even when she is asleep. But Eve's resting metabolic rate is just a part of the picture. During an ordinary day, even a sedentary person moves around, and some so-called sedentary people move around a whole lot more or less than do others. Some people don't sit still. Some can't sit still. They fidget, or they're leg shakers, or they pace, or they work standing up. It can actually matter whether Eve is a leg-shaker. After all, we're talking about small differences of 24 to 115 calories per day over extended periods. But that's still not the end of the metabolic calculation. Eating food by itself causes a person's metabolism to rise. Some researchers say that naturally lean people get a bigger *thermic effect of food* (or *TEF*) than others.[36] You give them a pint of chocolate-chip ice cream and a dozen dough-nuts, and their thermic effect kicks in. When Eve ate dough-nuts, her metabolism went up, too, but perhaps by a smaller amount. One way or another, two people of the same weight can have very different daily energy expenditures, even when they're not exercising.[37]

Many researchers believe that extreme dieting itself slows one's baseline metabolism. If Eve restricts her fuel intake suffi-ciently, she'll have to rely upon her stored carbo- and fat-fuels and, if necessary, on her own muscle proteins, which can be internally converted into the burnable fuels. If she starts to break down her own muscles to use protein, then she's in *nega-tive nitrogen balance.* (To prevent this from happening, very low calorie diets are supposed to have protein supplements.) If Eve's negative nitrogen balance persists, her body may down-shift into first gear in order to avoid further muscle erosion. Even her TEF may drop off. While this phenomenon may not occur to the same extent and at the same degree of caloric restriction in every person, it would be one reason why Eve turned out to be *diet-resistant.*[38] As I'll explain shortly, this diet-induced metabolic slowdown may be one reason that people regain weight rapidly when the dietary program is over.[39]

If Eve's baseline metabolism were on the low side, couldn't she boost it with exercise? The short answer is probably yes, but the long answer is not so simple. Let's forget about putting Eve in a walking program, and send her instead into Tamar's bench-stepping aerobics class. If we got Eve accustomed to working out with arms and legs on a six-inch bench, she'd get to about the 3.7 CHP level. At 162 pounds, that's 600 calories per hour, or 300 per half-hour session. At three step classes per week, she'd be putting out about 130 extra calories per day. Wouldn't that do it? The problem, as we learned from

Stephen's choice in chapter 3, is that exercise is a long-term proposition. To burn as many calories as she overconsumed during her internship, Eve would need to keep up with regular step aerobics for an entire year. If she dropped out, she'd be back at square one.

There is no more agreement on the role of exercise in weight control than there is on the role of dietary restriction.[40] When overweight people engage in regular exercise but maintain unrestricted diets, they don't always lose weight. In short-term research studies, people who both exercise and restrict their calories are sometimes but not always more successful than dieters alone. There are almost as many explanations and prescribed exercise/diet combinations as there are authorities. Some researchers believe that calorie restriction by itself will not work unless the dieter exercises concurrently. The idea is that exercise stops the metabolic slowdown that occurs during extreme fuel restriction. Others believe that dietary control is essential to weight loss, and that exercise somehow prevents relapse and weight regain. In this view, it's exercise after dieting, rather than concurrently, that really counts. An alternative explanation is that exercise doesn't help prevent relapse at all. It's just that a person with the self-discipline to exercise is exactly the kind of person who can stay on a diet. Still other authorities believe that exercise is really the key to weight loss, but, without concomitant dietary restriction, some people just eat more. Some scientists believe that exercise can stop the tendency of some obese people preferentially to convert dietary fuels into stored body fat. Some researchers believe that strength training works better than aerobics, while others believe the opposite.[41]

My reading of this superabundance of studies is that, when it comes to weight control, the *intensity* of exercise is what really counts. In particular, the intensity of physical activity affects the mix of fuels that Eve's body burns while she is exercising. It also affects the degree to which Eve's metabolism stays revved up after she stops exercising.

When Eve is at total bed rest (and provided she isn't running a fever), her body burns about 2 calories of fat-fuel for every 1 calorie of carbo-fuel. As she moves around, the ratio gets closer to 1:1. When she exercises moderately, but well below her physical limits, the fuel-mix ratio reverses and she burns about 2 calories of carbo-fuel for every 1 calorie of fat-fuel. With a sufficiently intense workout, Eve will burn virtually all her calories as carbo-fuel.

When Eve engages in a walking program, she's probably performing an activity that gets her muscles going and her heart pumping, but doesn't push her even close to her physical limits—that is, well below her V-Dot-O_2-Max. The weight-control philosophy underlying such low-intensity exercise is that it tends to burn a significant proportion of fat-fuel.[42] As Eve starts walking, she uses the fatty acids that are circulating in her bloodstream. As she continues walking for a certain number of minutes—ten, twenty, or thirty minutes, depending on who you read—she begins to extract triglycerides from storage. In other words, she burns her own body fat. Since this low-intensity form of exercise burns calories relatively slowly, and since it can take a while before one starts extracting fat-fuel from storage, Eve will likely have to exercise for a long time.

But this form of low-intensity, high-volume exercise doesn't always work, even when a person concurrently diets. Some people, it appears, guard their fat-fuel stores. They'll use up their ingested and circulating carbo-fuels and fat-fuels, as well as their glycogen carbo-fuel stores, but even after a half-hour of low-intensity exercise, they still won't burn very much stored body fat. For these body fat–"defenders," the key to fat loss may be the proportion of fat-fuels in the diet, and not just the total number of calories consumed. These people are, in my classification, combination fat-restricters and high-volume exercisers.

Eve is thirty years old. She's got borderline hypertension and a mildly elevated blood sugar. She's on the road to heart and circulatory problems, but she's probably not there yet. Her knees, hips, and back bother her, but nobody said anything about a slipped disc or arthritis or torn ligaments. So, in the course of Eve's walking program, we begin to introduce some higher-intensity exercise. If she can take it even for five minutes, we'll have her walk faster or walk uphill or jog. If she can jog, we'll get her to run. The idea is to push her into the discomfort zone enough to get her adrenaline really going, but not so much as to hurt her or get her to quit.

While Eve is intensely exercising, she's burning almost

entirely carbohydrates. Her muscles are grabbing up the glycogen that's stored in them. And because she can't intensively
exercise for too long, she's not really burning all that many
calories, at least while she's exercising. But in some people—
and Eve might be one of them—intense exercise revs up the
body's metabolism, even after exercising stops. This is partly
because intense exercise is not just a heart-lung workout. It's
also a form of muscle building. The muscle building in turn
enhances one's resting metabolism. It's also because intense
exercise gets adrenaline going, and the adrenaline appears to
keep the metabolic rate elevated for several hours after one
stops, a phenomenon called "excess postexercise oxygen consumption," or EPOC. Of course, the effects of high-intensity
exercise are subject to detraining, just like any other effect of
physical activity. But that doesn't change the main point. Persistent low-volume, high-intensity exercise may work for Eve.[43]

What can Eve take away from this extraordinary divergence
of views on the effects of diet and exercise on weight control?
Is Eve really going to have to try different combinations of
calorie restriction, fat restriction, and high-volume and high-
intensity exercise until she finds the combination that's right
for her? It will take forever, won't it? And in the end, nothing
might work. Isn't there some laboratory test that can circum-
vent all the trial and error? With the current state of the art,
the answer is probably not.

There are lots of measurements that we could take on Eve's
body in an attempt to assess, at least in theory, why and how
she has gained weight. We could obtain food journals to assess
her current daily caloric intake, as well as the fat, carbohydrate, and protein composition of her diet. We'd see how
often Eve eats at home, and how often she consumes high-fat,
calorie-dense foods at various fast food restaurants. We'd see
whether she skips breakfast, or whether she eats one huge
meal daily. From physical activity logs, we'd see whether Eve
takes the elevator or the stairs. We could consult a fellow psychiatrist to see whether Eve eats to satisfy particular needs. We
could retain a behavioral psychologist to see whether Eve eats
on the road, or after work, or in front of the television.

Equipped with these consultants' reports, we could bring
Eve into the hospital metabolic ward, put her in a breathing
chamber, and measure her resting energy expenditure, as well

as her rate of calorie burning during a typical sedentary day. In the process, we'd observe what percentage of her calories are burned from fat-fuel. Then we'd have her eat something and measure the thermic effect of food. Then we could put Eve on a treadmill to see how her fuel-burning mix changed with exercise. After that, we could determine whether her metabolic rate remained elevated after exercising. Then we could perform an overfeeding experiment and see what happens to her metabolism.

We could get even fancier and measure the number and size of her fat cells, and how much of her fat is so-called brown fat. Then we could measure a host of hormone levels: thyroid, insulin, C-peptide, growth hormone, prolactin, and lipoprotein lipase. Perhaps Eve has a disorder of satiety. Maybe her stomach and intestines don't send the right signals to her brain when she's full. So, we'll get gut hormone levels, like cholecystokinin and bombesin, not to mention glucagon. Of course, it would be desirable to repeat these measurements in several months. It wouldn't be a bad idea to study some immediate family members, too.

If you and I were consultants on Eve's case, and if we had unlimited time and resources, we'd probably like to have all these measurements. In the final analysis, however, there are so many different styles of overweight, and the factors that distinguish one style from another are so difficult to identify and measure, that the best approach will still be the empirical one. In short, Eve has no choice but to navigate, to try to find her way.

Eve may fail. She could try every reasonable combination of weight-loss strategies and still, for reasons unexplained, not drop one pound. Or she could achieve a six- or twelve-pound weight loss, or even a thirty-pound weight loss, and then gain it all back. Or she could go through repeated cycles of weight loss and regain. Not only are these failures at weight control psychologically painful, but they might make Eve's overall health even worse.

I do not have a magic formula that will tell Eve in advance whether her weight-control efforts will be a waste of time. The fact that Eve's BMI of 27 points is already giving her medical troubles is an indicator that the stakes are high. It tips her hand into trying something, but it is not all-controlling. If there is any principle that can govern Eve's and Everywoman's decision, it is this: Move in small increments. Don't go for big weight changes. Go for one or two BMI points at a time. Small weight cycles are less dangerous than wide swings in weight. And if Eve keeps the weight off, she will have made a significant accomplishment. After all, those were the most hazardous pounds that Eve has gained thus far.

What is weight cycling about, anyway? The idea is that every time Eve loses X number of pounds and then gains X pounds back, she ends up weighing the same number of pounds but she has actually gotten fatter.

Just like Everywoman, Eve has fat from head to toe. When she pinches the back of her upper arm, she can feel the *subcutaneous fat* that is attached directly under her skin. Her thighs contain not only subcutaneous fat, which Eve might call cellulite, but also fat that is layered between her leg muscles, which is termed *intramuscular fat*. Eve's midsection contains not only subcutaneous fat, which she might be able to pinch as a "love handle" or "spare tire," but also fatty tissues attached to the organs within her abdominal cavity, which is called *intra-abdominal fat*. As the amount of Eve's intra-abdominal fat increases, her belly will protrude. These are Eve's primary fat stores, but not the only ones. She has a pad of fat, for example, surrounding her heart. The total weight of all the fatty tissues in Eve's body is called her *fat weight*. Everything else (including muscle, bone, teeth, lung, intestine, ovaries, brains, and other organs, as well as her blood and other body fluids) is Eve's *lean weight*. When we divide Eve's fat weight by her body weight, we get her *percentage body fat*.

There are many simple ways to gauge Eve's fat weight and percentage body fat, as well as the distribution of her body fat. One simple, commonplace method is to pinch Eve's skin at three or four standard places, use calipers to measure the thickness of each skin fold, and then look up the combined skin-fold thickness in a chart. While this pinch method actually measures the thickness of the fat under Eve's skin, the amount of subcutaneous fat is still a reasonable gauge of her total fat weight. To get a separate indicator of Eve's intra-abdominal fat, it is commonplace to measure her girth at the waist and to compare it to the circumference at her hips. If her *waist-to-hip ratio* exceeded 0.80 (or 0.95 for an adult man), we would ordinarily say that Eve had some degree of *central obesity*.

Of course, we could get much fancier. To gauge her total body fat, we could subject Eve to DPA (dual photon absorptiometry) or DEXA (dual emission X-ray absorptiometry), among others. If we weren't so high-tech, we could weigh Eve while she and her scale were immersed under water. (The idea is that fat floats.) To assess the degree of Eve's central obesity, we could get a CAT (computerized axial tomographic) scan or an MRI (magnetic resonance imaging) scan of her insides at the level of her lumbar vertebrae.

We could measure Eve's body fat twenty different ways, but what really counts is the path that her fatness has taken over the last twelve years. So, let's just say that when Eve graduated from high school at the age of eighteen, she had 33 ½ pounds of fat. Now, as chief resident at thirty years of age, Eve has 53 pounds of fat weight. In the process of gaining 30 pounds, Eve acquired 19 ½ pounds of fat and 10 ½ pounds of new muscle. Say that again? Eve gained 10 ½ pounds of new muscle? But she didn't go near the gym. She didn't even take the stairs. All true. But Eve did acquire extra fat, and in the process she developed extra muscles to carry the extra fat. Eve, literally, got stronger. In other words, Eve's weight gain was *partitioned* as 65 percent fat and 35 percent lean.

Now we get to the weight-cycling part. Let's say that Eve goes on a crash diet and loses the entire 30 pounds in a year. Does that mean the process goes backward? If she loses weight, she'll lose muscle, too. Actually, the problem is that she may lose even more muscle than she gained. The idea is illustrated in figure 4.3. The horizontal scale measures Eve's BMI. The vertical scale measures her percentage body fat. Each point on the diagram represents a particular BMI-fat combination. It might be helpful to think of the diagram as a map of Eve's travels over her adult life. When Eve travels east, her BMI goes up, and when she travels west, her BMI goes down. When Eve travels north, her percent fat goes up, and when she travels south, her percent fat goes down.

From her high school graduation to her chief residency in psychiatry, Eve traveled northeast. She gained 30 pounds, raising her BMI from 22 to 27, and she increased her body fat from 25.4 to 32.7 percent. Over the next year, Eve travels

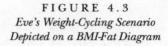

FIGURE 4.3
Eve's Weight-Cycling Scenario
Depicted on a BMI-Fat Diagram

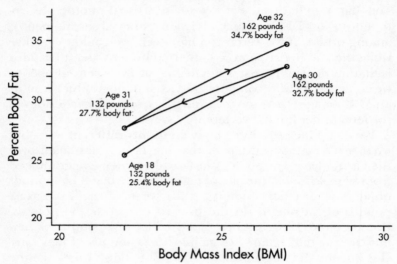

southwest. By age thirty-one, she's back down to 132 pounds, or a BMI of 22. But her body fat is now 27.7 percent. Eve's fat weight is now 36 ½ pounds, instead of the 33 ½ pounds of fat she had in high school. While Eve's long-term 30-pound weight gain consisted of 65 percent fat and 35 percent lean, her crash 30-pound weight loss consisted of 55 percent fat and 45 percent lean. Her crash diet threw her into negative nitrogen balance. She lost weight, but she lost muscle, too.

Let's suppose that Eve regains the weight in another year. She travels northeast again. When she regains the 30 pounds that she had just lost, it comes back on as 65 percent fat and 35 percent lean. When she completes the cycle, Eve is 34.7 percent body fat. She weighs 162 pounds again, but she now has three pounds more body fat. Maybe the extra three pounds is spread out under her skin. But there's a good chance that they're in her abdomen. She's the same weight, but she's converted three pounds of muscle into three pounds of belly fat.

Every time Eve goes through one of these 30-pound cycles, she'll convert another three pounds of lean into three pounds of fat. On the other hand, if Eve had initially lost only 12 pounds, then a subsequent 12-pound weight regain would not be so devastating. She'd be back at 162 pounds, but she'd have converted only 1.2 pounds from lean to fat. She'd still take a zigzag on the BMI-fat diagram, but the size of the excursion would be a lot smaller.

People are very different. In Dinah's choice, not every HIV-infected man is a superinfecter, and not every uninfected woman is supersusceptible. In Stephen's choice, not every person responds the same way to a physical training stimulus. In Eve's choice, not every person responds the same way to calorie or fat restriction, or high-intensity versus high-volume exercise. All three will have to navigate their way, to learn empirically, to adapt. In a sense, they are all engaged in lifetime careers of taking chances, making mistakes, bouncing back, and trying again.

"Now, doctor, what kinds of patients do you treat? People with a hundred pounds to lose? Fifty pounds?"

"I'm not calling for my patients."

"What's your specialty?"

"Psychiatry. Eating disorders, specifically."

"Then you'd be interested in our new instructional video entitled 'Self-esteem, Self-reward, Self-control.' Now, doctor, if you ordered the video in bulk quantity—"

"You don't understand. It's not for my patients."

"We'd be happy to send you samples of our prepackaged flavored powders, along with detailed brochures showing individual constituents and—"

"I'm not sure I need those yet."

"We have special prepared meals for your patients, planned according to our low-calorie, high-fiber—"

"But it's for me."

"Perhaps you're interested in our Pacing Program. It's a semi-supervised walking program that incorporates—"

"I haven't walked much, especially since the back spasms."

"Doctor, are you inquiring about our services for yourself? Hold the line. Let me connect—"

"I'll call back later."

"If you can just give us your name and office address, we'll at least send you our catalogue, doctor."

"My name is Eve. I'm a fat psychiatrist."

"Really? You don't sound fat. How much do you weigh?"

"None of your business."

"Hold the line, and I'll connect you with—"

"Wait a second. I changed my mind. I am calling for my patients. Send me the catalogue. Send me the video. Send me the brochures and the samples. Send me everything."

5

The Good Minus the Bad

Cholesterol

It is late Friday afternoon, and the American financial markets have closed. Gideon, the sixty-two-year-old manager of a hugely successful billion-dollar equity fund, is treating his junior colleague James to a late lunch at a new French restaurant. The mâitre d' has seated them at a nonsmoking table, près de la fenêtre, and both have declined an apéritif, explicitly stating their joint intent to have wine with the entrée. James, being a snap decision maker, has chosen quiche lorraine, la spécialité du jour. It is Gideon's turn to order.

Earlier that morning, before the markets opened, Gideon's internist informed him that his fasting blood-cholesterol level was 239. After nine difficult months, Gideon had managed to get it down from a high value of 257. As close as he and his protégé have become, Gideon has never disclosed his cholesterol problem to James. Spindling the wine list, Gideon nervously tells the young waiter that he needs more time.

Lest you're on the edge of your seat, Gideon will not inquire about the availability of gas-free kidney beans. Nor will he make a special request to have his quiche prepared with cholesterol-free egg substitute, low-fat cheese, skim milk, and hold the bacon, please.

"Speaking of transportation stocks," says James, picking up from an earlier conversation, "I've been looking into that international truck-

ing conglomerate. The stock has a favorable price-earnings multiple, but the company's mired in shareholder litigation. The truckers' union hasn't exactly boosted profits either."

"Every stock," says Gideon, "has a bad side and a good side."

"Excellent point," says James to his mentor.

Cholesterol, too, has a bad side and a good side, Gideon thinks to himself. That's what is making him so nervous. His "bad cholesterol" has come down from 182 to 166. But at the same time, his "good cholesterol" has come down, from 45 to only 35. Gideon's internist tried not to make too much of it. But for someone who has made his livelihood from small up-and-down movements in numbers, Gideon is, to put it delicately, afraid.

Virtually every American has heard the message that cholesterol is bad. Yet tens of millions of Americans regularly walk out of their doctors' offices having been told about their so-called good cholesterol and bad cholesterol. If cholesterol is really so bad, then how can it be good, too?

The term *good cholesterol* is a poorly chosen misnomer for a specific blood test called an HDL-cholesterol level. *Bad cholesterol* is likewise a misnomer for a blood test called an LDL-cholesterol level. As I shall explain shortly, there is a genuine sense in which a high blood level of HDL cholesterol is beneficial for you and a high blood level of LDL cholesterol is deleterious to you. But, again, language matters. The oxymoron *good cholesterol* is the thread on the fuse of the bomb that has blown open the credibility of the American message on diet, cholesterol, and the prevention of heart disease.

"James," asks Gideon, "what's your cholesterol level?"

"My cholesterol? Beats me. What's yours?"

"Two hundred thirty something," answers Gideon.

"Come on, Gideon, you're not into that cholesterol stuff, are you? Stress causes heart attacks, not cholesterol. Look, the French eat wads of Brie cheese, and they outlast us anyway. You think General de Gaulle skimped on omelettes? No way. Here, let's share some goose liver pâté."

"But the Chinese eat a low-fat diet," Gideon interjects, "and they rarely have heart attacks. I read it someplace."

"Let me take a look at that menu. Here, why don't you have the gâteau de crêpes filled with cream cheese, spinach—"

"James, don't you realize that cream cheese is loaded with cholesterol and saturated fat?"

"How about salade de moules? Fish is good for you, right?"

"Yeah, but they're mussels, and who knows which kind of oil they're marinated in."

"How about tournedos Henri IV? It's got filet steaks with artichoke hearts and béarnaise sauce. Now, Gideon, you can't sit there and tell me that artichokes have cholesterol."

"Artichokes have a lot of fiber, but the béarnaise sauce is made with egg yolks and butter, and the steaks have—"

"That settles it. Garçon, I mean, Monsieur," James calls out. "Mon confrère is all set to order."

The waiter approaches, pen and pad cocked and ready.

There's more to Gideon's choice than a single steak on a Friday afternoon, just as there was more to Stephen's choice than a single step-aerobics class. Even if Gideon had chosen the crêpes, he wouldn't have dropped dead after lunch from the 63 milligrams of cholesterol and 13 grams of saturated fat contained in two measly ounces of cream cheese. As perplexed as he may be about the latest down-ticks in his "good" and "bad" cholesterol numbers, Gideon does have perspective. He knows that there's a bigger picture. Still, Gideon's choice is a quintessentially deadly one. For Gideon also knows that each high-cholesterol, high-fat meal may push his body one extra fraction of an inch toward death's door. Every quiche kills, ever so slightly.

How can French people eat Brie cheese and goose liver pâté, but still have lower coronary rates than Americans? The short answer is that the French eat lots of other disease-preventing foods—especially fruits and vegetables—that tend to cancel out any deleterious effects of cheese and liver pâté. Why have Gideon's persistent dietary efforts yielded such ambiguous results? The short answer is basically the same. When Gideon cut back on cholesterol and saturated fats, he failed to substitute the right foods in their place. By focusing too heavily on avoiding the negatives, Gideon failed to accentuate the positives. The population of France does exactly the opposite.

For Gideon, food is no longer food, not anymore. Food has become a drug, with dosages, indications and contraindications, side effects, and benefits. Yes, cholesterol is a chemical constituent of food that can, in many people, enhance the risk of coronary heart disease. So, too, is the monounsaturated (and probably beneficial) oleic acid in the olive oil in which the mussels were marinated. So are the omega-3 polyunsaturated (and possibly beneficial) fatty acids in the mussels themselves. So is the Vitamin C in the artichokes in tournedos Henri IV. So are the antioxidant beta-carotene and Vitamin E in the spinach within the cream cheese–laden filling of the gâteau de crêpes. But anyone who's tasted challah, gazpacho, or chicken curry—let alone tournedos Henri IV—knows that food is a not merely a collection of nutrients and toxins. Food is a reflection of culture.

I shall do my best in this chapter to explain that there is indeed a good cholesterol and a bad cholesterol. But we don't eat good cholesterol and bad cholesterol. We eat better food and worse food. That's the message. The cholesterol diet-coronary heart disease paradigm has been misframed as: Accomplish Good by systematically teasing out and eliminating Bad. The problem, properly framed, is: Make Good by doing, on balance, more Good than Bad. There will probably never be such a thing as the coronary-perfect food or the cancer-perfect cuisine, with all Good and absolutely no Bad. There are, and there will continue to be, only better foods and better cuisines. There is no undeadly, perfect choice.

So much for moralizing. What did Gideon order? Was the senior portfolio manager intimidated by his junior colleague? Having little taste for suspense, I shall tell you now that Gideon took a deep breath and got the tournedos Henri IV. James ordered a bottle of burgundy, but Gideon drank none. As for dessert, you will have to wait, because it's now time for biochemistry.

Cholesterol is a basic building-block chemical that is found throughout the bodies of virtually every animal species, including human beings. Being a fatty substance, cholesterol does not dissolve easily in water. In order to circulate in the watery bloodstream, cholesterol attaches itself to specialized proteins. When cholesterol and other fatty substances attach to these specialized proteins, they form particles. These particles circulate in the blood. They come in many different sizes. As a class, they are called *lipoprotein particles*.

The Good Minus the Bad

Some lipoprotein particles are heavy and dense. If placed in a glass of water, they would tend to sink to the bottom. At the other extreme, some lipoprotein particles are light and fluffy. They would tend to float to the top. It's a continuum from the most dense to the fluffiest. Lipoprotein particles are classified by their density into three major groups: *high*-density lipoprotein (HDL); *low*-density lipoprotein (LDL); and *very low* density lipoprotein (VLDL). This is a slight oversimplification. There is another group of very fluffy, extremely low density lipoprotein particles that temporarily circulate in the bloodstream after a meal. But if Gideon got his blood test after an overnight fast, these lipoproteins would be out of the picture.

When Gideon gets a fasting blood cholesterol test, the result shows the *total cholesterol* in his blood, regardless of which type of lipoprotein particle the cholesterol was attached to. The amount of cholesterol that is specifically attached to HDL particles is called the *HDL cholesterol*. The amount of cholesterol that is specifically attached to LDL particles is called the *LDL cholesterol*. The remaining cholesterol is attached to VLDL particles, and is called the *VLDL cholesterol*. From this point on, I will abbreviate the total amount of cholesterol in the blood as C; the HDL cholesterol as H; the LDL cholesterol as L; and the VLDL cholesterol as V. Accordingly, we have a simple cholesterol partitioning equation: $C = H + L + V$.

Now let's tear a page from the waiter's notepad, and write down Gideon's present and past blood test results, as well as the change:

	Present	Past	Change
C	239	257	-18
H	35	45	-10
L	166	182	-16
V	38	30	+ 8
T	190	150	+40

Gideon's story didn't mention his blood level of VLDL cholesterol. But I computed it from the basic cholesterol equation, by subtracting his H and his L together from his C. The tabulation also contains an unidentified quantity, denoted by T. That's Gideon's blood *triglyceride level*. I put it up there so that we could have all Gideon's numbers in one place. $T = V \times 5$. I'll come back to T later.

So, what do these numbers mean? For now, let's just say that Gideon's past C of 257 placed him at about the eighty-ninth percentile of American men aged sixty to sixty-four, while his present C of 239 puts him at about the seventy-eighth percentile.[1] Put differently, in a cholesterol-lowering competition among 100 *American* men in the same age group, Gideon has moved from eighty-seventh place to seventy-eighth place, but he is still way in the back of the pack. I emphasize American, because if Gideon were competing internationally against men from China, he'd be much farther behind.

But those are only the statistics for Gideon's C, and not his H, L, and V. At this point, it's worth noting that most of Gideon's total cholesterol is attached to his LDL particles. Of the three individual components that add up to C, the L component is by far the biggest. That's enough biochemistry for now. It's time for some pathology.

You have already read about coronary heart disease. You saw a chart of heart attack rates in chapter 3 and a graph of the risk of a heart attack or coronary death in chapter 4. Now I need to explain what coronary heart disease actually is.

Arteries are blood vessels that carry blood from the heart. (Veins carry blood back to the heart.) *Atherosclerosis* is a chronic disease that can affect the arteries in virtually every part of the human body, including the carotid arteries, which supply blood to the brain; the iliac and femoral arteries, which carry blood to the legs; the aorta, the large artery that comes directly from the heart's main pumping chamber; and the relatively small *coronary arteries*, which branch from the root of the aorta to supply blood to the heart muscle itself.

In atherosclerosis, abnormal patches called *plaques* develop within the walls of the affected arteries. As the plaques enlarge, the artery becomes narrowed and blood flow is reduced. If the affected artery carries blood to the leg, then the person will feel calf pain when walking (called *claudication*). If blood flow to the brain is reduced, the person will suffer neurological symptoms, such as fainting or loss of vision, movement, or speech (called *transient ischemic attacks*). If the affected artery carries blood to a man's penis, then impotence can result (that is, he cannot maintain an erection sufficient for sexual intercourse). If the narrowed artery is a coronary artery that carries blood to the heart, then chest pain on exertion (*angina*) can occur.

A sufficiently narrowed artery is susceptible to complete blockage by a blood clot, which develops within the opening of the artery at the site of a plaque. A blockage of an artery supplying a limb can produce gangrene. A blockage to the arteries supplying the brain can cause a stroke. If the blocked artery is a coronary artery that carries blood to the heart, then a heart attack can result.

The most important form of atherosclerosis in the United States is atherosclerosis of the coronary arteries. Its manifestations, which include angina, heart attack, heart failure, and sudden death, are described by the inclusive term *coronary heart disease*. Atherosclerosis involving the arteries supplying the brain is a form of *cerebrovascular disease*. Atherosclerosis involving the arteries to the limbs is called *peripheral vascular disease*.

Atherosclerotic plaques take years to develop. The earliest lesion is called a *fatty streak*, which consists of deposits of cholesterol within the arterial wall. These fatty streaks can be observed in young people with no symptoms, and even in children. The body reacts to these fatty deposits by producing a type of chronic progressive inflammation. Over time, fibrous debris, muscle cells, and more fatty deposits are incorporated into the developing plaque. As the plaque enlarges and "matures," it transforms from a soft fatty streak into a hard knot.

How does a fatty streak get started? The fundamental event is the passage of LDL particles across the inner lining of the arterial wall. That's basically how the cholesterol gets inside the wall of an artery. Many important steps take place before and after the LDL particles get through. For example, there probably has to be some sort of scrape or scratch on the inner lining of the artery, something that roughens up its raw surface so that the LDL particles can enter. And once the LDL particles have gotten inside, they need to undergo certain chemical changes, including oxidation.[2] What's more, the progressive accumulation of material within the plaque, as well as the formation of a blood clot atop the plaque, has a lot to do with the process of blood coagulation. Still, the entry of LDL particles across the arterial wall is the essential step. That's what makes LDL particles bad actors.

I cannot come up with the perfect analogy, but it's helpful to think of a person's artery as an expressway that carries vehicular traffic. Inspired by James's interest in trucking companies, I ask you to imagine that a particular type of vehicle, called an LDL Dump Truck, is laden with cholesterol. Ordinarily, the expressway has a continuous barrier that prevents vehicles from straying off the road. Wherever there is a break in the barrier, however, LDL Trucks run off the road, dumping their loads at roadside. As the LDL Trucks and their loads accumulate along the roadside plaque, assorted other vehicles are dragged into the pileup, including squad cars, backhoes, and eventually concrete mixers. As the plaque expands, it encroaches on the road itself. First the stopping lane is blocked. Then vehicles in the slow lane get hung up. Eventually, traffic is choked off.

Mixed within the flow of traffic, however, is another type of vehicle called an HDL Sanitation Truck. HDL Trucks are trash collectors. They pick up cholesterol from the roadside and transport it back to a Grand Central Truck Terminal called the liver. The liver, in turn, has HDL Truck-Unloading Docks, at which the cholesterol is extracted. Once cholesterol is unloaded at the liver, it can be dumped via the bile ducts into the intestines. The HDL Sanitation Trucks thus undo some of the bad work of the LDL Dump Trucks. They are the good guys.[3]

Of course, there have to be VLDL Trucks, too. They're big transport trucks, too big to get through gaps in the roadside barrier. The VLDL Transport Trucks carry not only cholesterol but also triglycerides, which are the fat-fuels I discussed in chapter 4. In most people, Gideon included, VLDL Transport Trucks have a fixed number of triglyceride slots. Once the VLDL Trucks have delivered their fat-fuel to the muscles and other tissues, they're stripped down into cholesterol-laden LDL Dump Trucks.

Having identified the three main types of cholesterol-transporting trucks, I can push the analogy even further. When Gideon gets the results of his fasting blood test from the laboratory, his C counts all the cholesterol in traffic. His H

measures the amount of cholesterol currently carried by circulating HDL Sanitation Trucks; his L measures the amount carried by circulating LDL Dump Trucks; and his V measures the cholesterol in traveling VLDL Transport Trucks. His T measures the amount of triglyceride in the blood, which is pretty much contained in VLDL Trucks. Since VLDL Trucks have a fixed number of triglyceride slots, and since most triglyceride is loaded onto VLDL Trucks, a person's T is basically proportional to his V. That's why Gideon's T equaled his V multiplied by a factor of 5.

None of these tests measures how much cholesterol is in the liver's central station, or how much is being dumped via the bile ducts, or how much is in roadside plaques. The tests don't tell us whether Gideon even has any roadside plaques. If he does, they still don't tell us how big the plaques are or how much vehicular traffic has so far been blocked. The tests gauge only the trafficking in cholesterol at the time the blood sample was drawn. In other words, the fasting blood cholesterol tests provide Gideon with information that is obviously relevant to his risk of coronary heart disease. But they don't tell him whether he's actually got coronary heart disease. And even if he's got it, the cholesterol tests don't tell Gideon how severe it is. It may seem totally obvious to a pathologist that a blood cholesterol test is not a diagnostic test for coronary heart disease. But it is a major source of confusion and concern among otherwise smart people, including Gideon.

I haven't told the entire story. The LDL Dump Trucks have their own separate Docking Stations at the Grand Central Truck Terminal in the liver. The cholesterol and fats in the foods one eats—quiche lorraine, goose liver pâté, artichoke hearts, béarnaise sauce—can affect the traffic flow of LDL Dump Trucks back to their Docking Stations. That's basically how food on the table affects a person's L and C. But that's enough pathology and biochemistry for now. On to some epidemiology.

"James, I've got to make a telephone call. Please order for me. The tournedos are just fine."

"You want the steak rare? How about the wine?"

"Whatever, James." Gideon is halfway to the pay phone.

"Dr. Karkor please . . . I'll hold . . . It's me again, doctor. Did I hear

you correctly when you said that my cholesterol level doesn't actually tell me whether I have heart disease? Uh-huh. . . . A risk factor? Uh-huh. . . . You really think I've cut my risk of heart disease by that much? Uh-huh. . . . But what about the 'good cholesterol' that went down, too? Uh-huh. . . . How many drinks a day? Mmmm. . . . You sure I don't need drugs? Uh-huh. . . . No, it's I who should be thanking you, doctor. . . . Bye."

In the first wave of the Harvard Alumni Study, discussed in chapter 3, researchers found that a man's physical inactivity in 1966 (or 1962) was a predictor of his risk of heart attack during the period from 1966 (or 1962) through 1972. In the Nurses' Health Study, discussed in chapter 4, researchers found that a woman's Body Mass Index and cigarette-smoking history in 1976 were predictors of her risk of heart attacks or coronary deaths during the period from 1976 through 1984.

These are examples of a more general principle. When researchers keep track of large groups of people over several years, they find that certain measurable personal characteristics are consistent predictors of a person's risks of coronary heart disease or other diseases. These predictors of disease are often called "risk factors," especially by epidemiologists, but also by toxicologists, blue-ribbon scientific panelists, and science journalists.

Unfortunately, next to the phrase *good cholesterol,* the term *risk factor* is about as bad a choice of words as one can possibly make. If I were a science czar, I'd banish the term from scientific discourse, and every writer who contemplated using it would be compelled instead to explain what he or she actually meant. But we don't want to reform the world. We just want to help Gideon. So we'll live with *risk factor,* and try to explain what we mean, too.

A person's age, for example, is a "risk factor" for coronary heart disease. That means that Gideon has a higher chance of having a heart attack this year than does James, even though James doesn't know his cholesterol level. It doesn't mean that aging *per se* causes heart attacks. Atherosclerosis develops over many years, so the older a person is, the greater the chance that the disease has advanced far enough to block a coronary artery. Likewise, male gender is a "risk factor" for coronary heart disease. This does not mean that maleness *per se* causes heart attacks. Still, the facts that women have lower rates of coronary heart disease, that their risk of coronary heart disease increases after menopause, and that postmenopausal estrogen replacement therapy reduces coronary risks indicate that sex hormones are somehow important in the development of the disease.

Elevated blood pressure is a "risk factor" for coronary heart disease (and for strokes). This does not mean that hypertension by itself causes coronary heart disease. However, higher pressures in the arterial system tend to damage the inner lining of the arteries, thus contributing to the development of plaque formation and, later, arterial narrowing and blockage. The Nurses' Health Study showed that a high BMI is a "risk factor" for coronary heart disease. This fact doesn't tell us why or how obesity affects the risks of coronary disease. However, the excess fat disrupts the body's internal controls over blood pressure, blood sugar, and blood cholesterol, and these changes in turn raise one's risk of coronary heart disease.

Cigarette smokers consistently have higher rates of coronary heart disease, stroke, peripheral vascular disease, and other atherosclerotic diseases. For people under age sixty-five, the risks can be doubled or tripled. Again, the assertion that cigarette smoking is a "risk factor" doesn't tell us how or why cigarette smokers get more of these diseases. It turns out that carbon monoxide in cigarette smoke can choke off the oxygen supply to the heart; that nicotine and other chemicals in cigarette smoke can cause injury to the arterial lining, thus promoting the passage of LDL particles across the arterial wall; that chemicals in cigarette smoke can enhance the oxidation of LDL cholesterol once it gets inside the arterial wall; that smoking can affect the formation of blood clots that block a narrowed artery. As we will see shortly, smokers have lower HDL-cholesterol levels, which also raises their coronary risks. Quitting smoking brings their H levels back up.

You have probably read something to the effect that Type A personality is a "risk factor" for coronary disease. Type A people are supposed to be always in a hurry, very ambitious, aggressive, and competitive, and easily provoked to anger and hostility by everyday problems. It was thought, at least for some time, that Type A people had higher rates of coronary disease. When that didn't pan out, researchers distinguished between

Type A aggressives and Type A hostiles. The former Type A people, the competitive ones who are always in a hurry, actually had lower coronary rates, provided they didn't channel their aggressive instincts into anger and hostility. It was the Type A hostile people who got heart attacks. As one proponent put it, "The rushing-around workaholic is not at risk as long as stress is not the stimulus for anger."[4] To prove that Type A hostile was a "risk factor," researchers attempted to show that a person's "Ho-score" (short for "hostility score") predicted coronary risk. Accordingly, if you are more than a little peeved for having spent your money to buy this book, you had better calm down.

There are standard, reasonably objective methods for measuring blood pressure, weight, height, age, sex, smoking practices, and blood cholesterol. But methods for quantifying different aspects of personality and emotions are, obviously, far less standard. So some researchers will inevitably say that such-and-such personality score is a "risk factor" and that so-and-so emotional index is not. What's worse, there will always be some score or index that predicts coronary disease, even if a researcher has to work backward to find out what it is. To see how serious the problem of working backward is, suppose you were a researcher, and suppose that you found your hostility score to be a better predictor of coronary disease if you gave "cynicism" a few extra points. Do you now say that supercynical hostility is a "risk factor" for coronary heart disease? The best one can reasonably conclude is that some aspects of emotional life influence the course of coronary heart disease. It is hardly clear that we know much more about it than James's pat assertion that "stress causes heart attacks."

Even if we just count age, male gender, smoking, obesity, high blood pressure, and physical activity, how can there be so many different "risk factors" for coronary heart disease? Atherosclerosis entails a sequence of pathological events that is staggered over many years. It would be a total surprise not to find so many different personal characteristics affecting the course of such a disease. As we'll see in chapter 7, the same goes for cancer.

You may recall seeing a front-page headline in February 1993 to the effect that a bald spot on the top of the head may predict heart attack risk.[5] This study involved 665 men, aged twenty-one to fifty-four, who had already had one heart attack. (Half of them were Stephen's age of forty-six or younger.) The researchers matched up these heart attack victims with 772 similarly aged men who had been hospitalized for other reasons, mostly for injuries and gastrointestinal problems, but not heart attacks.[6] Both the heart cases and the matched controls were then interviewed to assess the extent of their baldness. When the results were tabulated, there was a greater proportion of severely bald men in the heart attack cases than in the non–heart attack controls.

Because many heart attack victims had already left the hospital, the researchers had to rely upon the men's self-assessments of their baldness during a telephone interview. Although the interviewers were instructed not to tell the men that this was a study of baldness and heart attacks, it was probably hard to keep it a secret. ("Hello, Mr. Sychar. I hope you're up and about again after your heart attack. Now, let's see, you're forty-six years old. Did your father have a heart attack at such an early age? Oh, by the way, how bald are you?") One could argue that many self-conscious men, especially the non-heart attack controls, understated their degree of baldness. One could argue that the researchers had tried different possible comparisons of extreme, moderate, and minimal baldness until they found a correlation (another example of working backward). One could argue that the study applies only to young men, and therefore has less relevance to coronary heart disease in the general population. Finally, one could argue that a coronary/baldness connection has to be established in a large study that tracks bald and nonbald men over many years, in a manner similar to the Harvard Alumni or Nurses' Health Studies.

I am not sure any of the foregoing criticisms is terribly potent. But the critical issue is not whether male-pattern vertex baldness is a "risk factor" for coronary disease. After all, baldness has something to do with male hormones, and sex hormones have something to do with coronary heart disease. The key point is that this baldness study doesn't knock age, gender, smoking, blood pressure, or BMI out of the "risk factor" box. Baldness or no baldness, cigarette smoking is still a predictor of coronary risk. Baldness or no baldness, high blood pressure is still a predictor of coronary risk.

This is an extremely critical point that is easy to miss. Whatever I say about dietary fat and cholesterol in this chapter, one cannot go back to smoking with the thought that it's all in your food, that you can just eat Chinese and smoke cigarettes, too. Even if one takes seriously the evidence that Type A hostile people are predisposed to heart disease, that doesn't mean it's all "stress" and nothing else. If tonight, on the 11:00 news, a reporter announces the latest medical finding that, say, herpes virus infection is a "risk factor" for coronary heart disease, that doesn't mean a sedentary life-style is all right for your heart.

Now we come to cholesterol. Independent of smoking, high blood pressure, inactivity, and obesity, a high value of total blood cholesterol is a "risk factor" for coronary heart disease. In men and women, young and old, a higher value of C predicts a higher risk of coronary heart disease. A lower value of C predicts a lower risk. The relationship is continuous. There is really no numerical cutoff below which a person's total cholesterol level is "safe." (Researchers who worry about the possible health risks of blood cholesterol levels below 160 are actually concerned that a low C value is a "risk factor" for diseases other than coronary heart disease. The best explanation is that people with severe alcohol abuse, who die from liver and gastrointestinal diseases as well as accidents and violence, coincidentally have very low C levels.)[7] Still, for practical purposes, panels of experts have established standard cutoff points beyond which a person's blood cholesterol is "too high." In the United States, a person with a C of 200 or more is supposed to have a cholesterol problem. A C of 240 or more is considered a potentially serious cholesterol problem.[8]

These total cholesterol cutoffs have been established by panels of experts who presumed, for some reason, that most Americans would go to their family doctors or work-site screening programs and have just their C values measured, and not their H, L, and V as well. These experts were probably thinking that a total cholesterol test by itself was less expensive, more widely available, and probably more accurate than the individual lipoprotein cholesterol tests. They were probably also relying on an older scientific tradition, in which total cholesterol was foremost in importance. After all, it wasn't too long ago that scientists were still in the dark about the roles of the lipoprotein particles.

Actually, I'm not sure what the experts were thinking when they hung their hats on the total blood cholesterol alone. In any case, they got caught with their pants down. Once the experts set the C cutoff at 200 points, literally half of the forty-five-year-old men and women in the United States suddenly fell into the "borderline high" or "high" cholesterol range. Sixty-one percent of the men and 77 percent of the women in Gideon's sixty- to sixty-four-year age group suddenly had a "cholesterol problem." Tens of millions of these Americans probably never had their cholesterol levels checked at all. But tens of millions more did, and when they saw a cholesterol over 200, they didn't just say ho-hum, my cholesterol is two-hundred-whatever, and docilely pour fat-free salad dressing over everything in sight. They didn't have Gideon's wealth and financial sophistication, but they all went back anyway and had their HDL cholesterols and LDL cholesterols checked, too, and they all came out as perplexed and confused as Gideon. And don't assume that their physicians had it all figured out, either.

Nowadays, LDL-cholesterol and HDL-cholesterol levels are routinely measured. And it has become clear that a high LDL cholesterol is the real predictor of high coronary risk, and that a high value of C is just a stand-in for a high value of L. That makes sense. When there are large numbers of LDL Dump Trucks in traffic, lots of cholesterol can be deposited into roadside plaques. As we saw from Gideon's test results, LDL cholesterol is the major portion of one's total blood cholesterol. When L is high, C is usually high, too. But even if a person's C were under the 200-point cutoff, that person could still have a "cholesterol problem" if his or her L alone were up.[9]

Experts agree that a person's risk of coronary disease rises continuously as his or her LDL-cholesterol level rises. There is no preferred numerical formula for relating LDL cholesterol and coronary disease rates. As a reasonable first approximation, the risk goes up by about 1.0 to 1.5 percent for every one-point increase in L.[10] Since it is difficult to communicate the meaning of a percentage change in a person's coronary rate, experts have felt compelled to resort once again to artificial cutoff levels. Accordingly, the recommendation is that L values under 130 are "desirable," L values from 130 to 159 are "borderline high," L values of 160 to 189 are "high" risk, and L values of 190 or more are "super-high" risk. Although doctors' actual practices undoubtedly deviate from expert recommendations, patients with L values in the super-high range are supposed to take cholesterol-reducing drugs when diet alone doesn't work. People with L values in the high range of 160 to 189 are candidates for drug treatment if they already have coronary heart disease, or if they smoke cigarettes and have high blood pressure.[11]

Most authorities now acknowledge that a low level of HDL cholesterol is also "risk factor" for coronary heart disease, quite apart from the predictive power of a high blood level of LDL cholesterol. That also makes sense. When there are fewer HDL Sanitation Trucks in traffic, less cholesterol will be picked up from the roadside and returned to the liver's HDL Truck-Unloading Docks. Conversely, when H is high, it means that there are lots of HDL Sanitation Trucks in traffic, which are picking up lots of roadside cholesterol trash.

There is general agreement that a person's risk of coronary heart disease is continuously and negatively related to his or her HDL-cholesterol level.[12] As a reasonable first approximation, the risk goes down by 2 to 3 percent for every one-point increase in H.[13] As in the case of total cholesterol and LDL cholesterol, artificial cutoff levels for HDL cholesterol have been established. An H value less than 35 is "very high" risk; and an H value between 35 and 44 is "intermediate" risk. Expert recommendations about diet and cholesterol-lowering drugs are still anchored on a person's L value. But if an L value is only "borderline high," then a favorably high H value can tip the scales against drug treatment. As I'll explain below, H values can be influenced by things other than diet.

There is much less agreement on whether a person's VLDL-cholesterol level predicts his risk of coronary disease. VLDL Trucks transport triglycerides, delivering them to muscles for fat-fuel. Only after they have fully unloaded their triglycerides can VLDL Transport Trucks turn into LDL Dump Trucks. Accordingly, the number of VLDL Trucks on the road is only an indirect indicator of the number of LDL Trucks to come. The situation is complicated by the presence of other "transient" triglyceride-transporting lipoproteins that can also hold small amounts of cholesterol. After Gideon eats lunch, triglycerides from his food are temporarily transported to his liver via extremely low density lipoproteins called *chylomicrons*. If Gideon got a blood sample right after lunch, rather than after an overnight fast, the basic equation, $C = H + L + V$, wouldn't hold anymore, because there's some additional cholesterol on the short-lived chylomicrons. If I calculated V as $C - H - L$, as I did for Gideon, I'd get the wrong answer.[14]

It turns out that VLDL matters in certain people with very high blood triglyceride (T) levels, usually over 500. Actually, these are the very same people who have high BMIs, high blood pressure, and elevated blood sugars, whom I mentioned briefly in chapter 4. If Eve doesn't take prompt measures to halt her upward BMI trend, she might soon be one of them. In her case, we really didn't need to get involved with cholesterol and triglyceride blood tests. Her BMI, blood pressure, and blood sugar gave away her problem. Gideon's problem is different. His T values are under 200. Only LDL and HDL matter for him.

It is one thing to say that a high L predicts future coronary disease. It's quite another thing to say that reducing an already high L will lower a person's coronary risk. In fact, a gargantuan amount of scientific effort has gone into proving the proposition that treating high blood cholesterol, especially high L, has a measurable benefit. Just to throw out an impressive-sounding list of names, there's the Lipid Research Clinics Coronary Primary Prevention Trial, in which 1,900 men received the cholesterol-lowering drug cholestyramine and another 1,900 received a placebo;[15] the Coronary Drug Project, in which 1,100 men with diagnosed coronary disease received the drug clofibrate, 1,100 men received the drug nicotinic acid, and 2,800 received a placebo;[16] the Helsinki Heart Study, in which 2,000 middle-aged men received the drug gemfibrozil and another 2,000 received a placebo;[17] the NHLBI Type II Coronary Intervention Study of 115 men and 28 women with known coronary disease and very high L values, who, based on a coin flip, received either cholestyramine or a placebo;[18] the Cholesterol-Lowering Atherosclerosis Study, in which the treatment group received a combination of two drugs, colestipol and nicotinic acid;[19] and the Familial Atherosclerosis Treat-

ment Study, in which middle-aged men with known coronary
disease received either lovastatin or one of the aforementioned drugs.[20]

These "intervention studies," which covered thousands of
carefully monitored human subjects, convincingly showed that
lowering a previously high L value will reduce the risk of heart
attack, and even reduce the size of existing plaques, *so long as
drugs are used to get the LDL cholesterol down.* That doesn't mean
diet is useless in the treatment of high LDL cholesterol. It's just
that the researchers designed their studies to produce large
declines in L, so that they could then see what happens to coronary rates. It's much easier and more reliable to achieve a whop-
ping decline in L if you give a cholesterol-lowering drug to
someone who already has a high L. It's much more difficult to
get thousands of people to adhere to a sufficiently stringent
cholesterol-lowering diet for long enough to get major changes
in L.[21] Of course, there are some studies of diet without drugs.
In the Lifestyle Heart Trial, 28 people who ate an essentially veg-
etarian, extremely low-fat diet dropped their L values from 152
to 95.[22] These people appeared to have a reduction in the narrowing of their coronary arteries after one year on the diet. But
they also stopped smoking, took up exercise, and, for what it's
worth, had a course in stress management.

In plain terms, Gideon's blood cholesterol level is a super-
fluous number that serves only to confuse him. The two numbers that matter are his L and his H. Some people have to
worry about V and T, but not Gideon. For every one-point
drop in Gideon's L, his risk of coronary disease declines by 1.0
to 1.5 percent. For every one-point rise in his H, his risk of
coronary heart disease falls by 2 to 3 percent. Put differently,
it's desirable to have LDL cholesterol go down and HDL cholesterol go up. Here's how I look at it: *A two-point drop in LDL
cholesterol is about as potent in preventing heart disease as a one-point
rise in HDL cholesterol. Conversely, the coronary-preventive effect of a
two-point drop in LDL cholesterol would be canceled out by a one-point
rise in HDL cholesterol.*

Now, while Gideon is trudging back from the pay phone
toward his table near the window, let's look at his numbers.

You may very well be disappointed. Gideon's story started with
his total blood cholesterol. Then it was complicated by his so-

called bad and good cholesterols. What I've basically done is to throw out his cholesterol as irrelevant; to relabel the "bad" as L and the "good" as $H;$ to play down triglycerides, except in special cases; and then to suggest that, point for point, H is twice as potent as L. I started with one number but ended up with two numbers. Couldn't the whole thing be collapsed into one number?

I shall now invent a new index of risk that is not in the scientific literature on cholesterol and lipoproteins: Its symbol is J. To calculate J, start with L and subtract twice the value of H. In other words, $J = L - H - H$. Every one-point increase in J is associated with a 1.0 to 1.5 percent increase in coronary disease. Conversely, every one-point decrease in J is associated with a 1.0 to 1.5 percent decline in coronary risk. It's best to have your J value as low as possible.[23]

The expert panels recommend that Gideon's L value be kept at 130 or under. They also recommend that his H value stay at 45 or over. Since, $130 - 45 - 45$ equals 40, the experts are implicitly recommending that Gideon's J value be 40 or under. Likewise, they suggest that Gideon's L value becomes much riskier when it exceeds 160, and that his H value becomes much riskier when it falls below 35. Accordingly, if we accept these arbitrary cutoffs, then Gideon would be getting into trouble when his J value exceeded $160 - 35 - 35$, which equals 90. (The experts may object that you can't combine the L and H cutoffs in this manner unless L and H are statistically uncorrelated. Actually, L and H move pretty much independent across different people.)[24]

Nine months ago, Gideon's total cholesterol was 257. It has fallen to 239. If Gideon's internist adhered only to the expert panel recommendations on total cholesterol, she would conclude that Gideon has gone from having a serious cholesterol problem to merely having a cholesterol problem. If Dr. Karkor looked only at Gideon's LDL cholesterol, she would see a drop of 16 points, down to 166. That alone would represent a 16 to 24 percent decline in Gideon's coronary risk. If she ignored his HDL cholesterol entirely, then he'd look pretty good. While Gideon's LDL cholesterol would still be in the 160-plus danger range, the fact is that it's coming down without drugs. But Gideon's HDL cholesterol also went down by ten points. That alone would represent a 20 to 30 percent rise in his coronary risk. Computing Gideon's *J* index is a convenient way to summarize the combined changes in his blood tests. His *J* value went from 92 to 96. The four-point increase in *J* means that, in total, Gideon's risk of coronary heart disease actually went up by 4 to 6 percent. He's doing worse.

What has happened to Gideon in the past nine months is not supposed to happen. Gideon has adhered to a low-cholesterol, low-fat diet. At least he has tried to. Many people who go on such diets do achieve drops in both *L* and *H*. But their drop in *H* is usually relatively small, much less than half the drop in *L*. They come out better. In other words, their *J* goes down. But that didn't happen to Gideon. Gideon's *H* has plummeted, and his *J* has gone up. Is there something wrong with his diet? What happened?

Gideon's most recent blood tests could be a mistake. Or they could be accurate, while his past blood test was a mistake.[25] Actually, it's not so much a "mistake" as an "unexplained variation." The same individual can have a different cholesterol level at a different laboratory, or even in the same laboratory a week later. That goes, too, for LDL cholesterol, HDL cholesterol, VLDL cholesterol, as well as triglyceride levels. It is well known, at least among laboratory specialists, that most people's cholesterol levels vary with the seasons, being higher in the winter.[26] Your cholesterol level might even change when you stand up or perform a stressful task.[27] This intraindividual and interlaboratory variation is especially applicable to HDL cholesterol, the one laboratory measurement that is giving Gideon the biggest headache. While a ten-point movement in *H* is fairly large, it is not unheard of, and random variations of four or five points are common. Although Gideon and Dr. Karkor are obligated to take them seriously, the tests results need to be repeated and confirmed before we can reach solid conclusions.

On the other hand, the drop in Gideon's HDL cholesterol could be genuine, but the cause may have little or nothing to do with Gideon's low-fat diet. Cigarette smoking lowers HDL cholesterol, and quitting brings it back up.[28] It's quite conceivable that Gideon quit smoking a year ago and managed to stay off cigarettes, at least at the time of his first blood test. Unfortunately, as a gentleman named Andrew will attest in chapter

6, smoking relapse is very common, even months after an apparently successful attempt at quitting. Perhaps Gideon resumed smoking before he got his cholesterol test repeated.

Physical activity raises HDL cholesterol in both men and women. There is no clear agreement whether some or all types of physical activity raise a person's *H*. Even regular walking may work.[29] As we learned in chapter 3, however, the benefits of exercise are short-lived. They go away within weeks or months after a person stops. The *H*-raising effect of regular physical activity is no exception. It is quite conceivable, in fact, that Gideon stopped smoking *and* started regular walking a year ago. When people decide to make a change, they sometimes try everything at once. Whether this was the best strategy for Gideon is something only he can determine. If it wasn't, then on the next try, he'll navigate a different course. However, if he were a double recidivist at the time of his recent blood test, it would go even further toward explaining why the bottom dropped out of Gideon's *H*.

Weight gain can also lower HDL cholesterol. Usually this happens in people like Eve, where blood sugar, blood pressure, VLDL, and triglycerides are up. Gideon's *V* and *T* went up to some degree, but they were not really his problem. Still, weight gain could have contributed to Gideon's HDL decrease. In fact, we might even speculate that he had lost weight while he had been walking regularly last year, and has now cycled back to his former BMI. Gideon is a sixty-two-year-old man. If his wife, Bethany, had experienced a similar pattern in HDL cholesterol, we'd have to ask whether she had been taking estrogen replacement tablets for menopause. When taken by mouth, estrogens can raise HDL. That's one possible reason why postmenopausal women who take such replacement hormones have about half as much coronary heart disease as other women their age.[30] We'd have to ask whether Bethany's gynecologist may have given her estrogen in the past and whether she had stopped the tablets recently.

In some but not all people, moderate alcohol consumption raises HDL cholesterol. It usually doesn't take much to raise a person's *H*, perhaps two drinks per day.[31] There is hardly any disagreement that the widespread consumption of wine in France has at least something to do with that country's lower coronary rates.[32] Despite Dr. Karkor's recommendation that

Gideon have a few drinks, there's little agreement about whether alcoholic beverages should be routinely used to correct a low HDL cholesterol. Alcohol also raises blood pressure, and in people who already have coronary problems, it can lead to serious heart rhythm disturbances. And, of course, "moderate" amounts of alcohol can be consumed at the wrong time and place. And some people who attempt to consume only two drinks daily end up with many more. Still, in our inquiry as to the causes of Gideon's H drop, we might ask whether he has recently given up drinking. Gideon didn't seem terribly eager to choose the wine. Perhaps he has recently given up a regular glass or two with lunch.

After nine months of trying, Gideon's LDL cholesterol has dropped by sixteen points. But it's still in the experts' danger range of 160 to 189. We can try to explain away the unfavorable drop in his HDL cholesterol, and we can pat him on the back for going in the right direction. We can take the attitude, as we did for Eve, that the last few L points were the worst. We can emphasize, as we did for Stephen, that cholesterol control is a matter of lifelong persistence. But the question remains: With all his efforts, why hasn't Gideon done better? For all we know, his efforts at cholesterol control have driven his wife to a psychiatrist. Even if the HDL level was a mistake, was it all worth it for sixteen lousy LDL points?

Many people need to take cholesterol-lowering drugs. For others, such drugs are a discretionary but wise choice. In theory, diet alone should be enough to control most people's LDL cholesterol. The problem isn't theory, but practice. A growing scientific literature is documenting how difficult it is for people to stick with the standard low-cholesterol, low-fat, low-saturated fat diets that the expert panels have recommended.[33] Even when they stick with them, the diets don't always work. The fact that the major intervention studies all used drugs to get LDL cholesterol down is testimony to the impracticality of getting large numbers of people to do it on diet alone.

But all this just begs the question: Why can't Gideon do better? Gideon might be one of those unusual cases who eats all the right things, and does all the right things, but still gets the wrong result. What is most disturbing, however, is the genuine possibility that Gideon, a successful and seasoned man who wants to control his coronary destiny, might not have eaten the right things. In fact, he might have eaten the wrong things.

Exactly how does eating cholesterol-laden food, as well as food containing certain saturated fats, raise one's blood LDL cholesterol? Can certain foods adversely affect one's HDL-cholesterol level, too? The answers require our delving into a field of research that is now in virtual total flux. As I write this chapter, the oleic acid in olive oil is "definitely good" and trans fatty acids in margarine are somewhere between "probably bad" and "very bad." The EPA (eicosa-penta-enoic acid) and DHA (docosa-hexa-enoic acid) in the oils of certain fin fish and shellfish are "maybe good" but on the way out, while the linoleic and α-linoleic acids in walnuts and other nuts, which were formerly "good with qualifications," are now making a comeback.

The final word on dietary constituents and lipoproteins is likely to be far more complicated and tentative than even these provisional pronouncements. One reason, which I put forth at the start of this chapter, is that people like Gideon, Bethany, Eve, Stephen, you, and me eat food, not pure cholesterol and not pure fatty acids. A certain substance may be "not so good" for your LDL cholesterol when it is ingested all by itself. But the same chemical might become "pretty good" or perhaps "really bad" when ingested in combination with another substance. But that's what food is: a combination of substances, not just one at a time. In short, chemical interactions can matter. That's where we get into Truck Dockers' Union on the Grand Central Truck Station in the liver.

Most of the fat that Gideon eats comes in the form of triglycerides. After a meal, these triglycerides are ingested and absorbed into the bloodstream. They can then be sent via VLDL Transport Trucks to Gideon's muscles, to be converted into fatty acids, which serve as fat-fuels. As I explained in the last chapter, the unused triglycerides can be stowed away in his own body fat. Whether the triglycerides are in Gideon's food, carried on his VLDL particles, or stored in his body fat, they all contain three fatty acids.

We constantly read and hear about saturated fat. Gideon himself is worried about the saturated fat in cream cheese. (Soon, in compliance with new FDA and USDA regulations, labels for virtually all packaged foods will show, among other things, the quantities of total fat, cholesterol and saturated fat per standard serving.)[34] Saturated fat, polyunsaturated fat, and monounsaturated fat describe the different types of fatty acids that can go into a single triglyceride.

These fats are not the same as cholesterol. Cholesterol, a fatty substance found in animal foods, dairy products, and eggs but not in plant foods, is neither a triglyceride nor a fatty acid. While cholesterol counts as fat, it is by weight a small fraction of the total fat one eats. Tournedos, usually cut from the tenderloin section of a prime beef carcass, contain about 12 grams of fat per 100 grams of meat, of which 5 grams is saturated fat and 84 *milli*grams is cholesterol. By weight, cholesterol is thus only 0.7 percent of the fat. (A 100-gram portion weighs about 3 ½ ounces. One milligram is equal to one-thousandth of a gram.)

There are many ways to classify fatty acids, but it has become standard practice to distinguish between two basic kinds: saturated fatty acids and unsaturated fatty acids. *Saturated fatty acids* are generally solid at room temperature. When you look at the white marbling in red meats, or the visible fat in a strip of bacon, or the white layer of fat that congeals at the top of gravy left to cool overnight, or a stick of butter, you're looking at solid, saturated fat. These are examples of visible saturated fat in almost pure form. Some foods, such as whole milk, cheese, and ice cream, contain saturated fat that is invisible because it's mixed together with other substances.

Unsaturated fats generally form oily liquids at room temperature. There are two basic types of unsaturated fatty acids: *monounsaturated fatty acids* and *polyunsaturated fatty acids*. Olive oil and canola oil are high in monounsaturated fatty acids, while safflower oil, sunflower seed oil, corn oil, and soybean oil are high in polyunsaturated fatty acids. If saturated fats are mostly solid and unsaturated fats are mostly oily, and if corn oil has polyunsaturated fat, then how come corn oil margarine is solid at room temperature? That's the trans fatty acid part of the story, which I'll come to shortly.

In keeping with scientific parlance, I use the shorthand "Sats" for saturated fatty acids, "Polys" for polyunsaturated fatty acids, and "Monos" for monounsaturated fatty acids. Each term describes not a single chemical but a class of related chemicals. It is helpful to think of each fatty acid as having an identification number or serial number. The Sats all have serial numbers ending in "0" because they have zero "unsaturation." The Monos have serial numbers ending in "1" because they have a single "unsaturation." The Polys have serial numbers ending in 2, 3, 4, or higher.

For example, stearic acid (serial number 18:0), myristic acid (14:0), and palmitic acid (16:0) are but three examples of different Sats that are found in different proportions in beef fat, chicken fat, coconut oil, palm oil, and cocoa butter, which is used to make chocolate. (The digits "18" in the serial number for stearic acid mean that it's 18 carbons long.) Oleic acid (18:1) is a particular Mono that is found in olive oil. Linoleic acid (18:2) is a Poly found in corn oil and safflower oil; α-linoleic acid (18:3) and arachidonic acid (20:4) are also Polys. The fatty acid EPA (serial number 20:5) is found in the plankton eaten by small cold-water fish, which are in turn eaten by bigger fish. Most foods contain mixtures of these different fatty acids in various proportions. While olive oil contains a high proportion of Monos, it also contains lesser quantities of specific Sats and Polys. Peanuts contain Sats, Polys, and a high proportion of Monos. Even the subcutaneous fatty tissue under the skin of Gideon's buttocks contains Sats, Polys, and Monos.[35]

When Gideon eats cholesterol-containing food, the cholesterol is absorbed in his intestines and travels via his bloodstream to his liver, which is his Grand Central Truck Station. When the Truck Dockers' Union gets a big shipment of cholesterol from the diet, it shuts down the liver's LDL Truck Docking Stations.[36] The LDL Dump Trucks can't dock at the liver, so they keep circulating in traffic. That's how Gideon's intake of dietary cholesterol results in an increase in his L value. This phenomenon doesn't happen to the same degree in everyone. Some people can eat gobs of cholesterol-laden food but their LDL Truck Docks stay open, and so the blood L values don't change. On the other hand, others have an inherited condition in which their LDL Truck Docks are permanently shut down. These people comprise a significant portion of the population with sky-high cholesterol and correspondingly high risks of coronary disease.[37]

When Gideon eats certain fats, his LDL-cholesterol level

also goes up. In a manner similar to cholesterol, the Truck Dockers' Union shuts down the Docks when it gets large shipments of fatty acids with certain serial numbers.[38] Some of these dietary fats are much more effective in shutting off the LDL Trucking Docks, and thus raising a person's LDL cholesterol, than is dietary cholesterol itself, and Gideon is probably no exception to this rule.[39] In other words, the fat in the cream cheese in the gâteau de crêpes may be more effective, ounce for ounce, in raising Gideon's blood L value than the cholesterol in the egg yolks of the béarnaise sauce.

For a long time, it was thought that all the saturated fats were cholesterol-raising and all the unsaturated fats were cholesterol-lowering. In other words, when the Truck Dockers' Union saw a zero at the end of a shipment of fat, it shut down the person's LDL Truck Docks. When it saw any other serial number ("1" for Monos and "2" or more for Polys), it did the opposite. That simple conclusion led authorities to the recommendation that people like Gideon, whose blood cholesterol appears to be diet-sensitive, should cut down on both dietary cholesterol and saturated fats.

It now appears, however, that the relationship between dietary fats and lipoproteins isn't so simple, and that the Sat versus Poly versus Mono classification scheme is far from perfect. Certain Sats, such as lauric acid (12:0), myristic acid (14:0), and probably palmitic acid (16:0) do raise a person's cholesterol, at least when they're given separately in the diet.[40] But other Sats don't do all that much to cholesterol, and one Sat—stearic acid (18:0)—seems to lower rather than raise a person's LDL cholesterol.[41] Stearic acid, in particular, is contained in fairly high proportions in beef fat, including tournedos Henri IV, as well as in cocoa butter. What's more, certain Polys, such as linoleic acid (18:2), may lower *both* the deleterious LDL cholesterol and the beneficial HDL cholesterol, while certain Monos, such as oleic acid (18:1), may lower LDL cholesterol without lowering HDL cholesterol.[42]

As if it were any surprise to you at this juncture in this book, people vary considerably in their individual responses to these fats.[43] People with normal blood cholesterol levels do not always respond to different fats in the same way as people with high blood cholesterol. Their Truck Dockers just don't shut down or open up their LDL Docks in the same ways. Many of the research studies that concluded that certain fats raised or lowered LDL cholesterol were performed on human subjects with normal cholesterol levels. These studies may have to be repeated in people with high cholesterol levels before scientists can be sure of their relevance to the prevention of coronary heart disease.

But that is not the end of the story. To an increasing degree, American food has a unique chemical constituent called a trans fatty acid. As I have explained, unsaturated fats tend to be liquid oils at room temperature. Their liquid state renders them a poor choice in mass food production. For example, corn oil has a lot of polyunsaturated fat. It's an oil, so you can use it for cooking or salad dressing. But it will not make solid corn-oil margarine. To make corn oil solid, food manufacturers "partially hydrogenate" it. They transform it.

If you pick up a box of any processed food you can find, there's a good chance that it contains "partially hydrogenated" corn oil, soybean oil, cottonseed oil, or some other naturally unsaturated fat oil. But, once again, language matters. In order of appearance, we have had "good cholesterol," "risk factor," and now "partially hydrogenated." Actually, "partially hydrogenated" means "partially saturated." The naturally occurring saturated fat is removed, and unsaturated fat is used in its place. Then the unsaturated fat is resaturated; it's transformed. In the process of partial hydrogenation, certain trans fatty acids are formed.[44] These trans fats aren't just in margarine. They're in many imitation cheeses, frozen fish sticks, ready-made frostings, candies, fast-food oils and spreads, french fries, and chicken nuggets.

The manufacturers may still designate these fatty acids by a "1" or a "2" at the end of their serial numbers, but the Truck Dockers in the liver appear to know better. There is now strong evidence that these "trans fats" raise LDL cholesterol and lower HDL cholesterol. First came the Dutch study of August 1990, explained in one of the clippings I had saved.[45] This study was later criticized because the Dutch researchers used a process of hydrogenation different than that used in the United States and because they tested diets that were uncharacteristically high in trans fats.[46] But new studies confirmed the LDL-raising and HDL-lower effects of American-style trans fats.[47] What's more, new data reported from the

Nurses' Health Study indicate that women who ate foods higher in trans-fats had higher coronary disease rates.[48] While some authorities still believe that the trans fats raise LDL and lower HDL to a smaller extent than the saturated fats do, and that margarine is thus still safer than butter, the plain fact is that there isn't enough evidence to be sure.

Nutrition experts have acknowledged that beef fat and butter fat may contain stearic acid, but they note that these foods also contain many other cholesterol-raising Sats. They also acknowledge that many processed foods and spreads contain trans fats. Their view is that all fat should be reduced in the diet, with the greatest reductions still in Sats. If one is going to consume fats, they say, then one should still eat Polys and Monos, although there is some disagreement over the relative amounts of each, partly because Polys may cause cancer.[49]

But that still isn't the end of the story. When people cut down on the fat-fuels in their diets, they substitute carbo-fuels instead. Lower-fat diets therefore mean higher-carbohydrate diets. There is serious contention in the scientific community that low-fat, high-carbohydrate diets produce a deleterious lowering of HDL cholesterol.[50] The extra carbos apparently decrease the production of HDL Sanitation Trucks off the assembly line.[51] Some researchers argue that the drop in HDL is usually pretty small, not enough to offset the drop in LDL. They argue that the drop in HDL can be ignored. But that's not always the case.[52] Again, people are different. In studies of the effects of low-fat, high-carbo diets, there are usually people whose HDL falls out the bottom. With each point of HDL worth two points of LDL on the coronary risk scale, I do not see how the HDL-lowering effect of a low-fat, high-carbo diet can be ignored. In fact, some researchers have rejected the ultra-low-fat diet philosophy. Their view is that Monos should be a major source of fat-fuel, and that we shouldn't be filling up on carbo-fuels. The Mediterrean diet, for example, derives a huge proportion of its fuel from olive oil, which, as we now know, is high in oleic acid (18:1), a Mono that does not lower HDL. Some researchers, however, believe that the superiority of the Mediterranean diet in bolstering HDL is overstated.[53]

Still others have suggested that if we can only sort out once and for all which fats are *L*-raising, which are *L*-lowering, which are *H*-raising and lowering, then we could label all foods exactly. Your can of olive oil would have a large "18:1" on it, with perhaps a "smile" logo to show its beneficial properties; while a container of coconut shreds would have a large "12:0" with a big "frown" logo; and a box of milk chocolate would have a big "16:0" and "18:0" on it, with a small frown. This idea would actually be no less confusing than labels that show Fat, Sat, Poly, Mono, and Trans. But that's not the problem. The difficulty is that these constituents combine together in food. And even if one eats pure 18:1, that food combines with others in one's intestines.

Researchers are now beginning to pay more serious attention not to individual fatty acids and individual oils but to real food. They are studying the effects of food not in the laboratory but under ordinary living conditions. For example, eggs do have a lot of cholesterol, but they are not a big source of Sats. One whole large egg may contain well over twice the amount of cholesterol as 100 grams of prime tenderloin beef, but less than half as much saturated fat. In fact, recent studies suggest that, on balance, L doesn't go up when people eat moderate amounts of eggs.[54]

Researchers have become increasingly worried that fish oils contain the wrong kinds of polyunsaturated fats. But when scientists were gung-ho on fish oils several years ago, their enthusiasm derived not from laboratory studies of human subjects who ate fish oils but from long-term follow-up studies of people who ate fish.[55]

Nuts contain a lot of fuel, but most of it is fat-fuel. While most of the fat-fuel is composed of Monos, authorities have cautioned not to eat too many peanuts and walnuts because, in the final analysis, they still contain a lot of fat. New evidence, however, suggests that a diet high in walnuts may lower cholesterol and blood pressure.[56] The amount of LDL-cholesterol lowering could not have been predicted from a chemical analysis of the individual components of walnuts. The researchers suggested, in fact, that almonds and hazelnuts have similar properties. What's more, in a long-term study of Seventh Day Adventists in California, designed in a manner similar to the Harvard Alumni and Nurses' Health studies, researchers found that men and women who ate nuts of all kinds had lower coronary rates.[57] Peanuts are a good dietary source of the antioxidant Vitamin E.

Now we're getting to the crucial point. People like Gideon and James don't eat cholesterol, Sats, Polys, and Monos. They don't eat 12:0, 16:0, and 18:2. They eat food. When Gideon and James decided to go out for a late lunch, they didn't decide whether to eat stearic or oleic or palmitic or linoleic, but whether to eat Chinese or French. In fact, while Gideon may be fretting this Friday afternoon over Brie, mussels, and goose liver pâté in a French restaurant, the rest of the week he eats American.

Somewhere out there, in space and time, between the Northwest Territories and Papua New Guinea, between the Ice Age and This Age, there was or is the perfect coronary-free human diet. Perhaps we could piece together such an ideal diet, borrowing from the berries picked by early humans; the grains cultivated by the first Nile farmers; the fish eaten by the Eskimos; the olive oil pressed along the Mediterranean coast; the bean curd of Oriental cuisine; and a few sips of cabernet.

Wherever that ideal diet is, and whenever it was, it isn't the typical American diet now. In fact, when it comes to atherosclerosis and coronary heart disease, the typical American diet has all the wrong things in it. There is too much fat. Whatever one wants to say about stearic acid and Monos, there is still too much saturated fat and too much trans fat. But far more important, there aren't enough fresh fruits and vegetables. Far more important, the grainy food is overly processed, degrained, too smooth. Far more important, there isn't enough fiber.

From their restaurant window, Gideon and James can see another restaurant that offers high-fat, low-fiber, highly processed fare. These days, the same restaurant may also have special offerings for fat-conscious customers. These fat-conscious foods are a prototypical American invention. They are high-fat food with the fat taken out. They are high-calorie foods with the calories taken out. They are low-vitamin foods with the vitamins put back in. They are dietetically correct. They are an amalgam, an alloy of gums, fillers, colors, and texturizers. On the other side of the street, Gideon and James can also see a grocery store, loaded with more low-cal nonfat neo-food. This is not French food. If it were, then the idea of a nonfat diet quiche wouldn't be such a joke. This is not Chinese food. If it were, you could get diet nonfat moo-shi shrimp in Canton Province. This isn't Mediterranean food. If it were, you could get gnocchi fortified with beta-carotene in Venice.

Antioxidants prevent oxidation. Once the LDL particles cross the arterial wall, they get oxidized. The oxidation is part of the process of plaque formation. The antioxidants may stop it. Some of these antioxidants are vitamins. Whatever type of chemical they are, they're found in abundance in fresh fruits and raw vegetables. Some authorities believe that the French have lower coronary rates because they consume a lot of antioxidants. They point out that the Scots, for example, eat few fruits and vegetables and have high coronary rates.[58] These arguments are not airtight. Some scientists think that antioxidation is a minor phenomenon, an unimportant sideshow. I doubt it. But one thing is for sure. The highly processed, partially hydrogenated, trans fat–loaded, neo-American diet is painfully low in fresh fruits and raw vegetables.[59]

Gideon has tried to take the leap from the standard American fare to the imaginary, ideal cuisine. But in taking the leap, he may have stumbled and fallen flat. Gideon, like tens of millions of well-meaning Americans, is trying to eat properly. He is told to eat French because the French don't have as many heart attacks. He is told to eat Chinese, for basically the same reason. He is told to eat Mediterrean, or Eskimo, or Neanderthal, for basically the same reason.

Gideon surely knows that eating French isn't the same as being French. But if there is anything to the argument that the French diet is cardio-protective, then Gideon may lose out trying to second-guess all the bad foods on the menu. At least in traditional cuisines, most foods are part good and part bad. If Gideon wants to get anywhere, he should focus on the good foods on the menu. We cannot advise Gideon to put slabs of cream cheese on bagels, to wolf down strips of fat-laden roast beef, to gorge on cheese and eggs. But we can at least help him by changing his perspective.

"How is everything, Monsieur?" asks the maître d'. "Would you like to see our desserts?"

"Everything was delicious," answers James. "Gideon, look at that charlotte malakoff. What's in it?"

"It's charlotte malakoff au chocolat, Monsieur. First we make a

cream from powdered sugar, orange liqueur, crushed almonds, semi-sweet chocolate, and coffee. We layer it on—how do you say—Ladyfingers, alternating with crème anglais."

"James," interrupts Gideon, "you know I can't have that."

"Gideon, you're torturing yourself," James answers. "For all you know, that chocolate is good for you. And the crushed almonds? Aren't nuts good for you, too?"

"James," says Gideon, getting up from the table, "you order dessert. I've got to make one more call." Gideon heads to the pay phone.

"It's me again, doctor. I hope you don't mind. . . . Do you think I could have that fasting cholesterol test repeated? Yes, along with my good—Oh, sure. . . . I'll get there as soon as the lab opens, at the crack of—Really, the firm's donation was just a small token of—Uh-huh. . . . Okay, see you."

"So, James, what did you get?"

"Brie with fruit and french bread. Yum."

"Fruit? What fruit? James, you ate all the fruit."

"We'll get another order. Oh, Monsieur," James calls. The waiter approaches. "Encore des fruits."

"Café?" asks the waiter. "A brandy perhaps?"

"I need to make another call," says Gideon, arising.

"Coffee for me," says James. "Boy, am I full. I'm sure my friend will have nothing, Monsieur. You don't have to ask him. He didn't touch the wine."

6

Smoking and Nothingness
Cigarettes

Andrew, a fifty-three-and-a-half-year-old acclaimed novelist, is about to appear on nationally syndicated TalkLine Radio to promote his latest book. He is preparing to light another cigarette when Judith, the show's host, signals that it's airtime. After a few introductory remarks, Judith begins the interview.

JUDITH: *Glad to have you back with us at TalkLine, Andy.*
ANDREW: *Kuf-kuf-kuf, ahem.*
JUDITH: *Still got that signature cough of yours.*
ANDREW: *Kuf-kuf-kah, ahem. I hate it.*
JUDITH: *How long have you been smoking?*
ANDREW: *Kuf-kaf, ahem. Since I was thirteen and a half, two packs a day.*
JUDITH: *Ever tried to quit?*
ANDREW: *During the past three years, Judy, I have tried unsuccessfully to quit at least nine times, and if one counted each and every halfhearted resolution and half-smoked rod, the number of attempts would surpass ninety.*
JUDITH: *I quit when I had my son. Haven't smoked another—*
ANDREW: *It infuriates me when other people testify how easy it was to stop. Hell is other people who have quit smoking.*
JUDITH: *We have a caller. Go ahead, you're on TalkLine.*
CALLER: *Ever tried cutting down gradually?*

*ANDREW: Whenever I have tried to cut down, my novels and plays
    are filled with scenes of torture.*

CALLER: How about hypnosis?

*ANDREW: Hypnosis worked once for a week, and I'm not paying for
    that again. Acupuncture is definitely out.*

CALLER: How about nicotine gum or the new nicotine patch?

*ANDREW: Against doctor's orders, I smoked between pieces of gum.
    And I'm not going to pay for that skin patch. My health insurance
    won't cover it. Anyway, you can't smoke with the patch in place.
    Kuf-kuf. Mind if I light up?*

JUDITH: Well, our producer wouldn't exactly be thrilled—

*ANDREW: You know, Judith [lighting up], it's so ontological. When I
    reach for a cigarette and it's not there,—*

CALLER: Health insurance doesn't cover cigarettes, either.

*ANDREW: —it's very different from the way in which spinach is not
    there, or the president is not there. When a cigarette is not there,
    nothing is there.*

*CALLER: Keep trying. Eat lots of celery and carrots. Don't drink too
    much coffee or alcohol.*

*ANDREW: It's the ultimate boundary situation. Other smokers are free
    to quit, while I am condemned to be a slave to my cigarettes. I merely
    pretend that I am free to smoke or not to smoke. I am conditioned,
    addicted, so completely trapped that without a smoke, I am nothing-
    ized. [Puffs, exhales.] I will never escape from my cigarettes, nor
    will I ever escape from my need to quit smoking. In my cigarette-by-
    cigarette anguish, I do not do what I want, yet I am responsible for
    what I do.*

JUDITH: Well put.

CALLER: If you stop smoking, I'll buy your book.

*JUDITH: Interesting proposition. We could lauch a "Get Andrew to
    Stop" campaign—G.A.S.—right here on TalkLine Radio. What do
    you say, Andy?*

ANDREW: Kuf-kuf-kaf.

Andrew has been put to the challenge. If a half-million otherwise loyal readers joined G.A.S., and if his royalties were $2 per
copy sold, then we're talking $1,000,000 on the nose. Of
course, we couldn't just have Andrew quit for a day or two, as
he's done so many times before. We'd have to set ground
rules. Members of G.A.S. would buy Andrew's book only after
he'd abstained completely for a month, and they'd return the

book for a full refund if he relapsed before a year was up. Andrew would be obligated to appear every week on TalkLine, swearing to a live nationwide audience, hand upon Bible, that he had used no tobacco products whatsoever. He'd have to produce notarized results of laboratory tests of the levels of carbon monoxide in his exhaled breath, thiocyanate (a cyanide by-product) in his saliva, and cotinine (a nicotine by-product) in his urine. The cost of his laboratory tests probably wouldn't be covered by Andrew's health insurance, either. But his publisher, having paid him an arm and a leg as an advance, would no doubt agree to foot the bill.

Forty-six million American adults smoke cigarettes, including 24 million men and 22 million women.[1] At least 15 million smokers make a serious but unsuccessful attempt to quit smoking each year.[2] About 38 million have tried to stop at one time or another.[3] Most have tried several times. To each of these Americans, not just Andrew, I ask the same question: *If you were paid $1,000,000 to quit smoking now, how would you do it?* I have begun to ask this question of my patients who smoke, especially those who express sentiments like Andrew's. It's one of those unrealistic, hypothetical questions that helps to focus the mind, to get the essence of a choice that Andrew, my patients, and tens of millions of smokers make, on average, thirty times per day—namely, whether or not this cigarette will be the very last one. If you don't smoke, then ask the question of someone who does, someone whom you care about. With 46 million, there is no shortage of people to ask.

This book is about choices, difficult choices. Yet there are special cases where there is only one choice. Granted, quitting smoking isn't all good and no bad, just as Gideon's dietary choices weren't all good and no bad. No two smokers are exactly the same, just as (in Eve's case) no two overweight people are the same. Different smokers have to be matched up to different quitting strategies. One cannot predict whether a particular quitting strategy will succeed, just as (in Dinah's case) one can never have perfect knowledge of any choice. The task of quitting smoking entails persistence, just as Stephen's task was one of persistence. What matters is not a single cigarette but the lifelong summation of smoked and forgone cigarettes. The smoker has to be empirical, to learn which quitting strategy works for him, just as all our decision makers have had to navigate, to find their ways. That said, when it comes to smoking, there is just one choice: how to quit.

Andrew is caught up in the illusion of his uniqueness. He is as distinctive as his cough, so he thinks. Only he is trapped, enslaved, so he thinks. Everyone else, he thinks, is free to quit, can easily quit, and has quit. He hates them for it. Only he has tried and failed nine times, ninety times. For other people, there is life beyond cigarettes. For Andrew, cigarettes have deeper, special meaning. For Andrew, when a cigarette is not there, nothing is there.

But Andrew is not alone. We may all be different, but we can carry those differences only so far. Tens of millions of smokers feel that they cannot do it, either. Tens of millions of smokers think that they, too, are different; that they derive a unique benefit from smoking; that they are especially incapable of quitting; and perhaps that they may be singularly immune to tobacco's ill-health consequences. Andrew and those tens of millions who can't quit have something in common. They are enslaved not by cigarettes but by a single chemical, $C_{10}H_{14}N_2$, or nicotine. When cigarettes are not there, nicotine is not there.

All is not hopeless. In fact, as I shall explain in this chapter, new technologies are now available to quit smoking that go well beyond Andrew's expectations. Andrew may have no choice but to quit smoking, but he has and will have many choices about how. He needs merely to do his best. We cannot ask any more of him. So, just this once, let's pay him $1,000,000 and see if he can do it.

Andrew has a lot of money at stake. Having heard about the advice that you offered Eve, he seeks your competent medical counsel. Okay, you're the doctor again. What would you advise? To begin with, let's see if we can scare Andrew into trying once again to quit. Once he's off cigarettes, at least temporarily, we can decide how best to keep him from relapsing.

You may protest that scare tactics don't work. Not exactly. Recrimination and scolding don't work. Intimidation won't, either. But gentle, subtle scaring, when properly timed, does work. That's my experience. In fact, there is compelling evidence that when a physician suggests to a patient, one on one, with the office door closed, that it's time he quit, the patient goes home and actually tries to stop smoking.[4] Unfortunately, while seven in ten Americans seek medical attention at least once a year, no more than half the smokers can remember ever receiving any physician-initiated advice. That family doctors and specialists alike have not universally adopted such a practice, that they spend more time filling out insurance forms and taking manifold precautions lest they be sued, is one of the albatrosses of modern preventive medicine. Perhaps doctors would spend fifteen minutes counseling their patients about smoking if they got paid for that, too.

But we're not here to reform the system. Let the insurers and government health-care financiers pay chest surgeons thousands for cleanly resecting a wedge of Andrew's tumor-laden lung. Let them pay primary-care doctors pennies on the surgeon's dollar for taking a quarter-hour, behind closed office doors, to give Andrew a few facts. All we want is to help Andrew. So let's get him into the office, close the door, take a medical history, and perform a physical examination. We'll get some routine lab work, as we did for Eve, but only after we've had a chance to talk.

"I understand you've been smoking for forty years," you start off.

"I know it's no good for me," Andrew responds in classic fashion.

"After forty years, it's probably done you some harm. But smoking doesn't kill everybody. Some smokers live to be a hundred." As his doctor, you need to say that first, before Andrew has a chance to. "You know, Andrew, you could be one of those people who aren't terribly susceptible to cigarette smoke. After all, everybody's different. Let's take a history and do a physical and see if we can find out." By suggesting to Andrew that he may be singularly immune to cigarette smoke, you have implicitly suggested the opposite, that he may be especially susceptible. Perhaps you're beginning to see what I mean by gentle, subtle scaring.

"I feel fine," says Andrew. "I just have this cough."

"You probably have a touch of chronic bronchitis, and small-airways disease, too," you interject. "But that doesn't mean you've got full-blown emphysema. Anyway, you're not about to compete in the hundred-meter dash." Obviously,

Andrew isn't about to take up track and field. What you're really saying is that Andrew has a respiratory impairment, the full extent of which you have left to his imagination.

"Small-airways disease?" Andrew asks.

"In the early years after a child or teenager starts to smoke, he may report no symptoms, not even a cough. Even at this early stage, however, special breathing tests often show blockages in the small airways at the outer edges of the lung,[5] and these abnormalities have been directly observed by pathologists who performed autopsies on young smokers who died from accidents and violence.[6] By the time a smoker gets into his or her twenties, researchers can detect a relationship between the degree of abnormality in lung function tests and the number of cigarettes smoked per day. It's quite common. Anywhere from 17 to 60 percent of smokers under age fifty-five have small-airways disease."[7]

"Do I have it?" Andrew asks.

"Probably, but perhaps you don't have it too badly. Maybe you don't inhale." Of course, at two packs per day for forty years, with so many unsuccessful quits, you know that he certainly does inhale. But you're giving him something to latch on to, if only for a few minutes. It's a matter of timing. "Anyway," you continue, "if you stopped smoking early enough, before you developed chronic obstruction, it would probably go away."[8]

"Chronic obstruction?"

"After twenty or more years of cigarette use, a smoker develops chronic changes in his respiratory system. There are basically three types of pathology. First, there is a chronic cough and phlegm, especially when he gets up in the morning. It sounds as if you've got that already."

"Uh-huh." He is holding back his cough.

"Tell me, how much mucus do you bring up in the morning? Less than a teaspoonful?" you ask.

"Maybe a tablespoonful," Andrew says.

"I see." You say this with body language that shows consternation, as if you're a bit taken back by "a tablespoonful." But your words still have an upbeat tone. "Anyway," you go on, "after that comes the actual chronic obstruction of the flow of air in the main breathing passages of the lung, especially when you try to exhale rapidly. The tubes have basically become thickened and narrowed. But it doesn't happen in every smoker, and lately I've been seeing it happen more in women than in men." That, of course, is irrelevant. But you're again giving him a straw to grasp. "And then, finally, there's emphysema. That's where the walls between the little air sacs have been destroyed, and the lung has lost its rubber band–like elasticity, and the airflow gets really stuck. That's bad news."

"But you don't think I've got that, do you?"

"We can get some breathing tests and a chest X ray and see. If you had full-blown *chronic obstructive lung disease,* you'd have all three: the chronic cough and phlegm, the airflow obstruction, and the emphysema. But only a minority of smokers go that far."

"But I could still have it, you're saying."

"Some chronic deterioration in lung function will take place in most people who have smoked as long as you. But whether it's the cough and phlegm part of it, or the asthma-like obstruction, or the emphysema, or some combination of the three, depends on the individual smoker. Let's see, now, you've smoked two packs per day for forty years. That's eighty pack-years. We'd pretty much expect some irreversible chronic lung disease. But don't worry—there's still time to halt its progression.[9] You're still all right on three or four flights of stairs, aren't you?"

"Well, I take it easy," answers Andrew.

"Uh-huh," you answer, again with body language. You have now made the transition from the hundred-meter dash to ordinary stair climbing. You have raised doubts that Andrew can engage in normal physical activities without ever actually denying that he can. "I take it you don't have heart trouble," you continue.

"Not that I know of," says Andrew. "Except for my cough, I'm fine."

"You don't have diabetes or high blood pressure, do you?"

"Not that I know of."

"Your parents are still alive?" you ask him.

"My father died suddenly when he was fifty-nine. We never knew why. Mother is just strapping fine."

"It's possible that your father had a sudden death from a heart attack, but even if he did, you could very well not have inherited his predisposition for coronary heart disease. Or he could have died from a sudden brain hemorrhage. But again, even if he did, you may not have inherited a tendency toward strokes before age sixty. After all, you probably have your mother's eyes."

"I have my father's eyes."

"Did he smoke?" you ask.

"Yes."

"Cigarette smokers get atherosclerosis in just about every artery in the body, and they get more strokes, too. He might have been one of the more smoking-sensitive people. Still, you could just as well have inherited your mother's cardiac constitution."

"What do you mean by 'just about every artery in the body'?"

"Well, arteries carry blood to a man's penis. If he has severe enough atherosclerosis in those arteries, he will eventually lose his ability to attain or maintain an erection.[10] I've seen smokers regain their potency after they quit." When it comes to this delicate subject matter, you speak only in the third person, carefully avoiding second-person phrases such as "your erection" or "your penis" or "your impotence." And you don't linger, either. Keep moving. Change the subject. "Do you have cholesterol problems?" you ask.

"I haven't bothered with that recently. But I'm not overweight."

"We'll check your waist-hip ratio during your physical," you say.

"You mean my pants size?"

"Smokers weigh less than nonsmokers on average, but they may have extra body fat. Some researchers now think that smokers, even 'thin' smokers, actually have too much abdominal or central body fat, and that this form of fat is the most dangerous to them.[11] If your girth at your waist is larger than your girth at your hips, you might be in that situation. Don't worry. We'll check it."

"But if I quit smoking, I'd get even heavier," says Andrew.

"Actually, researchers believe that most of the weight you gain after you quit smoking doesn't end up in your abdominal fat stores. Don't worry. We'll talk about that later."

"But I can't quit," says Andrew. "I've already tried so many times. Nothing works."

"What's the longest you ever stayed off cigarettes?" you ask.

"Once I stayed off for two months," he answers.

"Two months is great. For those two months, you might have cut your heart attack risk by a third, maybe by half. That's terrific. This is going to be a piece of cake," you say. "No sweat."

"You mean I was doing myself some good by merely staying off cigarettes for two months?"

"When it comes to heart attacks, you certainly were. Your risk of heart attack probably starts to fall the day after you stop smoking, and it will have definitely fallen after a year of abstinence. It takes perhaps five to ten years before your risk comes down all the way. That seems to apply to men and women alike."[12]

"You mean I'm back to normal after two months?"

"That's not what I meant. Cigarette smoke has many different chemicals that can influence various stages in the lifelong process of atherosclerosis in your coronary arteries. Some of those chemicals are working from the very beginning, enhancing the development of fatty streaks and cholesterol-containing plaques. That's one reason I asked about your past blood cholesterol tests, because your beneficial HDL-cholesterol level might be down as a result of your smoking. But don't worry. We'll get it back up when you quit. You've heard of antioxidant vitamins, haven't you?"

"Like Vitamins C and E and beta-carotene?"

"Yes. We'll have to consider your taking supplements of these vitamins so long as you smoke, because cigarette smoke contains oxidant chemicals, some of which may promote the passage of cholesterol into the developing plaque in your arteries. And the nicotine in cigarette smoke seems to damage the inner lining of the arteries, and this also helps to let the LDL cholesterol get through.[13] But that's not why quitting smoking helps immediately. There are also chemicals in cigarette smoke that can induce a heart attack by promoting the complete blockage of an artery that's already partially obstructed. Nicotine also affects your pulse rate. It tightens up the blood vessels in your arms and legs. The carbon monoxide in smoke gets into your red blood cells and binds to the hemoglobin, which prevents the cells from carrying oxygen. You know how some football players breathe oxygen between downs?"

"They keep an oxygen tank at the sidelines. They're trying to fill the players' blood with oxygen."

"Basically, the carbon monoxide in cigarette smoke does the opposite. The smoke has a much higher level of carbon monoxide than you'd get from all but the most intense traffic pollution."

"So that's why the laboratory wants to test the carbon monoxide in my exhaled breath before I go on TalkLine Radio," says Andrew, referring to the rules of the G.A.S. campaign.

"Exactly. A high concentration of carbon monoxide in one's breath is basically diagnostic for smoking. Anyway, there are other chemicals in cigarette smoke that affect the blood platelets, which are important in forming the blood clot that finally blocks a narrowed coronary artery.[14] I could go on, of course. Cigarette smoke can also cause spasm of the coronary arteries. Whether it's the nicotine, or the hydrogen cyanide in smoke, or the nitrogen oxides—"

"But I thought all that stuff about heart attacks and cancer was just statistics," he interrupts.

"When scientists determine which chemicals in cigarette smoke are responsible for individual steps in the development of disease," you explain, "I wouldn't call it 'just statistics.'"

"But if I can cut my heart attack risk almost immediately, why do I have to stop smoking now?" Andrew asks. "I've got plenty of time."

"Not for cancer, unfortunately," you answer. "The risk of lung cancer gradually declines after you quit, but it could take twenty years or more before your risk is the same as if you never smoked, and it may never come back to baseline.[15] The same is likely to be true for all the other cancers caused by smoking: cancers of the mouth, voice box, the esophagus that carries food to the stomach, pancreas, kidney, bladder, possibly leukemia—"

"Smoking couldn't possibly cause all those diseases," Andrew interrupts.

"Cigarette smoke is a complicated chemical mixture. It shouldn't be a surprise that smoking has so many different effects on human health. In fact, it would be a surprise if the opposite were true, if a mixture that contained nicotine, hydrogen cyanide, formaldehyde, oxides of nitrogen, carbon monoxide, and over three dozen chemicals considered to cause cancer in humans or animals *didn't* do anything."

"But even if smokers get into trouble," Andrew suggests, "most don't get lung cancer."

"In 1985, about 256,000 American men died from their past or present cigarette smoking. That figure doesn't count cigarette-related residential fire deaths, or deaths of newborns and infants due to smoking during pregnancy, or deaths from lung cancer in nonsmokers due to passive smoking. And it doesn't count another 127,000 American women who died in the same year from their smoking. Lung cancer was the main cause of 30 percent of those male deaths, and if you group smoking-related cancers together, it comes to about 38 percent. For women, about 24 percent of smoking-attributable deaths were caused by lung cancer, and for all cancers combined, it's about 32 percent."[16]

"That means that 38 percent of the men who died from their smoking had cancer."

"That's right, and the rest had chronic obstructive pulmonary disease, coronary heart disease and other forms of atherosclerosis, and strokes, too. Of course, coronary heart disease and other heart and circulatory diseases are still the biggest health problems of smokers. But as more and more people have quit smoking, and as more and more smokers have controlled their blood pressure and their cholesterol levels, their risks of these circulatory diseases have fallen. Since it takes longer for a person's risk of cancer to fall after he quits smoking, you would expect cancer to become a more important problem. That's pretty much where we stand with you, Andrew. We can expect your risk of heart attack to go down pretty soon after you quit, but we'll just have to keep an eye out for cancer."

"I can get chest X rays, right?" Andrew asks.

"Chest X rays are not terribly good screening tests for lung cancer. It's not like mammograms, which can pick up many breast cancers at an early stage. By the time the radiologist sees a nodule in an X ray of your lungs, there's a good chance it's already spread. And lung cancer treatment isn't nearly so successful as breast cancer treatment."

"Who cares, anyway?" asks Andrew rhetorically. "Who cares if I live an extra year or two? I don't want to quit smoking just so I can sit on my rocking chair at seventy, incontinent, immobile, enfeebled, and with half my memory gone, staring out in space through cataract lenses."

"Andrew, life at age seventy, even at age eighty, is getting better and better. By the time you reached eighty, Andrew, in another quarter-century, I wouldn't count on being senile and incapacitated. These days, lots of older people are becoming more physically active. I saw this one article where people in their nineties were lifting weights. In a study of Harvard alumni, men of your age who quit smoking and took up sports during the 1960s and 1970s increased their life expectancy by two or three years.[17] But we do have the paperwork for living wills out in the reception area. If you got lung cancer, we wouldn't operate, not if you didn't want it. It's controversial, but you could even ask to be euthanized at age seventy, if that's what you want."

"But two or three extra years of life isn't all that much. Instead of dying at eighty, I'll just die at seventy-seven or seventy-eight. Big deal."

"Forget about age eighty. Let's just focus on age seventy. Andrew, if you keep smoking, your chances of surviving to your seventieth birthday are about 69 percent. If you quit smoking now, your survival rate would rise to about 79 percent. If you hadn't smoked at all, your chances of living to age seventy would have been about 89 percent.[18] Nobody's guaranteeing that you're going to live through the week, smoking or not smoking. Still, by quitting, you're adding an extra 10 percent to the chances that you'll live to age seventy. You're recovering about half the 20 percent gain in survival that you would have achieved if you had not smoked at all."

"But that doesn't count the weight gain," says Andrew.

"Good point," you say. Even when Andrew is wrong, you cannot insult his intelligence. "But not exactly. When epidemiologists determine that quitters are likely to live longer than continuing smokers, they're saying that the quitters may indeed have gained weight but they're living longer nonetheless. As I was saying before, most smokers who quit actually improve their body fat and cholesterol profiles.[19] Of course, these conclusions apply to typical smokers with typical amounts of postcessation weight gain. If you gained a whole lot of weight, we'd have to take special measures. I have some in mind, in fact. We might even consider putting you on diet pills after you quit. We'll get to that later."

"But my creativity will be stifled. I can't explain it. But that's what happened when I quit for two months," Andrew explains. "I just couldn't write. I'd sit in front of the word processor, and before you know it, I was ready to take a nap. If I heard the slightest noise, if I had the slightest interruption, if I had to answer the phone for an unsolicited call, I'd be paralyzed. I couldn't think of a single new sentence. My daily page quota went to pot."

"Now you're getting to the essence of the problem, Andrew."

Once someone has decided to stop smoking, the problem of how to quit boils down to one essential task: the management of *nicotine withdrawal*. This phenomenon happens predictably when a regular smoker stops smoking, even if the abstinence is involuntary. Despite dozens of research studies and scientific reviews, despite chapters on nicotine dependence in periodic surgeon general's reports on smoking,[20] despite the inclusion of Nicotine Withdrawal in official manuals of psychiatric diagnosis,[21] I continue to find that most nonsmokers, even the nonsmoking spouses of long-standing smokers, are baffled by the existence of such a well-defined condition. Even some of my patients who smoke, typically those who haven't tried seriously to quit, are not tuned in to their own symptoms. In fact, some of them who, like Andrew, have tried and failed are still not entirely sure what's happening to them when they stop.

They quit smoking for a day, only to find themselves tangled in an argument, or unable to concentrate, or prone to outbursts, or endlessly yearning for sweets, or repeatedly waking up at 2:00, 3:00, and 4:00 A.M., and then they blame their relapses and subpar performance on all sorts of contingencies. When I ask them why they went back to cigarettes after two hours or two days, they say that they got a traffic ticket, or their electricity was shut off, or they had a deadline to meet. They became impatient or frustrated or anxious or nervous or restless, so they had to bum a cigarette. They go through an experience that is nearly universal among millions of people every

time they try to quit. They have the well-documented symptoms of a recognized medical syndrome. Yet their explanation
for relapse is that, basically, life is difficult.

With all the research studies and personal accounts, I still
can find no better description of nicotine withdrawal than a
paper presented to a branch of the Chicago Medical Society in
1931 by Dr. Jerome Head, who described his attempt to stop
smoking for two months:

> About an hour after I have had a cigarette I develop a pecu-
> liar sensation in my mouth. . . . I feel like sucking my
> cheeks, biting my lips, and scraping my tongue over my
> teeth. . . .
>
> During the second hour and soon after the appearance of
> the mouth symptoms, I begin to be conscious of my legs and
> arms—in fact of my whole body. It is difficult to describe
> these sensations accurately, for there is no other feeling like
> it. It is not so much a pain as an awareness of every muscle
> and nerve in the body. This is the true urge to [smoke]
> another cigarette and disappears with the first puff. . . .
>
> As the desire to smoke increases I become mentally dull.
> I cannot work or concentrate. If I keep awake I cannot sit
> still but have to walk about or do something. All I can think
> of is smoking. . . .
>
> After the first day, and as soon as I had convinced myself
> that I would not give in to my desire, the discomfort was less
> bothersome. It was not absent, but I simply went about my
> business and frequently forgot about it. . . . The discomfort
> and desire [were] not constant. On some days I would
> notice them very little and again they would come back as
> strongly as ever and for long periods the thought of smok-
> ing was constantly in my mind. Waves of desire to smoke
> were associated usually with lack of sleep or worry. The last
> week of the two months was the most difficult for the
> thought that I would soon be able to smoke was constantly
> with me. . . .
>
> Finally the great day arrived and I hurried through my
> breakfast and sighed with relief as I lit a cigarette. I was to be
> normal again. I was unpleasantly surprised. Not only did the
> smoke taste like that from an old rag but on attempting to
> inhale I was choked up as I had been when I was learning. It
> was evident that I would have to learn to smoke again. . . .

That was three months ago. By gradually increasing the dose I have again become a smoker and can inhale regular cigarettes like a regular fellow.[22]

Perhaps the misunderstanding about nicotine withdrawal is yet another problem with the use and interpretation of language. Not everyone is going to be as articulate as Dr. Head when he spoke of waves of desire to smoke, or Andrew when he says that his creativity was stifled. Some patients will say, "I'm not sure exactly why, but I had this indescribable urge to have a cigarette." Others won't be able to put it into words, but when I suggest it's nicotine withdrawal, they nod knowingly. Others just don't want to talk about it. It's a secret. It's personal, a bodily function like belching or flatulence. We talk and talk, and in the end I'm not sure they know that every other smoker feels the same things.

Nonsmokers suffer a much larger language gap. To say to a nonsmoker that Andrew relapsed nine times because he experienced cigarette craving or nicotine withdrawal is to accuse Andrew of a loss of control. They don't see it. To them, the word *withdrawal* conjures up images of drenching sweats, tremulousness, delirium and seizures. The confusion is even worse for the word *addiction,* which in one sense is used to imply that a person would sell sex and commit crimes for a fix, and at the other extreme is used casually, as in addictions to Porsches, golf, or Chinese food. I have tried other phrases, such as "cigarette/nicotine dependence,"[23] but the word *dependence* likewise has too many other meanings. To call smoking a "tobacco abuse disorder" gets us right back to the "disorder" problem of chapter 4. In the end, there is no better way to say it: Without some form of nicotine replacement—such as nicotine gum, a nicotine skin patch, or a nicotine nasal spray or inhaler—virtually every regular smoker who abstains from cigarettes will go through his or her own version of nicotine withdrawal.

Not every smoker has the same nicotine-withdrawal experience, however. Some researchers have suggested, in fact, that nicotine-withdrawal symptoms are much more variable than are other forms of drug withdrawal.[24] The problem, I believe, is that many people aren't sure what to expect when they stop smoking, and they're not sure what counts as withdrawal and what doesn't. In fact, some smokers are so unsure about the genuineness of their withdrawal experiences that researchers have tricked them into thinking that such-and-such a sensation is or isn't caused by withdrawal.[25] While some people begin to experience symptoms one to six waking hours after the last cigarette, the tide of restlessness, anxiety, impatience, and irritability seems to rise rapidly in the first or second day after quitting.[26] These mood changes, as well as impairments in performance, usually peak in the first two weeks after quitting and subside in about four or five weeks, but they can last for two or three months.[27] What most often persists beyond the five-week benchmark is an enhanced appetite and weight gain, as well as that nondescript, persistent feeling of needing to have a cigarette.[28]

There are many theories of smoking relapse. Some psychologists emphasize smokers' feelings of self-efficacy or their sense of control over their bodies and their lives. When an abstaining smoker backslips and has even a single cigarette, they suggest, his sense of failure and disempowerment can doom his efforts. Other researchers talk about stress-coping skills. They argue that the smoker who formerly relied on cigarettes to cope with anxiety and stress must now learn new ways to cope. Some psychologists will say that the traffic ticket, the electricity shutoff, and the pressure of the deadline were environmental cues for which the smoker was behaviorally conditioned to smoke. Others will say that the impatience or restlessness were personality traits that had been suppressed or controlled by nicotine but that emerged once nicotine was withdrawn.

These explanations may have merit, but they are unnecessarily complicated. They don't get to the essence of the problem any more than my patients' simple explanations about life being difficult do. When it comes down to it, what caused my patients' symptoms and what precipitated their relapse was their inability to manage their nicotine-withdrawal symptoms. The mountains of insightful psychologizing do little more than detract from the central fact that quitting smokers are trying to wean themselves from a drug.

Psychologists acknowledge that when smokers are tracked in their attempts to quit, the severity of their initial withdrawal symptoms predicts the likelihood of relapse.[29] But they protest that something else, called "degree of dependence," causes both severe withdrawal and relapse. These abstractions are actually worse than my patients' concrete explanations about traffic tickets, power shutdowns, and deadlines. Other researchers will legitimately point out that a smoker who overcomes the initial withdrawal symptoms has no ultimate guarantee of success in quitting. Many smokers who have stayed off cigarettes for six months, they point out, can still relapse. So it can't be all nicotine withdrawal, they say. But the observation that smoking cessation and relapse aren't 100 percent nicotine withdrawal hardly demolishes the main point. In fact, as I am about to show, only 3 percent of all relapses occur after the smoker has stayed off cigarettes for six months.

In figure 6.1, I have graphed the "success curve" for a single attempt to quit smoking. The horizontal axis measures the time (in weeks) from the start of the smoker's attempt to quit.

FIGURE 6.1
Success Curve for a Single Attempt to Quit Smoking

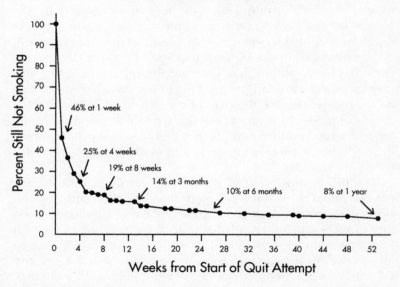

SOURCE: Based on reports of 7,510 current and recent former smokers polled in the 1978–80 National Health Interview Surveys. See also National Center for Health Statistics, "Current Estimates from the Health Interview Survey," app. 1. *Vital and Health Statistics* ser. 10 (1977), no. 11, and "Changes in Cigarette Smoking Practies Among Adults, United States, 1978," *Advance Data on Vital and Health Statistics* (1979), no. 52.

In essence, the clock is reset to zero and starts ticking as soon as the smoker says to herself, "That's the last cigarette—ever." The vertical axis measures the proportion of smokers who will still be abstinent at various points in time. Imagine that 100 smokers, who are in scattered locations and don't know one another, have all independently tried to quit at the same time on the same day. The curve shows how many are still off cigarettes as each successive week is ticked off on the calendar. If a smoker quit once, and then backslid and smoked a pack, and then started to quit again, that would count as two attempts.

The data I have used to construct the curve come from the National Health Interview Surveys of 1978 through 1980. My use of data more than a decade old may seem outmoded. But it is important to examine smokers' relapse patterns at a time before nicotine gum, nicotine skin patches, and other nicotine replacement treatments began to be prescribed. The curve does not come from a stop-smoking clinic or a psychologist's study of a few dozen or a few hundred volunteers. It comes from thousands of smokers who told interviewers, in the course of answering many questions about personal demographics and health, when they last tried to quit smoking and, if they relapsed, how long they managed to stay off cigarettes. Included in the survey data base are the reports of 2,105 "former" smokers who had been off cigarettes anywhere from one day to two years since the date of the interview. While there is a natural tendency in surveys of this type to overemphasize the longest, most serious attempts to quit, the success curve shown in the figure is picking up each and every attempt, even if it lasted just one day.[30]

The figure shows that by the end of one week, only 46 percent of smokers were still off cigarettes. Put differently, 54 percent of smokers relapsed within seven days of starting. Their rate of success dropped steadily until, by the end of a year, only 8 percent remained abstinent. If we were to extend the chart all the way out to two years, we'd be down to about 7.4 percent. Of course, some people resume smoking even after two years. But if we defined two years of continuous abstinence as "successful" quitting, then we're left to conclude that the vast majority of failures occur within a couple of weeks of quitting. Only one in eleven failures occurs after three months, and only one in thirty-two failures occurs after six months.

No amount of psychologizing could explain this curve. I will not accept the explanation that only 7 or 8 percent of all cigarette smokers have a sense of self-empowerment, or are capable of acquiring new personal strategies for stress management and temptation control, or can learn to use noncigarette means to suppress their innate restlessness and impatience. I will not yield to the possibility that, after two or three months, traffic tickets and power outages have actually become less frequent. If Andrew came back to your office and told you that he relapsed yet again after only three weeks, I suggest that you avoid explanations to the effect that he had not acquired the requisite coping skills or did not have adequate social supports. Do not, I beg you, tell him that he lacked sufficient motivation. To express empathy for Andrew, I suggest that you erase those rationalizations from your files and instead sit down with Andrew for another scantily compensated fifteen minutes, and tell him that you know what it's like and that you've got some new ideas that might help.

The most striking proof that nicotine withdrawal is the fundamental event in smoking cessation comes from a single, straightforward observation. If the smoker gets his nicotine back, his withdrawal symptoms go away and his relapse is aborted.[31] In the beginning, researchers weren't entirely sure of this conclusion. When they gave abstinent smokers nicotine chewing gum, they observed only partial alleviation of withdrawal symptoms. As I shall explain shortly, this was because the gum was delivering nicotine into the smoker's bloodstream at a rate less than half that of cigarette smoke. Now, scientists are developing more advanced technologies for delivering nicotine and controlling withdrawal symptoms. Now, when it comes to quitting, Andrew has choices.

In fact, in the sixty-plus years since Jerome Head offered his observations to his fellow physicians in Evanston, Illinois, on why the smoker "would walk more than a mile" for his cigarette, the only truly important advances in smoking cessation have been the development of nicotine replacement therapies, as well as other nonnicotine drug treatments to block or control nicotine-withdrawal symptoms.[32] One may cite the fact that Americans began to quit smoking in large numbers after the publication of the first surgeon general's report in 1964 and the ensuing antismoking publicity of the late 1960s.[33] But information about the risks of smoking merely gives people an incentive to try to quit. It doesn't tell them how to quit. That's what you were doing during Andrew's first office visit. You reinforced his motivation. When governments raise taxes on cigarettes and when manufacturers raise cigarette prices, smokers likewise try to quit.[34] That's an economic incentive at work. The same goes for Andrew's $1,000,000 reward for quitting. One may cite the fact that 90 percent of successful quitters have used so-called self-help quitting strategies, mostly by stopping abruptly.[35] That's like saying that 90 percent of people took trains and cars before there were jets. Or that 90 percent of Andrew's novels were typed on an old typewriter before he learned to use a word processor.

You may now be thinking that you know X number of smokers who tried nicotine gum or the patch, and it didn't work. I do not pretend to explain everything. I don't know whether the gum caused one smoker a stomach upset, or whether a second smoker couldn't learn how to chew it properly, or a third found it embarrassing to masticate during an important meeting, or whether a fourth felt itching under the skin patch, or a fifth had sleep disturbances with the patch, or the sixth's doctor wouldn't give her a prescription. Actually, we needn't go further than Andrew, who smoked between pieces of nicotine gum against doctor's orders and who won't even buy the patch because his health insurance won't pay for it.

Nor can I promise to cure everyone's smoking by a single, uniformly applicable method. As I'll explain shortly, smokers differ in their patterns of nicotine withdrawal, and therefore they will differ in their strategies for managing withdrawal. But let's focus solely on probabilities for now. Let's concede that we cannot definitely cure Andrew of smoking. Suppose we could merely improve his chances of successful quitting. After all, isn't that what Dinah wanted? She didn't ask for zero risk. She didn't expect perfection. She needed a means of assessing her partner's HIV infectivity so that she could reduce risk, not eliminate it. Likewise, what Andrew needs are methods to reduce materially his chances of relapse, not to guarantee pain-free abstinence.

If Andrew's success curve were the same as that of the smokers in the National Health Interview Survey, then his long-term chances of success on a single, unaided quit attempt would be only 7.4 percent. Even with nine tries, I wouldn't give Andrew any more than one-to-one odds of getting off cigarettes. But if we had some technology that could shift Andrew's success curve upward just a bit, if we could raise the chances of continued abstinence at three months from 14 percent to, say, 25 percent, then I'll take three-to-one odds on Andrew's kicking the habit in no more than nine tries. Of course, Andrew is atypical for having tried nine times in three years, which is about once every four months. In the National Health Interview Survey, the average quitter tried again every eight and a half months. But the message is the same: When unaided success rates in quitting are so low, any technology that can consistently improve a smoker's chances, even by a small amount, will greatly magnify the odds in favor of success in the long run.

Cigarette smoke is an aerosol, a chemical spray. It contains droplets of vapor and very tiny solid particles that are suspended in a mixture of various gases, such as carbon monoxide. The cigarette smoker puffs on the opposite end of the burning rod, drawing the smoke initially into his mouth. Then, as he inhales the puffed smoke, its droplets, particles, and gases go deep into his lungs. One of the chemicals on the tiny particles is nicotine. The particles can pass so deeply into the lung that the nicotine enters the bloodstream within seconds. From the blood, nicotine goes straight to the brain. Once every thirty to ninety seconds, with each puff, the smoker injects a bolus of nicotine into his lungs, through his bloodstream, and up to his brain.

After the smoker finishes each cigarette, the level of nicotine in the blood gradually falls over minutes and hours. How rapidly the nicotine level falls after a cigarette is finished will also depend upon the individual smoker. Finally, when the level of nicotine falls too low, it is time for another cigarette. The threshold level of nicotine below which another cigarette is needed also depends on the smoker. Accordingly, the number of cigarettes smoked in any one day will vary with each person.

Smokers smoke cigarettes differently. Each smoker has his own characteristic smoking style or "topography," which determines how much nicotine enters the blood. It is based on his depth of draw on the cigarette, the volume of smoke he takes in with each puff, the time he pauses between puffs, how deeply he inhales the smoke into his lungs, the number of puffs he takes on a given cigarette, and the number of cigarettes he smokes per day. The fact that a cigarette is labeled "low-tar" or "light" is by itself a poor indicator of the amount of nicotine a smoker actually absorbs.[36]

Despite these individual variations, the basic pattern of nicotine intake is the same. The drug is self-administered in a series of rapid-fire bursts, with gaps between individual cigarettes. If one were to draw a chart of the level of nicotine in a smoker's blood during the course of a waking day, you might think it looked like the seismic recording of a series of earthquakes: a rapid succession of shocks and aftershocks during the smoking of one cigarette, followed by calm between cigarettes, and then more shocks. This is the pattern of nicotine self-administration that the smoker has grown accustomed to. A smoker like Andrew, who takes perhaps ten puffs per cigarette, is therefore self-administering about four hundred dosages of nicotine per day, or over five million individual quanta of nicotine since he started smoking forty years ago.

When Andrew stops smoking, he experiences nicotine withdrawal. He can manage the withdrawal by self-administering nicotine in the form of a chewing gum, a skin patch, a nasal spray, or an inhaler. None of these forms of nicotine substitution, however, produces the exact rapid-fire pattern of nicotine absorption that occurs during cigarette smoking. Nor does each form necessarily deliver the same quantity of nicotine that a cigarette does. Moreover, Andrew has much more control over the exact dosage of nicotine during his cigarette smoking than he has with these alternate methods of nicotine self-administration.

To manage his nicotine withdrawal successfully, Andrew needs to use these nicotine substitutes to mimic his past nicotine profile, yet at the same time gradually wean himself from the drug. If all smokers had the same smoking topography, then there would be a standard dosage and frequency of these drugs that would fit everyone. It would be like taking a standard number of tablets of penicillin for a standard number of days to cure strep throat. But that's obviously not the case. It is absolutely critical for Andrew and his doctor to understand this. There is rock-solid evidence that nicotine-substitution therapies, such as the chewing gum[37] and the skin patch,[38] help a great many smokers to quit for good. But there are still many relapses. As I see it, nicotine substitution fails when the patient and his doctor do not appreciate the critical role played by individual differences, when they treat the gum and the patch like antibiotics.[39]

The therapeutic field of managing nicotine withdrawal is still burgeoning. A year or two after this book is published, the entire field may explode. From what we know so far, there are two critical dimensions to treatment: the *nicotine-dosing schedule* and the *weaning (or downtitration) schedule*. A third, more exploratory area is the use of *non-nicotine adjuvants*. These are not merely theoretical speculations by somebody in a laboratory. Andrew already has genuine choices to make.

Each form of nicotine substitution has a different nicotine delivery profile and can be used in a different manner. When a quitter uses a sixteen- or twenty-four-hour skin patch, for example, she can control the dose of nicotine in two basic ways: by deciding when and whether to change the patch, and by choosing a particular strength. Current versions of the patch come in two or three strengths—7, 14, and 21 milligrams, for example—which correspond to the respective total amounts of nicotine delivered by a patch over the prescribed time it remains on the skin. Once the strength is chosen and the patch is in place, the quitter has no other control over the nicotine-dosing schedule.

The patch is like a flat pastry with many very thin layers. Under the outer backing is an inner layer of nicotine filling, under which may be an adhesive layer that holds the patch in place. Because the nicotine is gradually absorbed through the skin, the patch produces a relatively smooth nicotine blood profile. A chart of the level of nicotine in the blood of a person who wore the patch (and didn't smoke) would look like a mountain, with a smooth, steep rise to a single peak after about four to ten hours, followed by a slower downward slope for the rest of the day.[40] This smooth mountainlike profile is completely different from the rapid-burst-and-pause nicotine profile that the smoker derives from cigarettes. Even at the peak of the mountain, the blood level of nicotine may be anywhere from 12 to 85 percent of the level that a smoker is accustomed to.[41]

If you, as Andrew's doctor, should choose to prescribe this technology, then it is critical that you and your patient understand these differences in nicotine delivery between the patch and his cigarettes. By itself, the patch cannot be used to produce an extra needed burst of nicotine just when Andrew's electricity is shut off, or the police officer writes him a ticket, or he needs to concentrate on writing a paragraph. What's more, your patient's withdrawal experience will depend critically on the extent of initial nicotine replacement. A relatively low degree of nicotine substitution—typically between 25 and 50 percent of the smoker's usual blood level—can alleviate many initial withdrawal symptoms, such as anxiety, restlessness, impatience, and insomnia. Higher percentages—typically over 50 percent—are sometimes required to overcome those indescribable "waves of desire to smoke" a cigarette, as well as enhanced appetite. Even with the higher percentage substitution, weight gain is often not prevented. At the other extreme, nicotine substitution rates below 25 percent may be too low, at least in the first week or two after quitting. You and your patient need to understand that just as each smoker has his own topography of smoking, so each smoker will have his own required level of nicotine-dosing.[42]

At present, nicotine chewing gum comes in one 2-milligram size,[43] although researchers have studied dosages ranging from 0.5 to 4 milligrams. A critical difference between the gum and the patch is that the quitter can use the gum ad lib. Although this form of nicotine self-administration has greater flexibility, it also is more liable to be abused.[44] When a quitter chews a 2-milligram piece once every hour, he gets a relatively flat nicotine blood profile, with a nicotine substitution rate somewhere between 16 and 60 percent.[45] While some earlier studies showed high relapse rates on the chewing gum,[46] it is becoming clear that the 2-milligram dosage can be too low for some smokers and that 4 milligrams may be required, at least initially.[47] Some authorities say that nicotine gum works only when the quitter concurrently joins a program that teaches her self-management and temptation-control skills. My view is that these quit-smoking groups, when they do help, show her how to use nicotine replacement correctly and to adjust the dosage to her individual needs. They're merely doing what you, as doctor, should have done in the first place.[48]

But these are only the more established forms of nicotine self-administration. Nicotine toothpicks and nicotine lozenges are now under study.[49] Two newer technologies, the nicotine nasal spray[50] and nicotine inhaler,[51] have recently received favorable evaluation. Both can be used ad lib. Both appear to produce levels of nicotine that peak in five to ten minutes after a single dosage, a pattern that more closely approximates the rapid-fire nicotine delivery of cigarettes. These technologies likewise do not guarantee smoking cessation. As do the more established methods of nicotine substitution, they can double or even triple the lowly 7 percent success rate that the smoker can otherwise expect from unaided attempts to quit. Future studies will undoubtedly evaluate combinations of fixed-dose nicotine patches and ad lib forms of nicotine replacement.

Once the smoker has found an initial schedule of nicotine replacement, the next step is to reduce the dosage of nicotine over time. Researchers have tried a great many different "downtitration," or weaning, schedules. In some protocols, smokers use a given dosage of patch for four weeks, then drop to a lower dosage for another four weeks, then perhaps to a still lower dosage for another four weeks. In other protocols, the subjects start out at 4-milligram nicotine gum for six weeks and then start weaning to 2-milligram gum, but the use of the gum can be continued for months.[52] In other studies, the tapering period for nicotine replacement didn't begin until three months after quitting. While the weaning schedule can depend on the form of nicotine replacement, my experience is that successful quitters learn how rapidly to wean themselves. What matters in practice is that they understand that some smokers can cut the dosage rapidly while others cannot.

Nicotine substitutes are not the only drugs currently under study for the management of nicotine withdrawal. This is a much more fluid area of research, with many scientists issuing promising preliminary reports. Some but not all researchers have found that clonidine, a prescription drug for high blood pressure, might alleviate the withdrawal symptoms from nicotine,[53] as well as from alcohol[54] and opiates such as morphine.[55] The initial optimism about clonidine, however, has been subdued by the drug's side effects, including dry mouth, drowsiness, and dizziness.[56] Buspirone, a new anti-anxiety drug, is under consideration for possible suppression of withdrawal symptoms.[57] So is the anti-anxiety, anti-depressant drug doxepin.[58] This is only the beginning. Now that nicotine withdrawal is becoming the accepted paradigm for studying quitting, researchers are seriously considering other nicotine blockers.[59]

When quitters use nicotine-replacement therapies to achieve at least 25 percent substitution, they can still gain weight, but not as rapidly as in unaided quitting.[60] Still, researchers are now beginning to study the concomitant use of the new generation of appetite-suppressant drugs. In one study, phenylpropanolamine, a drug found in many over-the-counter appetite suppressants and antihistamines, helped reduce weight gain from quitting smoking.[61] So did dextro-fenfluramine, an appetite-suppressant drug that is currently available by prescription in Europe.[62]

When I ask former smokers how they finally stopped, I don't receive scientific lectures on the management of nicotine withdrawal. Many patients, suffering from retrograde amnesia, tell me that they just quit, period. They don't recall the details. But others tell great stories, fantastic stories.

One young man bought ten new cartons, sat down at a curbside, and, one by one, tossed the shredded fragments of 1,999 freshly unwrapped filter-tipped cigarettes into the city sewer system. Then he smoked the 2,000th all the way down to the filter, and that, he explained, was it. What he didn't tell me about was the five other times he had tried before he finally devised this ritual. A young woman used the nicotine patch without the slightest side effects. She explained, however, that what really worked was a remark, unintentionally overheard from the hallway while a certain person was having sex with her roommate, that he would have dated her if only . . . well, I needn't go on.

Sure, people have all sorts of post hoc explanations for why and how they quit. They discard. They edit. They forget. It's not all that different from their manifold explanations for why they failed. Of course, after the fact, you as the doctor are entitled to tell them how they attained new stress-coping skills, how they achieved new levels of self-control and self-empowerment. You're not going to divulge to them that they managed, somehow, to beat a drug. That wouldn't be empathic. But if Andrew or any other patient comes to see you, closes the office door, and tells you he cannot quit, you have to keep hammering away at the same message. It's not over. You do have choices. Try again.

JUDITH: *Welcome back, Andy. It's your sixth monthly visit to Talk-Line. Did you bring your lab tests?*

ANDREW: *Right here, Judy. They did a blood carboxyhemoglobin level this time, just to be sure.*

JUDITH: *I understand that sales of your novel have soared. More people signed up for G.A.S. than we could have imagined. Looks like 750,000 readers have now asked for a refund if you resume smoking before the year's up.*

ANDREW: *Well, here's my Bible. I'm ready any time—*

JUDITH: *We've got a caller. Go ahead, you're on TalkLine.*

CALLER: *How did you quit? What's your secret?*

ANDREW: *In the beginning, I relied upon nicotine-replacement therapy. That I have to admit. But what really helped me is working hard on my new play, entitled "Door Slammed Shut."*

JUDITH: *Interesting title.*

ANDREW: *I got the idea in my doctor's office. My doctor slammed the office door shut and gave it to me straight out.*

CALLER: *Did you stay off coffee and alcohol?*

ANDREW: *It's a fairly simple plot. Three people are in Hell, two of them as a result of a mutual suicide pact. The third, Nicholas, smoked cigarettes up to the day he died suddenly at age fifty-nine. Nick's perpetual condemnation is the thought that, if only he had quit smoking—*

CALLER: *Sounds like the carrots and celery worked.*

7

Lump

Breast Cancer

RUTH: *Hello. May I help—*

SHARON: *I am so glad I didn't get your voice mailbox. You're the first person I wanted to call. I'm in a total panic.*

RUTH: *Uh-oh. The biopsy was positive?*

SHARON: *I'm going to have a double mastectomy and after that, plastic reconstructive—*

RUTH: *Double mastectomy? But it was just a tiny lump on one side, in one breast. They could barely feel it.*

SHARON: *Mom had breast cancer when she was fifty-nine, and it killed her. Now I've got it. The doctors think it hasn't spread, but they don't know for sure. I'm not taking any chances. Ruth, you're my baby sister. You've got to do it, too.*

RUTH: *But I had a mammogram just last—*

SHARON: *Mammograms don't work, especially if you're under fifty. There was an article in the paper. I saved it. I'll fax it to you. My lump didn't even show up in the mammogram.*

RUTH: *But I don't have a lump, and I just had my checkup.*

SHARON: *You already had one biopsy. That was quite a scare.*

RUTH: *That was four years ago. They said that was nothing.*

SHARON: *Nothing, my foot. How about the next checkup, or the next biopsy? That's just what happened to me. Every checkup was just fine. And then, out of nowhere, a lump.*

RUTH: *But they found the cancer while it was still in the early stages. You should be thankful for that.*

SHARON: *Early? You can say that again. I'm forty-four. I still have my period. I might take tamoxifen. And they're talking about using RU-486 for breast cancer. If there's a research study, I'll sign up. And you know what? Cousin Sarah—*

RUTH: *Sarah's got it, too?*

SHARON: *Ovarian cancer. How do you like that?*

RUTH: *That's terrible. She's only forty-two—*

SHARON: *And you're only forty, Ruthie.*

RUTH: *So you want me to get my ovaries out, too? I might still have children.*

SHARON: *Children? At forty? When did you get that idea?*

RUTH: *Buzz has been talking about it. I didn't tell you.*

SHARON: *Come on, Ruthie, at least talk to my oncologist.*

RUTH: *I've been taking daily multivitamins. Buzz says chestnuts have Vitamins C and E and selenium, and halibut has Vitamin A. And I'm on an ultra low-fat diet, with lots of—*

SHARON: *Ruth, honey, you're dreaming.*

RUTH: *Lots of fresh vegetables and high fiber and—*

SHARON: *That low-fat stuff won't work. There was an article in the paper. I saved it.*

RUTH: *I'm cutting out alcohol. I'm going to join a health club and slim down. There's this place called WestSide Fit—*

SHARON: *I'll fax you that low-fat article, too. You'll see. Ruthie, my surgeon is really great, and you could—*

RUTH: *No more faxes for personal matters. It's a new rule.*

SHARON: *I'm sending them anyway. We're talking about cancer, not some business deal, or whatever you do over there.*

RUTH: *We do strategic business planning. Our clients range from large corporations to—*

SHARON: *Let me give you the oncologist's telephone number—*

RUTH: *Uh-oh, I've got to run. I'll call you tonight.*

Put yourself in Ruth's situation. Suppose you had a high risk of developing breast cancer. You could virtually eliminate that risk by having both breasts removed. On each side, the surgeon would excise the underlying breast tissue, preserving the nipple and skin, and perhaps insert an implant. Would you consider the operation? How high would your risk of cancer have to be? Suppose you were "very likely" to get cancer. Is that enough? Suppose you were "almost certain" to contract cancer. Is there some level of risk at which you would have surgery?

Ruth's choice is difficult. It is so difficult that some women would ask someone else to make it for them. Not surprisingly, that someone else may be their own doctor. Yet many medical writers, including female physicians, find Ruth's choice so difficult that they, too, back off from an answer. Instead, they urge their readers to collect all the facts, weigh the options carefully, and make up their own minds. Of course, the medical writer's job is to educate and inform, not to give personalized medical advice. And then there is the ever-present problem of new medical developments. The writer's book, at some point, has to go to press. But when the patient asks her doctor for advice, she is also asking for a forecast. Don't just tell me the latest information, doctor. Tell me what the future holds for breast cancer diagnosis and treatment. Give me your best prediction.

I am not Ruth's doctor. I am not your doctor. But I will not shirk. I would advise Ruth not to have the bilateral prophylactic mastectomy, at least not right away. Here's my reasoning.

Ruth's mother had breast cancer at age fifty-nine. Her sister Sharon has cancer at age forty-four. Her cousin Sarah has ovarian cancer at age forty-two. In all likelihood, an inherited form of breast cancer runs in her family, just as certain other cancers (retinoblastoma of the eye, adenomatous polyps of the colon) run in families.[1] To be sure, Ruth's mother discovered her breast cancer in her late fifties, not in her forties or before her change of life. So her mother's breast cancer may have been *sporadic* rather than *familial*.[2] Even so, two breast cancers and one ovarian cancer are a bit too much to be sheer coincidence. But even if Sharon inherited a very high breast cancer susceptibility from her mother, that doesn't mean that Ruth, too, inherited it. It's basically no different from the proposition that Sharon may have inherited her Mom's eye color and hair texture, but Ruth didn't.

At present, there is no blood test to tell Ruth whether she has inherited a breast cancer gene. Not knowing any more than that Ruth *might* have the gene, I estimate that her chances of contracting breast cancer at some time over the next decade are 10 percent. Her chances of getting breast cancer at some time within the next twenty years are 18 percent. Her risk of having breast cancer during the coming three decades is 25 percent.[3] Those are pretty dismal odds. But as

Ruth's doctor, I'm betting that within ten years, and possibly five years, human genetics will advance to the point where a blood test will be available.[4] Quite apart from the cancer-gene blood test, scientists may find new ways for Ruth to reduce her breast cancer risk or to detect a cancer while it is still early. Even if no scientific advances are forthcoming, Ruth has options other than a prophylactic double mastectomy. For me, that's enough reason to tell Ruth that she can temporize, and see what happens, at least for now.

Whether or not Ruth has a familial form of breast cancer, her risk of contracting it depends on her own reproductive history.[5] That's because sex hormones, especially estrogen, play an important role in the development of breast cancer, even though scientists aren't exactly sure why. Once a young girl starts menstruating, her ovaries send the estrogen hormone throughout her body, including her breasts. The earlier she starts her period, the sooner her breasts are exposed to her own estrogens, and therefore the higher her cancer risk later in life.[6] As her doctor, I know that Ruth didn't start her menstrual periods until age fourteen, which is relatively late.[7] That's a mitigating factor. Had she started earlier, especially at twelve or younger, her future risk of breast cancer would be higher. That's true even if Ruth hasn't inherited a familial susceptibility to breast cancer.

Pregnancy also causes many important changes in the hormones in a woman's body. During pregnancy, a woman's body makes extra estrogen, and that may enhance her cancer risk in the short term. But for reasons that are likewise not entirely clear, pregnancy on balance tends to protect a woman's breasts against future cancer, especially after many years. Had Ruth gotten pregnant in her teens or early twenties, her cancer risk would thus be lower.[8] Ruth has never been pregnant, and that fact enhances her risk.

Ruth can't turn the clock back to age fourteen and somehow delay her period. She can't reverse time to get pregnant at age twenty. That's all past and gone, beyond control. Still, Ruth has many present and future options that can affect the sex hormones in her body and thus influence her breast cancer risk. For one thing, having her ovaries removed is a genuine option. Women who have their ovaries out before age thirty-five almost never get breast cancer, and Ruth is not that much older. The ovarectomy would be a much less extensive operation, and there would be no reconstructive plastic surgery involved. That way, Ruth would prevent ovarian cancer, which might also run in her family along with breast cancer,[9] and still keep her breasts. Yes, there's a downside. Once she lost her ovaries, she'd have a higher risk of heart disease and osteoporosis. But Ruth could defer the decision about ovary removal for a couple of years, to see whether a test for familial breast cancer becomes available. By that time, scientists may have learned whether hormone blockers such as tamoxifen might prevent breast cancer, especially in high-risk women.[10] She'd also have a chance to see whether she could get pregnant. That's right. She might even consider having the baby that her husband, Buzz, is talking about. Perhaps the extra estrogen hormones that her body produces during pregnancy will raise her risk of cancer. Perhaps it takes many years for pregnancy to have a protective effect on breast cancer risk. Even so, she could have her ovaries removed right after delivery.

I'd recommend that Ruth continue to do everything she has been doing. She should be sure to eat foods that contain Vitamins C, E, and selenium and beta-carotene. She might consider taking supplements of certain vitamins, but as her doctor, I'd have to watch for signs of vitamin overdose. No, I don't know whether any of these suspected anticancer micronutrients really prevents breast cancer, or the exact dosages that might be required. But in the next ten years, that information, too, may become available. I would ask Ruth to get exercise, to try to stay lean. Her body's fatty tissues make estrogenic hormones. The more body fat she has, the more hormone will be made.[11] Some scientists believe that excess body fat affects breast cancer risk. If it does, the influence is stronger in postmenopausal women, who tend to acquire more abdominal and upper body fat.[12] Still, Ruth has nothing to lose by trying. Other scientists have found that alcohol consumption is correlated with breast cancer risk.[13] There's no guarantee that these scientists are right. But the stakes are too high for Ruth not to consider abstinence from alcohol. I would likewise recommend that Ruth stay on a low-fat, high-fiber diet. Whatever Sharon's newspaper article says, we have to assume that something in a woman's diet matters. Perhaps within the next decade, scientists will know exactly what.[14]

Notwithstanding Sharon's newspaper article on mammography under age fifty, Ruth should definitely continue to get mammograms. As her doctor, I would make sure that she got the best-quality mammograms. In fact, I'd recommend she get a mammogram every six months. For women in their forties, cancer can show up in a mammogram about eighteen to twenty-four months before she or her nurse-practitioner can feel it. If Ruth had an inherited predisposition to cancer, the lead time might be even shorter.[15] That's right, I said nurse-practitioner. Ruth needs checkups by a medical provider who has been specifically trained in careful breast examination and who knows how to teach Ruth proper self-examination techniques. That person could just as well be a nurse as a physician. If I or a nurse or any other doctor felt a lump with even the slightest suspicious texture, or if Ruth's mammogram showed even a vague shadow, she should have it biopsied. If the pathologist said it was a precancerous lesion, she should seriously consider breast surgery. Perhaps limited surgery, maybe more.

If Ruth didn't contract breast cancer by age fifty, and she hadn't already had surgery on her breasts or her ovaries, then she should reassess her situation. By then, there may be blood tests for breast cancer susceptibility, or better information on the preventive value of diet and vitamins, or new data on the prophylactic effects of tamoxifen and other hormone blockers, or even new developments in immunotherapy of familial breast cancer. The fact that Ruth remained cancer-free throughout her forties would be at best a tentative sign that she hadn't inherited familial breast cancer. She wouldn't be off the hook.

Ruth wants to take control of her future. To submit to mastectomy before the arrival of cancer is, in her view, to relinquish control. Sharon may think differently, but Ruth sees surgery as capitulation, as a final admission that nothing else will work. If I were Ruth's doctor, I'd empathize. I wouldn't put the scalpel to Ruth's breasts merely to cut out her dread. I'd say to Ruth: Don't be so quick to give up. Try to take control. I'd say: Go ahead. Fight it.

Now what kind of medical advice is that? Much of what I just said was based on speculation about medical developments ten years from now. Even when my conclusions were based on more than just intuition, I knew only the odds. I was, in effect, betting against the odds that Ruth had familial breast cancer. I was relying upon preventive strategies that, in the long term, I really didn't know would work. We can't take a crapshoot over something as serious as cancer, can we?

Many readers will disagree with my recommendations. Some may violently disagree. They may think I have injected my own values into Ruth's decision, that my personal predilection toward breast preservation has slanted my forecasts; that I have pretended that vitamins might help, when no one really knows; that I have wishfully hoped that a practical blood test for familial cancer were in the offing, when no one really knows; that I have drummed up a statistic that Ruth has a 10 percent chance of cancer in the next ten years, when no one really knows. I would hope that most readers, having considered the choices faced by Dinah, Stephen, Eve, Gideon, and Andrew, would concede that no one *ever* really knows. No reader, I would hope, will disagree with the simple proposition that Ruth needs a plan, and that such a plan requires a forecast of the future, even if it's an educated guess.

If my medical predictions turned out to be wrong, it wouldn't be the first time. Nonetheless, we cannot get around the fact that prediction is necessary, that betting is necessary. Sharon might say to Ruth: "If I were you, I wouldn't bet that a blood test for inherited breast cancer will soon be available." Sharon instead is betting that RU-486, a drug that at this writing has been used for elective abortions and morning-after contraception, will show promise as breast cancer chemotherapy. Ruth's choice entails not a one-day forecast or a five-day forecast, but a ten-year forecast—in fact, a thirty-year forecast. In essence, Ruth has to formulate a long-term strategic plan. That's what I, as doctor, must do for my patient. After all, Ruth does it for her business clients. This time, the client is Ruth.

We all forecast, we all plan, and we all bet. We're all trying to take control. Ruth and Sharon may be in a super-high risk situation that applies to only one in forty American women. But they are not outliers, not really. Some women decline a screening mammogram because their mothers and sisters didn't have breast cancer. They're betting that they, too, won't get it. Other women who don't have a family history of breast cancer, who started menstruating later in life, who had babies early, are still getting mammograms because they're forecasting that they might get it anyway. Millions of women reacted with dismay at the widely publicized news that low-fat, high-fiber diets don't appear to prevent cancer.[16] Many women of all ages were likewise distraught by recent publicity that screening mammograms under age fifty are no longer to be recommended.[17] These women were unhappy because they were being sent a dismal message: You have lost yet another element of control over your life.

As much as Ruth, Sharon, you, and I want control of our destinies, there are limits to control. In the end, we are stuck with our genetics and family backgrounds. We cannot undo our own pasts. Nor can we escape the crucial role played by ordinary luck. No matter who our parents are, no matter what we did then or what we do now, some of us will be lucky and some will not. But before the ultimate winners and losers in the cancer sweepstakes are announced, we have no choice but to forecast, to plan, to make and execute strategies, to do our best.

Ruth is not a cancer surgeon. She cannot list exhaustively every known complication of mastectomy. Nor is she an oncologist. She cannot readily recite all the latest developments in cancer chemotherapy, or enumerate the side effects of tamoxifen. Ruth is not a radiologist. She cannot deliver a lecture on the technical value of X-ray grids in mammography, nor can she scrutinize the research studies on the value of screening mammograms under age fifty. Not being an epidemiologist either, she cannot conduct her own ten-year 100,000-woman research study of diet, exercise, and breast cancer.

Ruth is entitled to seek out the knowledge and counsel of all the aforementioned experts. But in the final analysis, she has to rely upon her own personal resources and, in a sense, her own expertise. Ruth's choice is her choice, not the experts' choice. It is fortunate that Ruth happens to be skilled in the one discipline that is most crucial to her choice: strategic planning. She needs only to ask herself: What advice would I, as a strategic planner, offer to a woman in exactly the same circumstances as I am?

In her seminars to corporate management, Ruth displays a
poster with the following imperatives:

- • DETERMINE YOUR OBJECTIVES.
- • MAKE A FORECAST.
- • DEVISE A PLAN.
- • BUILD A FOUNDATION.

Take the top line first: *Determine your objectives.* Week after
week, seminar after seminar, Ruth forces the officers and
directors of big companies to ask themselves the same simple
questions: What is my overarching goal? What's most important right now? What's secondary? What can wait? Ruth and
her consulting firm get paid top dollar for these seminars
because the managers of corporations rarely ask themselves
these important questions. But once her clients are yanked
from their daily responsibilities, transplanted to some distant
hotel retreat, and compelled to list and rank their corporate
objectives, they don't look to their technical experts for the
answer. They look within.

It's exactly the same for Ruth's personal choice. No expert
surgeon, oncologist, radiologist, or epidemiologist can tell
Ruth how important the preservation of her breasts are to her.
She won't find the answer in the newspaper articles that
Sharon faxed to her. Only Ruth knows whether she is the kind
of person who can bear the uncertainty of inheriting cancer or
the kind of person who wants to get it over with. Nor can the
experts tell Ruth how important it is to have, or even to try to
have, a biological child. The experts could help Ruth understand how her body might change upon the removal of her
ovaries. But only Ruth can answer the ultimate question: How
much do I care whether I am castrated at age forty?

This is totally obvious, you're saying to yourself. Everybody
knows that your goals have to be separated from the technical
means to achieve them. I beg to differ. Perhaps it's obvious
when we see it in another context. But it isn't always obvious to
millions of Americans who are continually barraged by
"expert" messages about their health and well-being. Over and
over, Dinah heard the message on sex and HIV: Abstinence.

Monogamy. Condoms. Yet only Dinah knew how much it meant for her to get remarried or how important it was for her children to have a stepfather. Ruth has been barraged by head-lines about dietary fat and breast cancer, about mammo-graphic screening under age fifty, about chemoprevention of breast cancer. Ruth needs to realize that the headlines are merely the voices of the corporation's technical staff. They can all leave their messages on Ruth's voice mailbox. They are not the voice inside her.

The second line in Ruth's poster reads: *Make a forecast.* Once they have formulated their objectives, Ruth advises her corporate clients to take an inventory of current information on technology, market trends, and so forth. Equipped with this data base, the client then produces a baseline forecast. Ruth explains that the data base will undoubtedly change, so the forecast will eventually need to be updated. But one has to start somewhere, she emphasizes. If the executives complain that technology is constantly in flux, Ruth explains how that's a flimsy excuse for not making a base forecast.

The same goes for Ruth's personal choice. She knows her family history of cancer and her own reproductive history. She knows that she's already had one breast biopsy. She doesn't know whether she inherited a familial breast cancer gene. She doesn't know whether diet or weight control will reduce her cancer risk. She doesn't know whether chemoprevention with tamoxifen will work. Still, she needs to ask herself: What are my chances of getting breast cancer? If she complains that the field is constantly in flux, that one day scientists say they can predict breast cancer spread and the next day mammography is no good, then she needs to remind herself: That's a poor reason not to make a base forecast of my cancer risks.

Another excursion into the obvious, you may argue. Not so. I began this chapter with grisly references to breast and ovar-ian cancers, followed by serial contemplation of double mas-tectomy, ovarectomy, mammograms, chemotherapy, and hor-mone blockers. It was only when I shifted to a less emotional, more mundane context that the need to make a base forecast became obvious. It is a central message that Ruth and all our decision makers need to learn. Eve might have complained that the evidence on the long-term success of weight-control programs isn't in. True, but she still needs a base forecast. She still needs to have some idea how many more pounds she'd gain if she didn't take any action. She could still make a base prediction of the health consequences of her weight gain. Gideon could complain that nobody knows which foods lower LDL cholesterol without lowering HDL cholesterol, too. But that doesn't prevent him from asking: Based upon what I know now, what are my risks of coronary heart disease?

When Ruth gives strategic planning seminars, managers ask her how many years into the future they should forecast. Ruth explains that the forecast horizon depends on their expectations about new information, as well as their goals. If the company expects to wait two years to learn whether a pending patent is to be approved, then it needs to forecast *at least* two years out. If the client's goal is to be the leader in a certain market in five years, then he needs *at least* a five-year forecast.

The same goes for Ruth's personal choice. Within the next ten years, she'll probably have more information on breast cancer prevention through diet and hormone blockers, as well as a blood test for familial breast cancer. That means she needs to forecast her breast cancer risk for at least ten years. Of course, Ruth hopes to live past the age of fifty. She needs to ask herself, what are my chances of getting breast cancer in the next twenty or even thirty years? If I don't get breast cancer by age fifty, then does that mean I didn't inherit a cancer gene? The fact that the information base is changing doesn't mean one has to be myopic. Stephen could read one article that says exercise must be at 70 percent intensity for thirty minutes three times per week, and another that says walking is just fine. That doesn't change the need for long-term persistence.

In Ruth's seminars, managers complain that analysts in the major brokerage houses have already made sophisticated industry-wide forecasts. Why, they ask, should they invest in their own forecasting efforts? Ruth then brings up a key point: The managers have private information about their company that the market analysts don't have.

Dinah can't rely upon blanket predictions about HIV risk, such as: "Every HIV-infected person can infect someone." She had to evaluate her partner, based upon information that only she could glean. Eve cannot rely upon broad-based statistics about the success of weight-loss programs. She has to determine the success of her own weight-control strategies. Likewise, Ruth cannot rely upon experts' predictions concerning the breast cancer risks of American women generally. She has to think of herself as a special case, because Ruth knows more about Ruth than the experts can know. That doesn't stop Ruth from making her own personal risk assessment. In fact, it obligates her to make such an assessment.

We have not finished with Ruth's strategic planning chart. But we need to stop momentarily to ask: How can Ruth actually forecast her future risk of breast cancer? Clearly, Ruth can't rely upon general statements. She has a sister and a mother with breast cancer. That raises a harder question. Ruth is not the only woman who rightly regards herself as different. Every American woman is different, unique unto herself.

You have probably read somewhere that "Breast cancer strikes one in eight American women." It used to be one in ten American women, but the numbers have been updated.[18] You may also have read that this well-aired statistic is somehow deceptive, a fabrication of the cancer-funding establishment, a scare tactic. Here's my view: The one-in-eight statistic is not a scare tactic. It definitely isn't a fabrication. It is confusing, but not really deceptive. It is also nearly useless. The one-in-eight statistic is, in a very narrow sense, an accurate statement about the lifetime cancer risks of a "representative" American woman. Yet in point of fact, it applies to almost no individual woman in this country.

When biostatisticians say that breast cancer strikes one in eight American women, they don't just count up the women with breast cancer and divide by the American female population. Instead, they estimate the chances that a "typical" woman will develop breast cancer over her hypothetical lifetime. I shall refer to this representative woman as "she," rather than by name, because she is a hypothetical construct, not an identifiable person like Ruth. Conceptually, the statisticians proceed year by year through her life, asking two questions: What are her chances of getting breast cancer in the coming year? And what are the chances of her dying in the coming year from any cause other than breast cancer? If neither event occurs, then they proceed to the next year and ask the same two questions. What the biostatisticians are saying is that over her lifetime, the chances are one in eight that she will get breast cancer before she dies of another cause. Equivalently, the chances are seven out of eight that she will die from some other cause, having never had breast cancer.

When biostatisticians actually make the one-in-eight calculation, they construct a composite lifetime, an amalgam to which American females of all ages have contributed. When she reaches age thirty, for example, the statisticians ask: What are her chances of developing breast cancer before age thirty-one? To answer this question, they use the latest data on the annual *diagnosis rate* of breast cancer among thirty-year-old American women. Then they ask: What are her chances of dying from another cause before her thirty-first birthday? To answer this question, they use the latest data on the annual *mortality rate* of thirty-year-olds, subtracting out their death rate from breast cancer. When she reaches age forty, the statisticians use the current breast cancer diagnosis rates and nonbreast-cancer mortality rates of American women aged forty.

Many different criticisms have been leveled at the one-in-eight statistic. Some critics cite the fact that the lifetime breast cancer risk keeps jumping around. In the space of a few years, it went from one in ten to one in eight women. Accordingly, the underlying vital data are unreliable, or at least unstable. As a matter of fact, from 1982 to 1987, the number of newly diagnosed breast cancer cases in the United States shot up abruptly. When the biostatisticians projected these latest diagnosis rates over the "representative" American woman's lifetime, her overall lifetime risk rose from 10 percent (or one in ten) to 12.5 percent (or one in eight).

Researchers now understand that the jump in breast cancer diagnoses was caused by the widespread adoption of a new generation of supersensitive mammography machines.[19] The new breast X-ray machines allowed women and their doctors to catch many small cancers at an early stage. In fact, the surge in breast cancer diagnoses from 1982 to 1987 came entirely from small tumors that measured no larger than three-quarters of an inch. At the same time, the diagnosis rate for larger tumors was falling. By 1988 and 1989, the diagnosis rates of breast cancers of all sizes had peaked and appeared to be headed back down. That's exactly what one would predict if mammography were identifying new breast cancers sooner than they might have been caught by manual examination alone.[20] Women who were supposed to have their cancers in the late 1980s already had their cancers identified in the early and mid-1980s. If the diagnosis rates continue to come down, then biostatisticians will have to readjust the one-in-eight statistic, possibly to one in nine, maybe back to one in ten.

One can imagine the confusion that this statistical roller coaster has created. When the lifetime risk of breast cancer rose from one in ten to one in eight, the apparently ominous news actually represented an improvement in women's health. That's because radiologists were catching breast cancers earlier, before the cancers had a chance to spread. In 1982, for example, nearly half of all newly diagnosed breast cancers had already spread "regionally" to the lymph nodes in the woman's armpit or "distantly" to the bones and other organs. By 1987, the proportion had fallen to less than one-third.[21] When statisticians eventually announce that the one-in-eight statistic is back down to one in ten, the public will sigh with relief, when in fact the proportional mix of metastatic versus nonspreading cancers will remain unchanged.

The 1980s temporary upstroke in breast cancer diagnosis rates is but a blip in a slowly rising trend that goes back at least to 1940, when the "representative" American woman's lifetime risk was actually closer to one in sixteen. A combination of hormonal effects may explain part of this long-term trend. During the first half of this century, American girls were starting to menstruate at progressively early ages. The average American mother has had progressively fewer full-term pregnancies, and has first become pregnant at an increasingly older age. Still, it's unclear how much of the secular rise in breast cancer can be explained by these trends. Postmenopausal estrogen replacement therapy was popular for a time. But not all researchers agree that it had a major effect on breast cancer risk.[22] Something else might be going on, possibly a long-term change in the American diet, possibly a trend in the average weight or percentage body fat of American women.

Some critics have argued that the one-in-eight statistic is a misleading by-product of long-term improvements in the longevity of American women. What's really happening, they say, is that women are living longer.[23] They've got to die from something, so it's going to be breast cancer. This criticism is only marginally accurate. Women are indeed living longer. But the decline in mortality rates explains only a small piece of the action. The "typical" American woman's risk has gone from one in sixteen in 1940, to one in eight today, mostly because her risk of a breast cancer diagnosis has gone up and not because her risk of dying from other causes has gone down.

Other critics take a different line of attack. They say that the one-in-eight calculation falsely assumes that a woman will live to 100 (or sometimes to 110).[24] This criticism may be well intended, but it's a misunderstanding of the way the calculation works. When biostatisticians proceed year by year through the "typical" American woman's lifetime, they usually pick a stopping point, such as age 100 or age 110. They're being practical. They're saying: In theory, we could keep going to age 150. But in practice, we don't have terribly good information on breast cancer diagnosis rates or mortality rates after age 100, and it doesn't matter too much anyway, because a woman is quite unlikely to live past 100.

As always, there is a problem in the use and interpretation of language. In effect, the biostatisticians are saying: The "representative" American woman, once she is born, has a one-in-eight chance of getting breast cancer *at some time* during the ensuing 100 years. If she doesn't get breast cancer during that time, then anything else could happen. She might be struck by a car as a child and die in the ambulance on the way to the hospital, or she could die from a stroke at age ninety-five. But she doesn't have to celebrate her centennial. The problem comes when the biostatisticians' statement is recast into ordinary language as: "One in eight American women will get breast cancer by age 100." The phrase "by age 100" gets misconstrued as "at age 100."

What these critics are trying to say is that many breast cancers occur later in life. If biostatisticians made their year-by-year lifetime calculation for the "representative" American woman, but arbitrarily stopped at age seventy-five, they wouldn't get a one-in-eight lifetime risk. Based on current diagnosis rates, they'd get a number closer to one in eleven. Then they would be saying: The "representative" American woman, once she is born, has a one-in-eleven chance of getting breast cancer at some time during the ensuing seventy-five years. Perhaps you are now comfortable reading that "Breast

cancer strikes one in eleven American women by the age of
seventy-five." But such a statement can engender no little confusion about what is assumed about her age of death.

Each of the aforementioned criticisms stems from a fundamental confusion about who the "representative" woman is,
and whom she's supposed to represent. When statisticians
computed that the "typical" American woman's lifetime risk
went from one in sixteen in 1940 to one in eight by the late
1980s, they didn't mean that a woman *born* in 1940 would have
a one-in-sixteen lifetime risk of breast cancer. Nor do they
imply that a female child *born* in 1987 will have a one-in-eight
lifetime risk. Instead, they're saying: When we performed the
1940-based analysis, we merely used the breast cancer diagnosis rates and mortality rates for women of all ages, as they were
reported in 1940. When we compute the lifetime risk for 1987,
we're merely using the rates that prevailed in 1987.

If the lifetime risks of 1940 don't apply to women born in
1940, don't they at least apply to some women who were alive
in 1940? Not at all. Let's say a woman was twenty-five years old
in 1940. By 1987, she'd be seventy-two. The breast cancer diagnosis rate for seventy-two-year-old American women in 1987 was
twice that reported in 1940. Any statistician who used 1940 rates
to forecast such a woman's future breast cancer risk would be off
by 100 percent. The same goes for today. If breast cancer rates
keep rising, any statistician who uses 1987 cancer rates to forecast
a woman's future cancer risk could be miles off the mark.

But if future breast cancer diagnosis rates stabilized, then
couldn't we use the biostatisticians' one-in-eight calculation to
help women gauge their cancer risks? Yes, if we could only find
a woman who had the same rates as the "representative" American woman. Who is that woman? It would probably have to be
a white American woman. Breast cancer diagnosis rates are
lower for African-American women,[25] even lower for Japanese-
American or Chinese-American women, and still lower for
Native American women. Come to think of it, when did the
"representative" woman start menstruating? When, if ever, did
she first become pregnant? Has she ever had a breast biopsy
for a suspicious lump? Does she have any first-degree relatives
with breast cancer? Who, in short, is she?

The one-in-eight statistic can at best be viewed as an average
risk. It is an average risk for some population of American

FIGURE 7.1

A 40-Year-Old American Woman Has a 1-in-16 Chance of Developing Breast
Cancer Over a Period of 30 Years

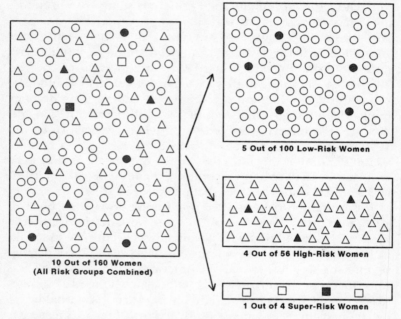

SOURCE: Based on tables in Mitchell H. Gail, Louise A. Brinton, David P. Byar, et al., "Projecting Individualized Probabilities of Developing Breast Cancer for White Females Who Are Being Examined Annually," *Journal of the National Cancer Institute* 81 (1989): 1879–86, as well as estimates of the distribution of "risk factors" in the Nurses' Health Study, as given in Jay R. Harris, Marc E. Lippman, Umberto Veronesi, and Walter Willett, "Breast Cancer," *New England Journal of Medicine* 327 (1992): 319–28.

women, although that population is rarely specified. Even if it's an accurate average for a group of women, it obscures the enormous variability of individual cancer risks.

Figure 7.1 shows my best estimate of the baseline breast cancer forecast for a forty-year-old American woman. The chart is not a "lifetime" calculation. I started at age forty, rather than birth, because breast cancer risks before age forty are now irrelevant to Ruth and her cohort. I have projected out thirty years, because that is Ruth's planning horizon. Anyway, I don't want to get entangled in a discussion of breast cancer risk at much older ages.[26] In my base scenario, breast cancer diagnosis rates will drift down toward the levels that prevailed before the 1980s mammography-related surge. You can complain that my base scenario is wrong, and therefore my base forecast is wrong. If so, then at least we're on the same wavelength. In my base scenario, nobody has yet discovered a test for a breast cancer gene. No one knows whether diet or hormone blockers will prevent breast cancer.

As the figure's title indicates, I estimate that 1 in 16 forty-year-old American women will develop breast cancer at some time in the next thirty years. One woman in 16 is the same as 10 in 160. Focus on the left-hand box momentarily. I count 160 symbols, one for each woman. Ten symbols have been darkened. Those are the ten women who will get breast cancer during our forecast horizon of thirty years. There are three types of women, corresponding to three different shapes. The circles are low-risk women. These women had *no* previous breast biopsy. They started their menstrual periods *after* age twelve. They have *no* relatives with breast cancer, and they had a baby *before* age thirty-five. In other words, they have none of the standard "risk factors" for breast cancer. The squares are the super-risk women at the other extreme. Like Ruth, they have multiple relatives with breast cancer and at least one other "risk factor," such as a previous breast biopsy, delayed pregnancy, or no pregnancies. The remaining high-risk women, represented by the triangles, have at least one "risk factor." They're not in the same category as the super-risk squares. All together, I count 100 low-risk circles, 56 high-risk triangles, and 4 super-risk squares inside the box on the left. That includes both the darkened and open symbols.

On the right-hand side of the chart, I have sorted the women into three separate boxes, corresponding to their risk categories. For the low-risk circles, the thirty-year breast cancer risk is 5 out of 100, or equivalently, 1 in 20. For the high-risk triangles, it's 4 out of 56, or equivalently, 1 in 14. And for the super-risk squares, it's 1 out of 4. That's where Ruth belongs. The figure shows that when we lump all the women together, it appears (on the left) as if each has a one-in-sixteen risk. As soon as we sort women by past medical and family history (on the right), not a single woman has a one-in-sixteen risk. Each has a different risk, either higher or lower.

Biostatistical nitpickers can tease my chart into shreds. They can complain that my baseline assumptions are wrong; or that I should have set the age-of-menarche cutoff at thirteen instead of twelve years; or that I don't have enough boxes on the right-hand side, because the fifty-six women in the high-risk group aren't all the same, either. But these criticisms do not belie the main point.

The chart illustrates a central idea that I have used repeatedly throughout this book. The constant barrage of messages about personal health—how to avoid HIV; how much to exercise; how to stop smoking; whether to have a mammogram or go on a low-fat diet to prevent breast cancer—is transmitted to us as if we belonged to an undifferentiated swarm, a faceless, nameless crowd. Yet we all have names. We are all different, and we know it. We have more data about ourselves than the senders of the messages can cope with. We need to learn how to use our private, personal data bases to make our own forecasts, our own bets, our own plans. The senders cannot do it.

The surgeon general can indeed issue a warning on sex and HIV. But the warning cannot contain a subparagraph entitled "To Dinah on the Sofa." A blue-ribbon committee of experts can announce that weight-loss programs don't work. But it cannot issue an appendix entitled "Special Considerations for Thirty-Year-Old Female Physicians Whose Body Mass Index Has Risen 5 Points in a Dozen Years and Whose Professional Career May Be at Stake." A panel of distinguished epidemiologists, convened to advise the U.S. government, can announce that mammograms are unproven for screening breast cancer in women under fifty years of age. But, sadly, it cannot leave a special message in Ruth's voice mailbox saying "We didn't mean you."

Look at the chart again. There are ten darkened symbols on the left, five of which are low-risk circles. In other words, half of the women who will ultimately get breast cancer have no identifiable "risk factors" for breast cancer. On the other hand, only one in ten breast cancer cases arise in super-risk women such as Ruth. This fact is not terribly important to Ruth. Her goal is to make a base forecast and to determine how her own risks differ from the average. Still, the chart illustrates how serious the problem of breast cancer prevention is. Ruth may be not be able to control her family background, but at least she knows that she is at high risk. Yet half of the 180,000 American women who each year receive a diagnosis of breast cancer will turn to their doctors and ask: Why me? Barring innovations in breast cancer prevention and risk identification, their doctors will have no answer.

Devise a plan: That was the next item on Ruth's strategic planning chart. If Ruth wants to preserve her breasts, and if she anticipates that a blood test for familial breast cancer will soon be available, then she needs a "holding strategy." This is not the first time we have encountered the term. In chapter 2, Dinah needed more time to find out about Caleb. She needed days, weeks, maybe months. In the present case, Ruth may need to temporize for five years, ten years, possibly longer. We can debate the effectiveness of diet and weight control, but there should be little doubt that careful breast self-examination, routine checkups by practitioners who are well trained in manual breast examination, and frequent mammography are important components of such a strategy.

At this writing, U.S. public health authorities are trying to retract an earlier recommendation that women in their forties should have regular screening mammograms. New evidence, the authorities say, raises questions about the value of mammography for women under the age of fifty.[27] MAMMOGRAPHY GUIDELINES FACE SCRUTINY ran the headline of an article that Sharon faxed to Ruth.[28] STUDIES SAY MAMMOGRAMS FAIL TO HELP MANY WOMEN ran another the next day.[29]

If I were writing a treatise on public health policy, I could spend pages explaining why retractions of this sort can be colossal blunders.[30] For years, the health authorities and private groups have urged mammography on American women. Yet only a third of women over forty years old say they get annual mammograms.[31] In recent surveys, only one-half to two-thirds of women over forty *ever* had a mammogram, and the rate drops to about one-third for women over sixty.[32] It is painfully obvious that many American women still don't ask their doctors for mammograms, and many doctors still don't press it upon their patients. In fact, if there is any group that is most concerned and educated about breast cancer, it is younger women. You'd think our public health authorities had their hands full educating fifty-, sixty-, and seventy-year-olds.

Yet they decide, on the basis of inconclusive negative research studies, to wave sayonara to their best customers. In another five years, more extensive research will likely show that screening mammograms are indeed valuable for women in their forties. By then, the health authorities will be committed to an untenable position.

But let's get back to Ruth's choice. When a woman with no palpable lumps and no symptoms gets a mammogram, she's getting a *screening test*. When a woman with a palpable lump gets a mammogram to see what the lump is, she's getting a *diagnostic test*. Ruth needs to understand that mammography is superior as a screening test and inferior as a diagnostic test.[33] In other words, you get the mammogram even if you don't feel a lump. You don't just wait to feel a lump and then get the mammogram to see what it is.

There are good reasons why mammograms are better at screening than diagnosis. When a woman or a medical practitioner feels for a lump, she is looking for certain characteristics of breast tissue—thickening, hardness, irregular shape, ill-defined borders, fixation of the mass to the skin or chest, dimpling or puckering of the overlying skin—that might signal the presence of a cancer. When a radiologist performs a mammogram, the X ray does not reveal the same breast tissue characteristics that the examiner can feel with her hands. In fact, that's exactly what happened to Sharon, who explained to Ruth that her lump didn't even show up on her mammogram. It is entirely possible for a palpable lump to turn out to be cancerous, even when there is no sign of cancer on the mammogram. Perhaps 10 or 20 percent of palpable breast cancers can be missed by mammography, and the "false negative" rate could conceivably be higher. Accordingly, if a lump feels suspicious on physical examination, it needs to be biopsied, regardless of the mammographic findings. In fact, if there is any role for mammography once a lump is found, it is in screening both breasts for other lesions.[34] This doesn't mean that manual breast examination is a better screening test than mammography. It means only that there are certain cancers that a well-trained hand will identify but an X ray will not. For that reason, a combination of routine manual examination and regular mammographic screening is recommended.

In women over fifty, mammograms can detect a cancer

about four years before a woman will be able to feel it. In women in their forties, the lead time between mammographic detection and self-discovery is thought to be about eighteen months to two years. This is not just a theoretical speculation. In the United States, as I have already explained, breast cancer diagnosis rates shot up in the 1980s after the advent and wide-spread adoption of sensitive mammography machines. Many more early-stage breast cancers were discovered. Even among women in their forties, the percentage of very early, "in situ" breast cancers doubled.[35]

There is no doubt that mammograms have been picking up many early breast cancers. Skeptics have argued, however, that early detection does not necessarily make a woman better off. Their argument has two prongs. First, mammography is merely giving a woman the inevitable bad news a few years ear-lier. I call this the "comet theory." If a comet were destined to strike and obliterate our planet in 2003, all our telescopes and satellites would accomplish is to tell us the bad news with a ten-year lead time. You may respond that my analogy is faulty. Even if you couldn't do anything about a comet, you can do something about breast cancer. There's surgery, irradiation, conventional chemotherapy, hormone blockers such as tamox-ifen, and soon immunotherapy. The skeptics answer: Prove it.

The second prong of their argument is that mammography is merely detecting small tumors that wouldn't have harmed a woman in the first place. These tumors may scare women and their doctors, but they're basically just false alarms. You may respond: Yes, but can't a pathologist tell whether a tumor is malignant or not? How could something that looks like can-cer not be cancer? The skeptics' answer is the same: Prove it. Show to us that mammography actually averts death from breast cancer.

To respond to these arguments, scientists have mounted a massive research effort to prove not only that mammograms detect early cancers but that mammograms also save lives. In cities across the globe, tens of thousands of women have been enrolled in studies that compared mammography plus check-ups with manual examination alone. Within the past decade, there has been the Swedish Two-County Study;[36] the Malmö Mammographic Screening Trial, also from Sweden;[37] the Canadian National Breast Cancer Screening Study;[38] and the

Edinburgh Trial of Screening for Breast Cancer, from Scotland;[39] as well as newer studies now under way.

These studies have turned out to be extremely difficult to execute and interpret. When a woman is enrolled, she can be assigned either to a "special intervention" program of mammographic screening or to her "usual care." For obvious ethical reasons, researchers cannot compel a woman in the "usual care" group to forgo mammograms. Nor can they force women in the "special intervention" group to show up for their X-ray appointments. In some of the studies, these "crossover" and "noncompliance" problems have been formidable. When researchers compare the intervention women with the usual-care women, they're not really comparing mammography to no-mammography.[40]

But that is hardly the end of the researchers' worries. A study of mammographic screening would have little relevance if the radiologists took inferior pictures. Yet each of these studies has been criticized for not using state-of-the-art mammographic techniques, including proper use of grids to prevent scattering of X rays; proper film processing; two views of the breast (as opposed to a single view); proper positioning of the woman; and proper breast compression to ensure that the film is as close to the breast as possible and thus is getting the sharpest picture.[41] What is more, the studies did not screen women annually. The Swedish Two-County Trial, for example, screened all women in their intervention group every two years, while the Malmö study screened every eighteen months. That's a reasonable screening frequency if you're only studying women in their fifties and sixties. Mammography in that age group, as I've explained, can pick up a cancer about four years before a woman can feel it. But for women in their forties, it won't do. If you want to see whether mammography can save their lives, you've got to study a program of annual examinations.

When researchers originally designed these screening trials, they never intended to test whether mammography specifically saves the lives of women in their forties. They enrolled women in a much wider age range (for example, forty-five to sixty-four years old in the Edinburgh study) with the intention of analyzing them as a single, combined group. Had they intended to break down their evaluation into separate ten-year age groups, they would have needed a much larger population. The researcher is basically thinking: If I want to see whether mammographic screening works in women aged forty-five to sixty-four, I've got to detect (say) five hundred women in that age range with early breast cancer, and then see whether they actually live longer. So, I'll use known information on breast cancer diagnosis rates to estimate how many forty-five- to sixty-four-year-old women I need to enroll in my study to find five hundred cancers. Of course, when the trial is completed, the researcher has five hundred breast cancer cases to study, but only a few dozen are in their forties. That's just too few to get statistically precise answers.

With all their difficulties, the two Swedish screening trials and the Edinburgh trial showed that mammography actually saves lives. No single study was perfect, but the overall picture seemed clear. Then came the publication of the Canadian National Breast Cancer Screening Study in November 1992.[42] Women in their forties *and* fifties did not benefit from mammography, the Canadians found. For women in their forties, the mammography group actually had a higher death rate. So the American public health authorities turned to the other researchers and asked: What can you tell us about forty- to forty-nine-year-old women? They answered: We didn't screen enough women in their forties to give a statistically precise answer. Still, the trend appears the same as for the other age groups.

Nobody has come up with a satisfactory explanation for the unexpected Canadian result that mammography is somehow detrimental to women in their forties. Researchers went back through their medical files to find women in their forties with mammographically detected breast cancer, to see whether they were somehow different. But they found the expected: Mammography detects cancers earlier, and women with early-stage cancers did better.[43] From what we know now, it is difficult to avoid the conclusion that mammography helps women in their forties, and not just in their fifties and beyond.

What can Ruth learn from this sequence of events? First, mammography, self-examination, and a regular checkup are all critical to her strategy of monitoring for early breast cancer. She cannot use mammography as a diagnostic tool only after a lump has been found. Second, she needs to get mammograms at least once per year, and probably every six months. For all women in their forties, the lead time is about one and a half to two years, but for her, the lead time could be much shorter. Most of all, Ruth needs to understand that the message in Sharon's news story does not address her special circumstances.

Even if Ruth reads ten news stories, she will probably learn little about the design, the findings, and the limitations of the major studies on mammography. Still, she can understand that mammography does detect cancers earlier, and that it's only sensible that early detection may save her life. The authorities still recommend that women over fifty have mammograms. It's just that they won't say the same for women in their forties. Apparently, the available evidence doesn't satisfy the authorities' standards of proof. Ruth needs to say to herself: I have a much higher risk than the average woman. So I need a different standard of proof. If it is reasonable that mammography will help me, then I'll do it. I don't need an assurance of certainty, because I have too much at stake.

When blue-ribbon panels and expert committees make public recommendations, they use a standard of proof that applies to the average-risk person. People with serious illnesses already appreciate this fact. They are willing to take experimental drugs, even though scientists aren't satisfied that they're safe or effective. Sharon herself is willing to sign up for a hormone-blocker research study. Even though Ruth has no serious illness, at least not yet, the same principle applies. Ruth may seem like a special super-high-risk case, like one of those four squares in my chart. But the principle just as well applies to the high-risk triangles. Some of those women have had a previous breast biopsy, or have a mother with breast cancer. They, too, need to read between the lines of the messages about mammography guidelines.

I do not know whether a low-fat, high-fiber diet reduces a woman's risk of breast cancer. I have read the same headlines that Sharon faxed to Ruth. And I have read the research studies upon which the headlines are based.[44] But I would advise Ruth nonetheless to adhere to a moderately, but not severely, low-fat diet. Perhaps there are other health advantages of such a diet. But that's not the issue here.

Researchers may still determine that a low-fat, high-fiber diet, or some aspect of a low-fat, high-fiber diet, offers a protective effect. They are quite unlikely to conclude that a high-fat, low-fiber diet will help. If and when scientists determine that a low-fat, high-fiber diet is protective, they will undoubtedly conclude that a woman's *cumulative* fat and *cumulative* fiber intake matter more than just last month's or last year's dietary composition. To prepare for that possibility, Ruth needs to start her diet now. In the words of her seminar poster, she needs to *build a foundation*.

The recent negative findings on diet and breast cancer were based upon the Nurses' Health Study, the same study that I relied upon in chapter 4. As well designed as that study was, it cannot be the final word. The researchers used two food questionnaires, four years apart, to gauge the nurses' intake of total fat, saturated fat, monounsaturated fat, and linoleic acid (18:2, you may recall), which is a specific polyunsaturated fatty acid. But, as we know from studying Gideon's choice, people eat food, not individual fatty acids. As sophisticated as researchers' food questionnaires have become, it is still much harder to measure a person's diet than her weight or smoking habits. Some scientists point to a separate finding from the Nurses' Health Study, in which dietary fat intake predicted colon cancer risk.[45] If the researchers could find a relation between diet and colon cancer, they argue, then their questionnaires must have some validity. But the fat–colon cancer relation was really a connection between saturated animal fats and cancer, while the fat–breast cancer relation may involve polyunsaturated vegetable fats, which are much harder to measure in diet questionnaires.[46] In any case, even the Nurses' Health Study found that alcohol intake was related to breast cancer risk, a finding that Ruth should also heed.

In chapter 4, I suggested that anytime the scientific community does not know the cause of a complex disease, there's a good bet that it's several diseases rolled into one. This conclusion is just as apt for breast cancer. In the next ten years, scientists will probably find out that there are perhaps a dozen different kinds of familial cancer genes, that some genes are strong predictors and others only weakly predispose a woman to breast cancer. Researchers have already found estrogen and progesterone "receptors" on the surfaces of breast cancer cells. They will undoubtedly find even more specific receptors and begin to design drugs that block these cell-surface receptors. As the different types of breast cancer are identified and classified, researchers will begin to make antibodies against tumors. Immunotherapy will be an option for some afflicted women. Pharmacologists will find estrogen blockers that are even more effective than tamoxifen, which will itself be found a form a chemoprevention.

Ruth cannot make these things happen on schedule by the force of her will. She cannot magically excise her cancer gene, if it's there, on chromosome #17, or maybe #10. She cannot control the future. She can only decide what she wants, make a plan, be prepared, take her chances, and do her best. The barrage of messages will not tell her how to do it. She has to learn herself.

SHARON: *Hello, Room 708.*
RUTH: *Hi, it's me.*
SHARON: *Oh, hi. Just a second. My surgeon is looking at my chart. I had a slight fever yesterday, but it's gone. . . . You mean I can go home tomorrow? Great! Thanks. . . . Ruth, did you hear that? I'm coming home—*
RUTH: *Sharon, I just want to say that I think you did the right thing.*
SHARON: *Ruth, what's wrong? Something is wrong.*
RUTH: *No, nothing's wrong. I read the articles you faxed me.*
SHARON: *In between your business clients, no doubt.*
RUTH: *They were very enlightening.*
SHARON: *Come on, what's wrong? You don't talk that way.*
RUTH: *I'll tell you when you get home from the hospital. Buzz can pick up your stuff. What time will they discharge you?*
SHARON: *Come on, Ruthie, what's wrong?*
RUTH: *I'm pregnant.*

Epilogue

I have tried to help Dinah, Stephen, Eve, Gideon, Andrew, and Ruth make their everyday deadly choices. I have tried to translate complicated scientific issues, to lay them open so that you, too, could choose. But I have tried to be more than just a popular translator. I have attempted to produce a philosophy, a way of thinking. Perhaps my point of view will stay with you long after every one of the scientific controversies in this book is settled.

How should you feel once you have finished this book? You may have found it difficult. If so, good. I did it on purpose. I wanted this book to be intellectually painless but psychologically exhausting. I started out with a headache at breakfast. That was nothing compared to the AIDS, heart attacks, bulimia, morbid obesity, emphysema, lung cancer, and double breast surgery that followed. I wanted to make you suffer along with my sufferers, just a little.

As a physician, my experience has been that when people confront their choices, they come away more composed, even when their problems remain unsolved. It's as if choosing is itself a form of therapy. After all, choosing is hard. Even thinking about hard choices is an accomplishment. It makes you feel better afterward, more optimistic.

My patients, my friends, and my scientific colleagues continue to express puzzlement and frustration over the constant barrage of health messages. They blame the messages for making their everyday lives more complicated, confusing, and dangerous. But the medical experts and the science writers did not create our choices. Our choices were already there. The blue-ribbon commissions and the government warnings did not make our choices difficult. They were difficult to begin with.

Yes, we are attacked from all sides by the ceaseless artillery fire of biomedical discoveries, health pronouncements, and product claims. But we cannot run for cover. We need to stand up to our assailants, without firing back aimlessly. Strewn among the mortar shells and shrapnel is important information that can improve our lives. We may need help finding it, but it is there. We are the beneficiaries of the health messages, not its victims, not its slaves. No, life isn't easy, but we have choices that can make it better. That's where optimism comes in.

Each of us is very different. We are as different on the inside as we appear on the outside. We cannot follow all the rules and recommendations exactly, because we each have our special circumstances. The medical messages have not been individually tailor-made for us, but that doesn't make them useless. We need to use the information in the messages to find our own niches along the continuum. Every day, we are told to do this and to avoid that. But, actually, our diversity gives us more choices. It hasn't been all decided for us. That's where optimism comes in.

Social critics have vilified our culture for being too health-conscious, too preoccupied with bodily functions and hazards. We are dancing the jig of the hypochondriacs, they say. On balance, their attacks are unfair. Whole segments of our society have been left out of the dance. We would all be better off if the ballroom doors were swung wide open and they, too, did the health fandango. I am optimistic, in fact, that the music of the messages will eventually do just that. We as a people are legitimately concerned about improving our health. Our culture sends messages that, by and large, are intended to do that. The problem is how to listen and learn from the messages. I hope I have helped you listen and learn, even a tiny bit.

Anyway, books are supposed to end where they start. It's morning again. It's breakfast time. And the newspaper is waiting for me.

Notes

CHAPTER 1: THE MARGARINE BATTLE BOOK

1. Dolores Kong, "Theory Links 'Good Cholesterol' to Breast Cancer," *Boston Globe,* 12 June 1990, p. 3.
2. Jane E. Brody, "Margarine, Too, Is Found to Have the Fat That Adds to Heart Risk," *New York Times,* 16 Aug. 1990.
3. "Vasectomies and Prostate Cancer: A Link?" *New York Times,* 1 Jan. 1991.
4. Lawrence K. Altman, "Two New Studies Link Vasectomy to Higher Prostate Cancer Risk," *New York Times,* 17 Feb. 1993, p. C12.
5. Sandra Blakeslee, "Electric Currents and Leukemia Show Puzzling Links in New Study," *New York Times,* 8 Feb. 1991; idem, "Electromagnetic Fields Are Being Scrutinized for Linkage to Cancer," *New York Times,* 2 April 1991, p. C3; William K. Stevens, "Major U.S. Study Finds No Miscarriage Risk from Video Terminals," *New York Times,* 14 March 1991, p. A22; Associated Press, "U.S. Overestimates Peril of Radon in Homes, New Study Says," *New York Times,* 29 March 1991; Elisabeth Rosenthal, "Inner-Ear Damage Linked to Jarring High-Impact Aerobics," *New York Times,* 6 Dec. 1990; Judy Foreman, "Cholesterol Curb Urged for Children over Two," *Boston Globe,* 9 April 1991, p. 1.
6. Jane E. Brody, "Panel Criticizes Weight-Loss Programs," *New York Times,* 2 April 1992, p. D22; idem, "Vitamin C Linked to

Heart Benefit: It May Also Help Prevent an Early Death from Other Diseases, Study Says," *New York Times,* 8 May 1992, p. A17; Associated Press, "Vitamin A Type May Lower Risk of Heart Trouble," *Boston Globe,* 14 Nov. 1990; Lawrence K. Altman, "High Level of Iron Tied to Heart Risk," *New York Times,* 8 Sept. 1992, p. A1.

7. Marian Burros, "Now What? U.S. Study Says Margarine May Be Harmful," *New York Times,* 7 Oct. 1992, p. A1.

8. Marian Burros, "U.S. Will Require New Labels on Health on Packaged Food," *New York Times,* 3 Dec. 1992, p. 1.

9. Dolores Kong, "Harvard Study Links Margarine to Higher Heart Disease Risk," *Boston Globe,* 5 March 1993, p. 13.

10. David B. Wilson, "Breakfast Bamboozlement," *Boston Globe,* 7 Feb. 1990.

11. Dave Barry, "Alarming News from the Bureau of Medical Alarm" (syndicated col.), *Santa Fe New Mexican,* 2 Sept. 1990.

12. Ann Landers, "Curb Anger, Live Longer," *Boston Globe,* 17 Jan. 1990, p. 66 ("Cereals are supposed to be wonderful, and millions of health nuts have become addicted to oat bran").

13. Russell Baker, "O.K., Julia, Drop the Salt," *New York Times,* 18 Aug. 1990, p. 25.

14. Betsy A. Lehman, "Two Studies Raise Doubts on Oats Fad," *Boston Globe,* 18 Jan. 1990, p. 1.

15. Associated Press, "Oatmeal Lowers Cholesterol, Study Affirms," *New York Times,* 11 April 1991, p. A16. See also Linda Van Horn, Alicia Moag-Stahlberg, Kiang Liu, et al., "Effects on Serum Lipids of Adding Instant Oats to Usual American Diets," *American Journal of Public Health* 81 (1991): 183–88.

16. "Trends in Prostate Cancer—United States, 1980–1988," *Morbidity and Mortality Weekly Report* 41 (1992): 401–4.

17. "An Aspirin Every Other Day Is Found to Reduce Migraines," *New York Times,* 3 Oct. 1990 (see also Julie E. Buring, Richard Peto, and Charles H. Hennekens, "Low-Dose Aspirin for Migraine Prophylaxis," *Journal of the American Medical Association* 264 [1990]: 1711–13); Associated Press, "Aspirin Found to Aid Some Pregnancies," *Boston Globe,* 14 June 1991.

18. Jane E. Brody, "In Pursuit of the Best Possible Odds of Preventing or Minimizing the Perils of Major Diseases," *New York Times,* 31 Jan. 1991, referring to the research of Dr. Gary Williams of the American Health Foundation.

19. Dolores Kong, "Reducing Fat May Cut Risk of Breast Cancer," *Boston Globe,* 18 Jan. 1990 (see also R. L. Prentice, D. Thompson, C. Clifford, et al., "Dietary Fat Reduction and Plasma Estra-

diol Concentration in Healthy Postmenopausal Women," *Journal of the National Cancer Institute* 82 [1990]: 129–34); Paul Recer, "Fiber Is Linked to Reduced Breast Cancer Risk," *Boston Globe,* 3 April 1991; Gina Kolata, "Big New Study Finds No Link Between Fat and Breast Cancer," *New York Times,* 21 Oct. 1992, health page. See also Dolores Kong, "Diet's Link to Breast Cancer Is Downplayed," *Boston Globe,* 21 Oct. 1992, p. 1.

20. Jane E. Brody, "Killer Trees? Is the Air Harmful? Don't Panic," *New York Times,* 24 Feb. 1993, p. C12.

21. L. Rosenberg, J. R. Palmer, A. G. Zauber, et al., "Vasectomy and the Risk of Prostate Cancer," *American Journal of Epidemiology* 132 (1990): 1051–55; C. Mettlin, N. Natarajan, and R. Huben, "Vasectomy and Prostate Cancer Risk"; and H. A. Guess, "Invited Commentary: Vasectomy and Prostate Cancer," *American Journal of Epidemiology* 132 (1990): 1056–61; 1062–65.

22. Edward Giovannucci, Alberto Ascherio, Eric B. Rimm, et al., "A Prospective Cohort Study of Vasectomy and Prostate Cancer in U.S. Men"; Edward Giovannucci, Tor D. Tosteson, Frank E. Speizer, et al., "A Retrospective Cohort Study of Vasectomy and Prostate Cancer in U.S. Men"; and Stuart S. Howards and Herbert B. Peterson, "Vasectomy and Prostate Cancer? Chance, Bias, or a Causal Relationship?" *Journal of the American Medical Association* 269 (1993): 873–77; 878–82; 913–14.

23. Ronald P. Mensink and Martijn B. Katan, "Effect of Dietary Trans Fatty Acids on High-Density and Low-Density Lipoprotein Cholesterol Levels in Healthy Subjects," and Scott M. Grundy, "Trans Monounsaturated Fatty Acids and Serum Cholesterol Levels" (editorial), *New England Journal of Medicine* 323 (1990): 439–45; 480–81.

24. Linda Van Horn et al., "Effects on Serum Lipids of Adding Instant Oats to Usual American Diets"; Charles G. Humble, "Oats and Cholesterol: The Prospects for Prevention of Heart Disease" (editorial), *American Journal of Public Health* 81 (1991): 159–60; Michael H. Davidson, Lynn D. Dugan, Julie H. Burns, et al., "The Hypocholesterolemic Effects of Beta-Glucan in Oatmeal and Oat Bran: A Dose-Controlled Study," *Journal of the American Medical Association* 265 (1991): 1833–39.

25. Daniel S. Greenberg, "Fickle Science?" *Boston Globe,* 9 Nov. 1992, p. 15; Editorial, "The VDT Miscarriage Scare," *New York Times,* 19 March 1991.

26. A. S. Geisel, *The Butter Battle Book, by Dr. Seuss* (New York: Random House, 1984).

CHAPTER 2: THE DEADLIEST CHOICE

1. "CDC Pushes 'Obscene' Test for New AIDS Messages," *The Nation's Health* (Sept. 1992): 5.
2. "Special Service Section: What Women Should Know About AIDS," *Cosmopolitan* (Nov. 1992): 108–9.
3. Jerry Adler et al., "Safer Sex," *Newsweek*, 9 Dec. 1991, pp. 52–56.
4. Earvin "Magic" Johnson, *What You Can Do to Avoid AIDS* (New York: Times Books, 1992), pp. 92–94.
5. Philip S. Rosenberg, Martin E. Levy, John F. Brundage, et al., "Population-Based Monitoring of an Urban HIV/AIDS Epidemic: Magnitude and Trends in the District of Columbia," *Journal of the American Medical Association* 268 (1992): 495–503.
6. Adam Nossiter, "Man Is the First Convicted in Louisiana for Putting Partner at Risk of HIV," *New York Times*, 28 Nov. 1992, p. 7.
7. Norman Hearst and Stephen B. Hulley, "Preventing the Heterosexual Spread of AIDS: Are We Giving Our Patients the Best Advice?" *Journal of the American Medical Association* 259 (1988): 2428–32; Willard Cates, Jr., and Alan R. Hinman, "AIDS and Absolutism," *New England Journal of Medicine* 327 (1992): 492–93; Correspondence, "AIDS and Absolutism," *New England Journal of Medicine* 327 (1992): 1460–61; Zena A. Stein, "Editorial: The Double Bind in Science Policy and the Protection of Women from HIV Infection," *American Journal of Public Health*, 82 (1992): 1471–72; Anke A. Ehrhardt, "Trends in Sexual Behavior and the HIV Pandemic," *American Journal of Public Health* 82 (1992): 1459–61.
8. Jeffrey E. Harris, "The Incubation Period for Human Immunodeficiency Virus (HIV-1)," in *AIDS 1988: AAAS Symposia Papers*, ed. Ruth Kulstad (Washington, D.C.: American Association for the Advancement of Science, 1989), pp. 67–74.
9. Alan R. Lifson, Paul M. O'Malley, Nancy A. Hessol, et al., "HIV Seroconversion in Two Homosexual Men After Receptive Oral Intercourse with Ejaculation: Implications for Counseling Concerning Safer Sexual Practices," *American Journal of Public Health* 80 (1990): 1509–11; H. Clifford Lane, Scott D. Holmberg, and Harold W. Jaffe, "HIV Seroconversion and Oral Intercourse" (letter), *American Journal of Public Health* 81 (1991): 658; W. Rozenbaum, S. Gharakhanian, B. Cardon, et al., "HIV Transmission by Oral Sex," *Lancet* 2 (1988): 1395; P. C. Spitzer and N. J. Weiner, "Transmission of HIV Infection from a Woman to a Man by Oral Sex," *New England Journal of Medicine* 320 (1989): 251.

10. Youth Behavioral Risk Survey. See "Sexual Behavior Among High School Students—United States, 1990," *Morbidity and Mortality Weekly Report* 40 (1992): 885–88; "Selected Behaviors That Increase Risk for HIV Infection Among High School Students—United States, 1990," *Morbidity and Mortality Weekly Report* 41 (1992): 231–40.

11. "HIV-Related Knowledge and Behaviors Among High School Students—Selected U.S. Sites, 1989," *Morbidity and Mortality Weekly Report* 39 (1990): 385–97; F. L. Sonenstein, J. H. Pleck, and L. C. Ku, "Sexual Activity, Condom Use, and AIDS Awareness Among Adolescent Males," *Family Planning Perspectives* 21 (1989): 152–60; "Selected Behaviors That Increase Risk for HIV Infection, Other Sexually Transmitted Diseases, and Unintended Pregnancy Among High School Students—United States, 1991," *Morbidity and Mortality Weekly Report* 41 (1992): 945–50. See also Tamar Lewin, "Promiscuity Growing for Teenage Girls," *New York Times,* 10 Dec. 1992, p. D20.

12. In the 1990 Youth Behavioral Risk Survey, 1 in 43 boys and 1 in 143 girls in the eleventh grade admitted to injecting illicit drugs. In that group, 72 percent of the boys and 54 percent of the girls had sex with four or more partners. But even among the eleventh graders who had never injected drugs, the four-partner cutoff was attained by 26 percent of boys and 14 percent of girls. Calculated from tables 1 and 3 and text of "Selected Behaviors That Increase Risk for HIV Infection Among High School Students—United States, 1990."

13. In the 1991 Youth Behavioral Risk Survey, rates of teenage condom use were still below 50 percent. See "HIV Instruction and Selected HIV-Risk Behaviors Among High School Students—United States, 1989–1991," *Morbidity and Mortality Weekly Report* 41 (1992): 866–68; J. E. Anderson, L. Kann, D. Holtzman, et al., "HIV/AIDS Knowledge and Sexual Behavior Among High School Students," *Family Planning Perspectives* 22 (1990): 252–55.

14. Ralph W. Hingson, Lee Strunin, Beth M. Berlin, and Timothy Heeren, "Beliefs About AIDS, Use of Alcohol and Drugs, and Unprotected Sex Among Massachusetts Adolescents," *American Journal of Public Health* 80 (1990): 295–99.

15. Lee Strunin and Ralph W. Hingson, "Acquired Immunodeficiency Syndrome and Adolescents: Knowledge, Beliefs, Attitudes and Behavior," *Pediatrics* 79 (1987): 825–28.

16. Ralph J. DiClemente, Mark M. Lanier, Patricia F. Horan, and Mark Lodico, "Comparison of AIDS Knowledge, Attitudes, and Behaviors Among Incarcerated Adolescents and a Public

School Sample in San Francisco," *American Journal of Public Health* 81 (1991): 628–30.

17. "HIV-Related Knowledge and Behaviors Among High School Students—Selected U.S. Sites, 1989," table 2.

18. "HIV Instruction and Selected HIV-Risk Behaviors Among High School Students—United States, 1989–1991."

19. "HIV Instruction and Selected HIV-Risk Behaviors Among High School Students—United States, 1989–1991."

20. "Characteristics of Parents Who Discuss AIDS with Their Children—United States, 1989," *Morbidity and Mortality Weekly Report* 40 (1991): 789–91.

21. Noni E. MacDonald, George A. Wells, William A. Fisher, et al., "High-Risk STD/HIV Behavior Among College Students," *Journal of the American Medical Association* 263 (1990): 3155–59; Erratum, *Journal of the American Medical Association* 264 (1990): 1661.

22. Barbara A. DeBuono, Stephen H. Zinner, Maxim Daamen, and William M. McCormack, "Sexual Behavior of College Women in 1975, 1986, and 1989," *New England Journal of Medicine* 322 (1990): 821–25.

23. In the 1988 installment of National Survey of Family Growth, one-quarter of all fifteen-year-old girls and three quarters of all nineteen-year-old women had engaged in premarital sex. In the 1980 installment, only one in six fifteen-year-old girls and two-thirds of nineteen-year-old women were sexually experienced. In 1970, fewer than one in twenty fifteen-year-old girls and fewer than half of all nineteen-year-old women had had sex with a man before marriage. See "Premarital Sexual Experience Among Adolescent Women—United States, 1970–1988," *Morbidity and Mortality Weekly Report* 39 (1991): 929–32; S. L. Hofferth, J. R. Kahn, and W. Baldwin, Jr., "Premarital Sexual Activity Among U.S. Teenage Women over the Past Three Decades," *Family Planning Perspectives* 19 (1987): 46–53. The proportion of college women who have had anal intercourse has remained at about 10 percent over the past fifteen years. See "Behavior Changes Key to STD Prevention in the 1990s," *STD Bulletin* 11 (February/March 1993): 3–4.

24. "Number of Sex Partners and Potential Risk of Sexual Exposure to Human Immunodeficiency Virus," *Morbidity and Mortality Weekly Report* 37 (1988): 565–68; J. D. Forrest and S. Singh, "The Sexual and Reproductive Behavior of American Women, 1982–1989," *Family Planning Perspectives* 22 (1990): 206–14; Sevgi O. Aral and Willard Cates, Jr., "The Multiple Dimensions of Sexual Behavior as Risk Factor for Sexually Transmitted Dis-

ease: The Sexually Experienced Are Not Necessarily Sexually Active," *Sexually Transmitted Diseases* 16 (1989): 173–77; James W. McNally and William D. Mosher, "AIDS-Related Knowledge and Behavior Among Women 15–44 Years of Age: United States, 1988," *Advance Data from Vital and Health Statistics* 200 (1991): 1–11; William D. Mosher, "Contraceptive Practice in the United States, 1982–1988," *Family Planning Perspectives* 22 (1990): 198–205; Sevgi O. Aral, "Sexual Behavior and Risk for Sexually Transmitted Infections, " *STD Bulletin* 10 (May 1991): 3–10; T. W. Smith, "Adult Sexual Behavior in 1989: Number of Partners, Frequency of Intercourse and Risk of AIDS," *Family Planning Perspectives* 23 (1991): 102–7.

25. Ann E. Biddlecom and Ann M. Hardy, "AIDS Knowledge and Attitudes of Hispanic Americans: United States, 1990," *Advance Data from Vital and Health Statistics* 207 (1991): 1–24; Ann M. Hardy and Ann E. Biddlecom, "AIDS Knowledge and Attitudes of Black Americans: United States, 1990," *Advance Data from Vital and Health Statistics* 206 (1991): 1–24; "HIV/AIDS Knowledge and Awareness of Testing and Treatment—Behavioral Risk Factor Surveillance System, 1990," *Morbidity and Mortality Weekly Report* 40 (1991): 794–804; "HIV-Infection Prevention Messages for Injecting Drug Users: Sources of Information and Use of Mass Media—Baltimore, 1989," *Morbidity and Mortality Weekly Report* 40 (1991): 465–69.

26. McNally and Mosher, "AIDS-Related Knowledge and Behavior Among Women 15–44 Years of Age: United States, 1988."

27. My calculations based upon M. Margaret Dolcini, Joseph A. Catania, Thomas J. Coates, et al., "Multiple Partnerships and Their Demographic Correlates: The National AIDS Behavioral Surveys (NABS)," *Family Planning Perspectives*, forthcoming, 1993. See also Joseph A. Catania, Thomas J. Coates, Ron Stall, et al., "Prevalence of AIDS-Related Risk Factors and Condom Use in the United States," *Science* 258 (1992): 1101–6.

28. Stuart N. Seidman, William D. Mosher, and Sevgi O. Aral, "Women with Multiple Sexual Partners: United States, 1988," *American Journal of Public Health* 82 (1992): 1388–94.

29. "Number of Sex Partners and Potential Risk"; T. Smith, "Adult Sexual Behavior in 1989: Number of Partners, Frequency of Intercourse and Risk of AIDS"; Aral, "Sexual Behavior and Risk."

30. John S. Moran, Harlan R. Janes, Thomas A. Peterman, and Katherine M. Stone, "Increase in Condom Sales Following AIDS Education and Publicity, United States," *American Journal*

of Public Health 80 (1990): 607–8; "AIDS Threat Continues to Fuel Condom Sales," *Rubber & Plastics News,* 1 Oct. 1990, p. 27; "Growth in Condom Category Means More Profit in the 90's," *Drug Store News,* 24 Sept. 1990, p. S16; "Condom Sales Up 20% due to STDs, AIDS," *Drug Store News,* 26 March 1990, p. IP14; "Condom Market Starts to Taper Off," *Chain Drug Review,* 1 Jan. 1990, p. 22; "AIDS Helps Condom Sales," *Chain Drug Review,* 13 March 1989, p. 56; "Condom Mania," *American Demographics,* June 1989, p. 17; "People Buying More Condoms as Results of AIDS Education," *AIDS Alert,* June 1989, p. 103; "Condom Use Leveling Off at About 22% of All Men," *MDDI Reports Gray Sheet,* 1 Feb. 1988, pp. 8–9; "Condom Market Grows Over 20% for '86," *Chain Drug Review,* 25 May 1987, pp. 18, 21.

31. Mosher, "Contraceptive Practice in the United States, 1982–1988."

32. When the National AIDS Behavioral Surveys polled heterosexuals who had practiced anal intercourse in the past six months, they found that 71 percent never used condoms and only 19 percent always did. See "Prevalence of AIDS-Related Risk Factors and Condom Use in the United States."

33. Joseph A. Catania, Thomas J. Coates, Susan Kegeles, et al., "Condom Use in Multi-Ethnic Neighborhoods of San Francisco: The Population-Based AMEN (AIDS in Multi-Ethnic Neighborhoods) Study," and Correspondence, *American Journal of Public Health* 82 (1992): 284–87; 1563–65.

34. "Condom Use Among Male Injecting-Drug Users—New York City, 1987–1990," *Morbidity and Mortality Weekly Report* 41 (1992): 617–20; "Risk Behaviors for HIV Transmission Among Intravenous-Drug Users Not in Drug Treatment—United States, 1987–1989," *Morbidity and Mortality Weekly Report* 39 (1990): 273–76; "Drug Use and Sexual Behaviors Among Sex Partners of Injecting-Drug Users—United States, 1988–1990," *Morbidity and Mortality Weekly Report* 40 (1991): 855–60; "HIV-Risk Behaviors of Sterilized and Nonsterilized Women in Drug-Treatment Programs—Philadelphia, 1989–1991," *Morbidity and Mortality Weekly Report* 41 (1992): 149–52; Jane McCusker, Beryl Koblin, Benjamin F. Lewis, and John Sullivan, "Demographic Characteristics, Risk Behaviors, and HIV Seroprevalence Among Intravenous Drug Users by Site of Contact: Results from a Community-wide HIV Surveillance Project," *American Journal of Public Health* 80 (1990): 1062–67; S. Magura, J. L. Shapiro, Q. Siddiqi, and D. S. Lipton, "Variables Influencing Condom Use Among Intravenous Drug Users," *American Journal of Public Health* 80

(1990): 82–84.

35. "Heterosexual Behaviors and Factors That Influence Condom Use Among Patients Attending a Sexually Transmitted Disease Clinic—San Francisco," *Morbidity and Mortality Weekly Report* 39 (1990): 685–89.

36. "Drug Use and Sexual Behaviors Among Sex Partners of Injecting-Drug Users—United States, 1988–1990;" A. S. Abdul-Quader, S. Tross, S. R. Friedman, et al., "Street-recruited Intravenous Drug Users and Sexual Risk Reduction in New York City," *AIDS* 4 (1990): 1075–79; S. O. Aral, V. Soskolne, L. S. Magder, and G. S. Bowen, "Condom Use by Women Seeking Family Planning Services (abstract)," *VI International Conference on AIDS* (San Francisco, June 20–24, 1990): vol. 2, p. 267; A. D'Aubigny, P. Berger, B. Bouhet, et al., "Comportements Sexuels et Précautions Face au SIDA dans la Région Rhone Alpes en 1989," *BEH* 6 (1990): 21–22; Laura Rodrigues, "HIV Transmission to Women in Stable Relationships" (letter), *New England Journal of Medicine* 325 (1991): 966.

37. C. Hooykaas, J. van der Pligt, G. J. van Doornum, et al., "Heterosexuals at Risk for HIV: Differences Between Private and Commercial Partners in Sexual Behaviour and Condom Use," *AIDS* 3 (1989): 525–32; S. Day, H. Ward and J. R. W. Harris, "Prostitute Women and Public Health," *British Medical Journal* 297 (1988): 1585.

38. L. Liskin, C. Wharton, and R. Blackburn, "The Gap Between Use and Need," *Population Reports (Johns Hopkins)* 18 (1990): 3–9.

39. The term *revirginalized* was used by Anke A. Ehrhardt in "Trends in Sexual Behavior and the HIV Pandemic."

40. C. R. Horsburgh, Jr., C. Y. Ou, J. Jason, et al., "Duration of Human Immunodeficiency Virus Infection Before Detection of Antibody," *Lancet* 2 (1989): 637–40; Stephen J. Clark, Michael S. Saag, W. Don Decker, et al., "High Titers of Cytopathic Virus in Plasma of Patients with Symptomatic Primary HIV-1 Infection," *New England Journal of Medicine* 324 (1991): 954–60; Susan L. Stramer, John S. Heller, Robert W. Coombs, et al., "Markers of HIV Infection Prior to IgG Antibody Seropositivity," *Journal of the American Medical Association* 262 (1989): 64–69.

41. The full quote is: "A negative test today doesn't give you any guarantee for tomorrow. Before you have unprotected sex, you must be absolutely sure that your partner is sexually faithful and is not sharing needles to inject drugs. Most of us can't be absolutely sure about someone else's behavior, so rather than

relying on a test result that may not tell the whole story, it's safest to take responsibility for what you do: If you have sex, use a latex condom. If you use needles, clean them with bleach and don't share. Don't rely on someone else's promise to protect your health." ("What Women Should Know About AIDS.")

42. Jay M. Fleisher, Howard L. Minkoff, Ruby T. Senie, and Robert E. Endias, "Assessing Prior History of Sexually Transmitted Disease (letter)," *Journal of the American Medical Association* 266 (1991): 1646; W. Penn Handwerker and Ross Jones, "STDs: To Clap, Add Leak, Coolant, and Bore (letter)," *Journal of the American Medical Association* 267 (1992): 1611.

43. The full quotation is: "If the partner says: 'You carry a condom around with you? You were planning to seduce me!' You can say: 'I always carry one with me because I care about myself. I have one with me tonight because I care about us both.'" From "How to Use a Condom," prepared by the editors of *Medical Aspects of Human Sexuality* in collaboration with Reed Adams, PH.D., Emanuel Fliegelman, D.O., and Alan Grieco, PH.D. (Secaucus, N.J.: Hospital Publications, July 1987).

44. Marlene Roberts, "Do We Need Expiration Dates for Condoms? You Bet We Do," *New York Times,* 14 March 1993, sec. 4, p. 16.

45. Susan M. Kegeles, Joseph A. Catania, and Thomas J. Coates, "Intentions to Communicate Positive HIV-Antibody Status to Sex Partners" (letter), *Journal of the American Medical Association* 259 (1988): 216–17; Gary Marks, Jean L. Richardson, and Norma Maldonado, "Self-disclosure of HIV Infection to Sexual Partners," *American Journal of Public Health* 81 (1991): 1321–22; L. Temoshok, R. M. Ellmer, J. M. Moulton, et al., "Youth at Risk for HIV: Knowledge, Sexual Practices, and Intentions to Inform Sexual Partners of HIV Status," *V International Conference on AIDS* (Montreal, Quebec, June 1989): Abstract T.D.O.29; J. L. Chervenak and S. H. Weiss, "Sexual Partner Notification: Attitudes and Actions of HIV-Infected Women," *V International Conference on AIDS* (Montreal, Quebec, June 1989): Abstract Th.D.P.4; R. Stempel, J. Moulton, P. Bacchetti and A. R. Moss, "Disclosure of HIV-Antibody Test Results and Reactions of Sexual Partners, Friends, Family, and Health Professionals," *V International Conference on AIDS* (Montreal, Quebec, June 1989): Abstract E.729.

46. "HIV Counseling and Testing Services from Public and Private Providers—United States, 1990," *Morbidity and Mortality Weekly Report* 41 (1992): 743–52; Ann M. Hardy, "AIDS Knowledge and

Attitudes for January–March 1991: Provisional Data from the National Health Interview Survey," *Advance Data from Vital and Health Statistics* 216 (1992).

47. "HIV Counseling and Testing Services from Public and Private Providers—United States, 1990."

48. A total of 5,957,000 HIV tests were performed at publicly funded sites through 1991, of which 259,000 were positive. See "Publicly Funded HIV Counseling and Testing—United States, 1985–1989," *Morbidity and Mortality Weekly Report* 39 (1990): 137–40; "Publicly Funded HIV Counseling and Testing—United States, 1990," *Morbidity and Mortality Weekly Report* 40 (1991): 666–75; "Publicly Funded HIV Counseling and Testing—United States, 1991," *Morbidity and Mortality Weekly Report* 41 (1992): 613–17. My estimates here assume that 19 percent of all HIV tests were repeat tests, while 8 percent of all positive tests were repeat tests. See also "Characteristics of, and HIV Infection Among, Women Served by Publicly Funded HIV Counseling and Testing Services—United States, 1989–1990," *Morbidity and Mortality Weekly Report* 40 (1991): 195–204.

49. "Testing for HIV in the Public and Private Sectors—Oregon, 1988–1991," *Morbidity and Mortality Weekly Report* 41 (1992): 581–84.

50. In 1989, an estimated one million Americans were HIV-infected, with 100,000 more HIV infections expected during 1990–1991. See: "HIV Prevalence Estimates and AIDS Case Projections for the United States: Report Based Upon a Workshop," *Morbidity and Mortality Weekly Report* 39 (1990, RR-16): 1–31; Ron Brookmeyer, "Reconstruction and Future Trends of the AIDS Epidemic in the United States," *Science* 253 (1991): 37–42.

51. Harry F. Hull, Carl J. Bettinger, Margaret M. Gallaher, et al., "Comparison of HIV-Antibody Prevalence in Patients Consenting to and Declining HIV-Antibody Testing in an STD Clinic," *Journal of the American Medical Association* 260 (1988): 935–38.

52. J. E. Anderson, A. M. Hardy, K. Cahill, et al., "HIV Counseling and Testing in the U.S.: Who Is Being Reached and Who Isn't?" *VII International Conference on AIDS* (Florence, Italy, June 1991): Abstracts vol.1, p. 383.

53. L. J. D'Angelo, P. R. Getson, N. L. C. Luban, et al., "Human Immunodeficiency Virus Infection in Urban Adolescents: Can We Predict Who Is at Risk?" *Pediatrics* 88 (1991): 982–86; K. G. Castro, A. R. Lifson, C. R. White, et al., "Investigations of AIDS Patients with No Previously Identified Risk Factors," *Journal of the American Medical Association* 259 (1988): 1338–42.

54. Steven B. Locke, Hollis B. Kowaloff, Robert G. Hoff, et al.,
"Computer-Based Interview for Screening Blood Donors for
Risk of HIV Transmission," *Journal of the American Medical Association* 268 (1992): 1301–5. Interview questions were obtained
from the authors.

55. Judy Foreman, "Degree of AIDS Risk to Some Questioned,"
Boston Globe, 29 June 1987, pp. 1,5; Steven Findlay, "Has the
Threat Been Exaggerated?" *U.S. News & World Report,* 29 Feb.
1988, p. 58. See also Jeffrey E. Harris, "The AIDS Epidemic:
Looking into the 1990s," *Technology Review* 90 (1987): 59–64;
Associated Press, "AIDS Risk Termed Low for Most Heterosexual Americans," wire story, 29 Sept. 1987.

56. Laura Rodrigues, "HIV Transmission to Women in Stable Relationships," *New England Journal of Medicine* 325 (1991): 966.

57. In some cases, the infected men were hemophiliacs. See J. K.
Kreiss, L. W. Kitchen, and H. E. Prince, "Antibody to Human
T-lymphotropic Virus Type III in Wives of Haemophiliacs: Evidence for Heterosexual Transmission," *Annals of Internal Medicine* 102 (1985): 623–26; J. M. Jason, J. S. McDouglas, G. Dixon,
et al., "HTLV-III/LAV Antibody and Immune Status of Household Contacts and Sexual Partners of Persons with Hemophilia," *Journal of the American Medical Association* 255 (1986):
212–15; J. P. Allain, "Prevalence of HTLV-III/LAV Antibodies
in Patients with Hemophilia and in their Sexual Partners in
France," *New England Journal of Medicine* 315 (1986): 517–18;
H. C. Kim, K. Raska, L. Clemow, et al., "Human Immunodeficiency Virus Infection in Sexually Active Wives of Infected
Hemophiliac Men," *American Journal of Medicine* 85 (1988):
472–76; M. E. Van der Ende, P. Rothbard, and J. Stibbe, "Heterosexual Transmission of HIV by Haemophiliacs," *British Medical Journal* 297 (1988): 1102–3. In other cases, the men had
received HIV via blood transfusion. See Thomas A. Peterman,
Rand L. Stoneburner, James R. Allen, et al., "Risk of Human
Immunodeficiency Virus Transmission from Heterosexual
Adults with Transfusion-Associated Infection," *Journal of the
American Medical Association* 259 (1988): 55–58 (erratum, *Journal
of the American Medical Association* 262 [1989]: 502). In still other
cases, the men were bisexual or injecting-drug users. See Nancy
Padian, Linda Marquis, Donald P. Francis, et al., "Male-to-
Female Transmission of Human Immunodeficiency Virus,"
Journal of the American Medical Association 258 (1987): 788–90;
Adriano Lazzarin, Alberto Saracco, Massimo Musicco, et al.,
"Man-to-Woman Sexual Transmission of the Human Immuno-

deficiency Virus: Risk Factors Related to Sexual Behavior, Man's Infectiousness, and Woman's Susceptibility," *Archives of Internal Medicine* 151 (1991): 2411–16 (erratum, *Archives of Internal Medicine* 152 [1992]: 876); Isabelle I. De Vincenzi and R. Ancelle-Park, "Heterosexual Transmission of HIV: A European Study, I: Male-to-Female Transmission," *V International Conference on AIDS* (Montreal, Quebec, June 1989): Abstracts, p. 115; idem, European Study Group on Heterosexual Transmission of HIV, "Comparison of Female-to-Male and Male-to-Female Transmission of HIV in 563 Stable Couples," *British Medical Journal* 304 (1992): 809–13.

58. Nancy S. Padian, "Sexual Histories of Heterosexual Couples with One HIV-Infected Partner," *American Journal of Public Health* 80 (1990): 990–91.

59. M. V. Ragni, L. A. Kingsley, P. Nimorwicz, et al., "HIV Heterosexual Transmission in Hemophilia Couples: Lack of Relation to T4 Number, Clinical Diagnosis or Duration of HIV Exposure," *Journal of Acquired Immune Deficiency Syndromes* 2 (1989): 557–63; N. Padian, S. Shiboski, "Heterogeneous Male-to-Female Transmission of Human Immunodeficiency Virus," *V International Conference on AIDS* (Montreal, Quebec, June 1989): Abstract T.A.O. 16; S. D. Holmberg, C. R. Horsburgh, Jr., J. W. Ward, and H. W. Jaffe, "AIDS Commentary: Biologic Factors in the Sexual Transmission of Human Immunodeficiency Virus," *Journal of Infectious Diseases* 160 (1989): 116–25.

60. A. M. Johnson, A. Petherick, S. Davidson, et al., "Transmission of HIV to Heterosexual Partners of Infected Men and Women," *IV International Conference on AIDS* (Stockholm, Sweden, June 1988): Abstract 4058; N. Padian, J. Wiley, S. Glass, et al., "Anomalies of Infectivity in the Heterosexual Transmission of HIV," *IV International Conference on AIDS* (Stockholm, Sweden, June, 1988): Abstract 4062.

61. Thomas A. Peterman, Rand L. Stoneburner, James R. Allen, et al., "Risk of Human Immunodeficiency Virus Transmission from Heterosexual Adults with Transfusion-Associated Infection," *Journal of the American Medical Association* 259 (1988): 55–58 (erratum, *Journal of the American Medical Association* 262 [1989]: 502).

62. Edward H. Kaplan, "Modeling HIV Infectivity: Must Sex Acts Be Counted?" *Journal of Acquired Immune Deficiency Syndromes* 3 (1990): 55–61.

63. Adriano Lazzarin, Alberto Saracco, Massimo Musicco, et al., "Man-to-Woman Sexual Transmission of the Human Immuno-

deficiency Virus: Risk Factors Related to Sexual Behavior, Man's Infectiousness, and Woman's Susceptibility," *Archives of Internal Medicine* 151 (1991): 2411–16 (erratum, *Archives of Internal Medicine* 152 [1992]: 876); De Vincenzi and Ancelle-Park, European Study Group, "Comparison of Female-to-Male and Male-to-Female Transmission"; Isabelle De Vincenzi, "Heterosexual Transmission of HIV" (letter), *Journal of the American Medical Association* 267 (1992): 1919; De Vincenzi and Ancelle-Park, "Heterosexual Transmission of HIV: A European Study"; J. J. Goedert, M. E. Eyster, B. J. Biggar, and W. A. Blattner, "Heterosexual Transmission of Human Immunodeficiency Virus: Association with Severe Depletion of T-helper Lymphocytes in Men with Hemophilia," *AIDS Research and Human Retroviruses* 3 (1987): 355–61; D. Osmond, P. Bacchetti, R. E. Chaisson, et al., "Time of Exposure and Risk of HIV Infection in Homosexual Partners of Men with AIDS," *American Journal of Public Health* 78 (1988): 944–48; Holmberg et al., "AIDS Commentary"; A. M. Johnson and M. Laga, "Heterosexual Transmission of HIV," *AIDS* 2 (1988): S49–S56.

64. Nathan Clumeck, Henri Taelman, Phillipe Hermans, et al., "A Cluster of HIV Infection Among Heterosexual People without Apparent Risk Factors," *New England Journal of Medicine* 321 (1989): 1460–62.

65. D. J. Anderson, J. A. Hill, "CD4+ Lymphocytes in Semen: Implication for the Transmission of AIDS," *Fertility and Sterility* 48 (1987): 703.

66. Deborah J. Anderson, Joseph A. Politch, A. Martinez, et al., "White Blood Cells and HIV-1 in Semen from Vasectomized Patients," *Lancet* 338 (1991): 573–74.

67. John N. Krieger, Robert W. Coombs, Ann C. Collier, et al., "Fertility Parameters in Men Infected with Human Immunodeficiency Virus," *Journal of Infectious Diseases* 164 (1991): 464–69; John N. Krieger, Robert W. Coombs, Ann C. Collier, et al., "Recovery of Human Immunodeficiency Virus Type 1 from Semen: Minimal Impact of Stage of Infection and Current Antiviral Chemotherapy," *Journal of Infectious Diseases* 163 (1991): 386–88.

68. Deborah J. Anderson, Thomas R. O'Brien, Joseph A. Politch, et al., "Effects of Disease Stage and Zidovudine Therapy on the Detection of Human Immunodeficiency Virus Type 1 in Semen," *Journal of the American Medical Association* 267 (1992): 2769–74.

69. It might also get through an open sore near the front of her

genitals. See P. Piot and M. Laga, "Genital Ulcers, Other Sexually Transmitted Diseases and Sexual Transmission of HIV," *British Medical Journal* 298 (1989): 623–24.

70. Bruce Voeller and Deborah J. Anderson, "Heterosexual Transmission of HIV" (letter), *Journal of the American Medical Association* 267 (1992): 1917–18.

71. G. B. Moss, D. Clemetson, L. DCosta, et al., "Association of Cervical Ectopy with Heterosexual Transmission of Human Immunodeficiency Virus: Results of a Study of Couples in Nairobi, Kenya," *Journal of Infectious Diseases* 164 (1991): 588–91.

72. Women in central Zaire insert a ball of rolled leaves or a fingerful of coarse powder into their vaginas with the intention of making them drier and tighter. See Richard C. Brown, Judith E. Brown, and Okako B. Ayowa, "Vaginal Inflammation in Africa" (letter), *New England Journal of Medicine* 327 (1992): 572. See also "More on Vaginal Inflammation in Africa" (correspondence), *New England Journal of Medicine* 328 (1993): 888–89.

73. D. A. Cooper, J. Gold, P. Maclean, et al., "Acute AIDS Retrovirus Infection," *Lancet* 1 (1985): 537–40; D. D. Ho, M. G. Sarngadharan, L. Resnick, et al., "Primary Human T-lymphotropic Virus Type III Infection," *Annals of Internal Medicine* 103 (1985): 8803; B. Tindall, S. Barker, B. Donovan, et al., "Characterization of the Acute Clinical Illness Associated with Human Immunodeficiency Virus Infection," *Archives of Internal Medicine* 148 (1988): 945–49.

74. John W. Ward, Timothy J. Bush, Herbert A. Perkins, et al., "The Natural History of Transfusion-Associated Infection with Human Immunodeficiency Virus," *New England Journal of Medicine* 321 (1989): 947–52.

75. Stephen J. Clark, Michael S. Saag, W. Don Decker, et al., "High Titers of Cytopathic Virus in Plasma of Patients with Symptomatic Primary HIV-1 Infection," *New England Journal of Medicine* 324 (1991): 954–60.

76. While medical researchers have studied mostly gay men, it appears that anyone can have the symptoms of primary HIV infection. See Susan L. Stramer, John S. Heller, Robert W. Coombs, et al., "Markers of HIV Infection Prior to IgG Antibody Seropositivity," *Journal of the American Medical Association* 262 (1989): 64–69; Ward et al., "The Natural History of Transfusion-Associated Infection with Human Immunodeficiency Virus"; C. R. Horsburgh, Jr., C. Y. Ou, J. Jason, et al., "Duration of Human Immunodeficiency Virus Infection Before Detection of Antibody," *Lancet* 2 (1989): 637–40.

77. M. von Sydow, H. Gaines, A. Sönnerborg, et al., "Antigen Detection in Primary HIV Infection," *British Medical Journal* 296 (1988): 238–40 (erratum, *British Medical Journal* 296 [1988]: 525); J. Albert, H. Gaines, A. Sönnerborg, et al., "Isolation of Human Immunodeficiency Virus (HIV) from Plasma During Primary HIV Infection," *Journal of Medical Virology* 23 (1987): 67–73; H. Gaines, M. von Sydow, A. Sönnerborg, et al., "Antibody Response in Primary Human Immunodeficiency Virus Infection," *Lancet* 1 (1987): 1249–53; H. Gaines, J. Albert, M. von Sydow, et al., "HIV Antigenaemia and Virus Isolation from Plasma During Primary HIV Infection," *Lancet* 1 (1987): 1317–18.

78. Horsburgh et al., "Duration of Human Immunodeficiency Virus Infection Before Detection of Antibody." See also J. E. Groopman, T. Caiazzo, M. A. Thomas, et al., "Lack of Evidence of Prolonged Human Immunodeficiency Virus Infection Before Antibody Seroconversion," *Blood* 71 (1988): 1752–54; D. T. Imagawa, M. H. Lee, S. M. Wolinsky, et al., "Human Immunodeficiency Virus Type 1 Infection in Homosexual Men Who Remain Seronegative for Prolonged Periods," *New England Journal of Medicine* 320 (1989): 1458–62.

79. David Baltimore and Mark B. Feinberg, "HIV Revealed: Toward a Natural History of HIV Infection" (editorial), *New England Journal of Medicine* 321 (1989): 1673–75; Guiseppe Pantaleo, Cecilia Graziosi, and Anthony Fauci, "The Immunopathogenesis of Human Immunodeficiency Virus Infection," *New England Journal of Medicine* 328 (1993): 327–35.

80. F. DeWolf, M. Roos, J. M. A. Lange, et al., "Decline in CD4+ Cell Numbers Reflects Increase in HIV-1 Replication," *AIDS Research and Human Retroviruses* 4 (1988): 433–40.

81. "Disease Progression and Early Predictors of AIDS in HIV-seroconverted Injecting Drug Users: The Italian Seroconversion Study," *AIDS* 6 (1992): 421–26; R. Zangerle, D. Fuchs, G. Reibnegger, et al., "Markers for Disease Progression in Intravenous Drug Users Infected with HIV-1," *AIDS* 5 (1991): 985–91; Nicholas Lange, Bradley P. Carlin, and Alan E. Gelfand, "Hierarchical Bayes Models for the Progression of HIV Infection Using Longitudinal CD4 T-Cell Numbers (with Comments)," *Journal of the American Statistical Association* 87 (1992): 615–32; Joseph B. Margolick, Alvaro Muñoz, David Vlahov, et al., "Changes in T-Lymphocyte Subsets in Intravenous Drug Users with HIV-1 Infection," *Journal of the American Medical Association* 267 (1992): 1631–36.

82. More precisely, normal people have 1,000 to 1,200 CD4 cells per cubic millimeter of blood, where a cubic millimeter is one five-thousandth of a teaspoon.

83. H. Masur, F. P. Ognibene, R. Yarchoan, et al., "CD4 Counts as Predictors of Opportunistic Pneumonias in Human Immunodeficiency Virus (HIV) Infection," *Annals of Internal Medicine* 111 (1989): 223–31; John Phair, Alvaro Muñoz, Roger Detels, et al., "The Risk of Pneumocystis Carinii Pneumonia Among Men Infected with Human Immunodeficiency Virus," *New England Journal of Medicine* 322 (1990): 161–65; Peter A. Selwyn, Philip Alcabes, Diana Hartel, et al., "Clinical Manifestations and Predictors of Disease Progression in Drug Users with Human Immunodeficiency Virus Infection," *New England Journal of Medicine* 327 (1992): 1697–1703.

84. Centers for Disease Control, "1993 Revised Classification System for HIV Infection and Expanded Surveillance Case Definition for AIDS Among Adolescents and Adults," *Morbidity and Mortality Weekly Report* 41 (1992, RR-17): 1–19.

85. Andrew N. Phillips, Jonathan Elford, Caroline Sabin, et al., "Immunodeficiency and the Risk of Death in HIV Infection," *Journal of the American Medical Association* 268 (1992): 2662–66. Currently available antiviral drugs, such as AZT and ddI, may prolong the time from primary HIV infection to AIDS. They may slow the decline in a person's CD4 count and they may postpone death once a person has developed AIDS, but they do not fundamentally alter this natural course of HIV disease. See Jeffrey E. Harris, "Improved Short-term Survival of AIDS Patients Initially Diagnosed with Pneumocystis Carinii Pneumonia, 1984 through 1987," *Journal of the American Medical Association* 263 (1990): 397–402.

86. S. M. Schnittman, M. C. Psallidopoulos, H. C. Lane, et al., "The Reservoir for HIV-1 in Human Peripheral Blood Is a T-cell That Maintains Expression of CD4," *Science* 245 (1989): 305–8.

87. M. S. Saag, M. J. Crain, W. D. Decker, et al., "High-level Viremia in Adults and Children Infected with Human Immunodeficiency Virus: Relation to Disease Stage and CD4+ Lymphocyte Levels," *Journal of Infectious Diseases* 164 (1991): 72–80; Robert W. Coombs, Ann C. Collier, Jean-P. Allain, et al., "Plasma Viremia in Human Immunodeficiency Virus Infection," *New England Journal of Medicine* 321 (1989): 1626–31; David D. Ho, Tarsem Moudgil, and Masud Alam, "Quantitation of Human Immunodeficiency Virus in the Blood of Infected Persons," *New England Journal of Medicine* 321 (1989): 1621–25; M. Piatak,

M. S. Saag, L. C. Yang, et al., "High Levels of HIV-1 in Plasma During All Stages of Infection Determined by Competitive PCR," *Science* 259 (1993): 1749–54.

88. J. Pudney and D. Anderson, "Orchitis and Human Immunodeficiency Virus Type 1 Infected Cells in Reproductive Tissues from Men with the Acquired Immune Deficiency Syndrome," *American Journal of Pathology* 139 (1991): 149–60; Anderson, O'Brien, Politch, et al., "Effects of Disease Stage and Zidovudine Therapy on the Detection of Human Immunodeficiency Virus Type 1 in Semen"; J. H. Mermin, M. Holodniy, D. A. Katzenstein, and T. C. Merigan, "Detection of Human Immunodeficiency Virus DNA and RNA in Semen by the Polymerase Chain Reaction," *Journal of Infectious Diseases* 164 (1991): 769–72.

89. Karen M. Farizo, James W. Buehler, Mary E. Chamberland, et al., "Spectrum of Disease in Persons with Human Immunodeficiency Virus Infection in the United States," *Journal of the American Medical Association* 267 (1992): 1798–1805; R. A. Kaslow, J. P. Phair, H. B. Friedman, et al., "Infection with the Human Immunodeficiency Virus: Clinical Manifestations and Their Relationship to Immune Deficiency. A Report from the Multicenter AIDS Cohort Study," *Annals of Internal Medicine* 107 (1987): 474–80.

90. J. S. Dover and R. A. Johnson, "Cutaneous Manifestations of Human Immunodeficiency Virus Infection," *Archives of Dermatology* 127 (1991): 1383–91, 1549–58.

91. Suzan E. Norman, Lionel Resnick, Martin A. Cohn, et al., "Sleep Disturbances in HIV-Seropositive Patients," *Journal of the American Medical Association* 260 (1988): 922.

92. D. D. Ho, D. E. Bredesen, H. V. Vinters and E. S. Daar, "The Acquired Immunodeficiency Syndrome (AIDS) Dementia Complex: Clinical Conference," *Annals of Internal Medicine* 111 (1991): 400–410.

93. S. M. de la Monte, D. H. Gabuzda, D. D. Ho, et al., "Peripheral Neuropathy in the Acquired Immunodeficiency Syndrome," *Annals of Neurology* 23 (1988): 485–92.

94. E. A. Schulten, R. W. ten-Kate, and I. van-der-Waal, "The Impact of Oral Examination on the Centers for Disease Control Classification of Subjects with Human Immunodeficiency Virus Infection," *Archives of Internal Medicine* 150 (1990): 1259–61; J. Howard, F. Sattler, R. Mahon, et al., "Clinical Features of 100 Human Immunodeficiency Virus Antibody-Positive Individuals from an Alternate Test Site," *Archives of Internal Medicine* 147 (1987): 2131–33.

95. John Phair, Alvaro Muñoz, Roger Detels, et al., "The Risk of Pneumocystis Carinii Pneumonia Among Men Infected with Human Immunodeficiency Virus," *New England Journal of Medicine* 322 (1990): 161–65; H. W. Murray, J. H. Godbold, K. B. Jurica, and R. B. Roberts, "Progression to AIDS in Patients with Lymphadenopathy or AIDS-Related Complex: Reappraisal of Risk and Predictive Factors," *American Journal of Medicine* 86 (1989): 533–38; A. R. Lifson, G. W. Rutherford, and H. W. Jaffe, "The Natural History of Human Immunodeficiency Virus Infection," *Journal of Infectious Diseases* 158 (1988): 1360–67.

96. Joanne L. Rhoads, D. Craig Wright, Robert R. Redfield, and Donald S. Burke, "Chronic Vaginal Candidiasis in Women with Human Immunodeficiency Virus," *Journal of the American Medical Association* 257 (1987): 3105–7; N. Imam, C. C. J. Carpenter, K. H. Mayer, et al., "Hierarchical Pattern of Mucosal Candidal Infections in HIV-Seropositive Women," *American Journal of Medicine* 89 (1990): 142–46.

97. "Risk for Cervical Disease in HIV-Infected Women—New York City," *Morbidity and Mortality Weekly Report* 39 (1990): 846–49; D. Provencher, B. Valme, H. E. Averette, et al., "HIV Status and Positive Papanicolau Screening: Identification of a High-Risk Population," *Gynecologic Oncology* 31 (1988): 184–88; S. H. Vermund, K. F. Kelley, R. S. Klein, et al., "High Risk of Human Papillomavirus Infection and Cervical Squamous Intraepithelial Lesions Among Women with Symptomatic Human Immunodeficiency Virus Infection," *American Journal of Obstetrics and Gynecology* 165 (1991): 392–400.

98. Donald R. Hoover, Alfred Saah, Helena Bacellar, et al., "The Progression of Untreated HIV-1 Infection Prior to AIDS," *American Journal of Public Health* 82 (1992): 1538–41; Peter A. Selwyn, Philip Alcabes, Diana Hartel, et al., "Clinical Manifestations and Predictors of Disease Progression in Drug Users with Human Immunodeficiency Virus Infection," *New England Journal of Medicine* 327 (1992): 1697–1703; Farizo, Buehler, Chamberland, et al., "Spectrum of Disease in Persons with Human Immunodeficiency Virus Infection in the United States"; Philip O. Renzullo, John G. McNeil, Lytt I. Gardner, and John F. Brundage, "Inpatient Morbidity Among HIV-Infected Male Soldiers Prior to Their Diagnosis of HIV Infection," *American Journal of Public Health* 81 (1991): 1280–84.

99. Hoover et al., "The Progression of Untreated HIV-1 Infection Prior to AIDS," table 1.

100. Farizo et al., "Spectrum of Disease."

101. J. H. Toogood, "Complications of Topical Steroid Therapy for Asthma," *American Review of Respiratory Diseases* 141 (1990): S89–S96; G. A. Salzman, and D. R. Pyszczynski, "Oropharyngeal Candidiasis in Patients Treated with Beclomethasone Dipropionate Delivered by Metered-Dose Inhaler Alone and with Aerochamber," *Journal of Allergy and Clinical Immunology* 81 (1988): 424–28; A. S. Rosemurgy, T. F. Drost, C. G. Murphy, et al., "Treatment of Candidosis in Severely Injured Adults with Short-course, Low-dose Amphotericin B," *Journal of Trauma* 30 (1990): 1521–23;. B. Rodu, J. T. Carpenter, and M. R. Jones, "The Pathogenesis and Clinical Significance of Cytologically Detectable Oral Candida in Acute Leukemia," *Cancer* 62 (1988): 2042–46.

102. Nancy S. Padian, Stephen C. Shiboski, and Nicholas P. Jewell, "Female-to-Male Transmission of Human Immunodeficiency Virus," *Journal of the American Medical Association* 266 (1991): 1664–67; D. W. Cameron, J. N. Simonsen, L. J. DCosta, et al., "Female-to-Male Transmission of Human Immunodeficiency Virus Type 1: Risk Factors for Seroconversion in Men," *Lancet* 2 (1989): 403–7; M. Al-Nozha, S. Ramia, A. Al-Frayh et al., "Female to Male: An Inefficient Mode of Transmission of Human Immunodeficiency Virus (HIV)," *Journal of Acquired Immune Deficiency Syndromes* 3 (1990): 193–94; A. M. Johnson, A. Petherick, S. Davidson, et al., "Transmission of HIV to Heterosexual Partners of Infected Men and Women," *AIDS* 3 (1989): 367–72; I. De Vincenzi, P. R. Ancelle, and European Study Group, "Heterosexual Transmission of HIV: a European Study, II: Female-to-Male Transmission," *V International Conference on AIDS* (Montreal, Quebec, June 8, 1989).

103. Nancy S. Padian, Stephen C. Shiboski, and Nicholas P. Jewell, "Heterosexual Transmission of HIV" (letter), *Journal of the American Medical Association* 267 (1992): 1917–19.

104. Stephen R. Tabet, Darwin L. Palmer, William H. Wiese, et al., "Seroprevalence of HIV-1 and Hepatitis B and C in Prostitutes in Albuquerque, New Mexico," *American Journal of Public Health* 82 (1992): 1151–54.

105. H. W. Haverkos and E. Steel, "Crack Cocaine, Fellatio, and the Transmission of HIV" (letter), *American Journal of Public Health* 81 (1991): 1078–79.

106. Padian, Shiboski, and Jewell, "Female-to-Male Transmission of Human Immunodeficiency Virus."

107. Michael J. Rosenberg and Erica L. Gollub, "Commentary: Methods Women Can Use That May Prevent Sexually Transmit-

ted Disease, Including HIV," *American Journal of Public Health* 82 (1992): 1473–78; Willard Cates, Jr, Felicia H. Stewart, and James Trussell, "Commentary: The Quest for Women's Prophylactic Methods—Hopes vs. Science," *American Journal of Public Health* 82 (1992): 1479–82; Michael J. Rosenberg, Arthur J. Davidson, Jian-Hua Chen, et al., "Barrier Contraceptives and Sexually Transmitted Diseases," *American Journal of Public Health* 82 (1992): 669–74; Katherine M. Stone and Herbert B. Peterson, "Spermicides, HIV, and the Vaginal Sponge" (editorial), *Journal of the American Medical Association* 268 (1992): 521–23; Mary E. Guinan, "HIV, Heterosexual Transmission, and Women" (commentary), *Journal of the American Medical Association* 268 (1992): 520–21; Zena A. Stein, "HIV Prevention: The Need for Methods Women Can Use," *American Journal of Public Health* 80 (1990): 460–62; E. L. Golub and Z. A. Stein, "Commentary: The New Female Condom—Item 1 on a Women's AIDS Prevention Agenda," *American Journal of Public Health* 83 (1993): 501–3.

108. Donald P. Francis, "Toward a Comprehensive HIV Prevention Program for the CDC and the Nation," *Journal of the American Medical Association* 268 (1992): 1444–47.

CHAPTER 3: SPRING TRAINING

1. Ralph S. Paffenbarger, Jr., Alvin L. Wing, and Robert T. Hyde, "Physical Activity as an Index of Heart Attack Risk in College Alumni," *American Journal of Epidemiology* 108 (1978): 161–75.

2. The heart attack rates are "age-adjusted"—that is, they are the rates that one would observe if the men in each physical activity category had the same mix of ages. To compute the age-adjusted rate for each physical activity category, the researchers first determined heart attack rates by five-year age interval (35–39, 40–44, and so forth up to 70–74 years). Then they computed a numerically weighted average of heart attack rates across age intervals, where the numerical weights were the same for each physical activity category.

3. Ralph S. Paffenbarger, Jr., Alvin L. Wing, Robert T. Hyde, and Dexter L. Jung, "Physical Activity and Incidence of Hypertension in College Alumni," *American Journal of Epidemiology* 117 (1983): 245–57; Ralph S. Paffenbarger, Jr., Robert T. Hyde, Alvin L. Wing, and Charles H. Steinmetz, "A Natural History of Athleticism and Cardiovascular Health," *Journal of the American Medical Association* 252 (1984): 491–95; Ralph S. Paffenbarger,

Jr., Robert T. Hyde, Alvin L. Wing, and Chung-Cheng Hsieh, "Physical Activity, All-Cause Mortality, and Longevity of College Alumni," *New England Journal of Medicine* 314 (1986): 605–13.

4. Gerald F. Fletcher, Victor F. Froelicher, Howard Hartley, et al., "Exercise Standards: A Statement for Health Professionals from the American Heart Association," *Circulation* 82 (1990): 2286–321; quotation on p. 2307.

5. Editorial, "Keep Moving," *New York Times,* 7 March 1986.

6. Ralph S. Paffenbarger, Jr., Robert T. Hyde, Alvin L. Wing, et al., "The Association of Changes in Physical-Activity Level and Other Lifestyle Characteristics with Mortality Among Men," *New England Journal of Medicine* 328 (1993): 538–45.

7. I-Min Lee, Ralph Seal Paffenbarger, Jr. and Chung-Cheng Hsieh, "Time Trends in Physical Activity Among College Alumni," *American Journal of Epidemiology* 135 (1992): 915–25.

8. Computed from table 3 in Paffenbarger et al., "The Association of Changes in Physical-Activity Level."

9. Linda E. Crozier Ghilarducci, Robert G. Holly, and Ezra A. Amsterdam, "Effects of High Resistance Training in Coronary Artery Disease," *American Journal of Cardiology* 64 (1989): 866–70; P. B. Sparling and J. D. Cantwell, "Strength Training Guidelines for Cardiac Patients," *Physician and Sportsmedicine* 17 (1989): 190–96; Frances Munnings, "Strength Training: Not Only for the Young," *Physician and Sportsmedicine* 21 (1993): 133–40.

10. Everett A. Harman, Richard M. Rosenstein, Peter N. Frykman, and George A. Nigro, "Effects of a Belt on Intra-Abdominal Pressure During Weight Lifting," *Medicine and Science in Sports and Exercise* 21 (1988): 186–90; Jeffrey E. Lander, R. Leslie Simonton, and Joel K. F. Giacobbe, "The Effectiveness of Weight-Belts During the Squat Exercise," *Medicine and Science in Sports and Exercise* 22 (1990): 117–26.

11. T. Jeff Changler, G. Dennis Wilson, and Michael H. Stone, "The Effect of the Squat Exercise on Knee Stability," *Medicine and Science in Sports and Exercise* 21 (1989): 299–303.

12. M. V. Narici, M. Bordini, and P. Cerretelli, "Effect of Aging on Human Adductor Pollicis Muscle Function," *Journal of Applied Physiology* 71 (1991): 1277–81.

13. Michael G. Bemben, Benjamin H. Massey, Debra A. Bemben, et al., "Isometric Muscle Force Production as a Function of Age in Healthy 20- to 70-Year-Old Men," *Medicine and Science in Sports and Exercise* 23 (1991): 1302–11.

14. A. Aniansson, G. Grimby, and A. Rundgren, "Isometric and Isoki-

netic Quadriceps Muscle Strength in 70-Year-Old Men and Women," *Scandinavian Journal of Rehabilitation Medicine* 12 (1980): 161–68; William J. Evans, "Exercise, Nutrition and Aging," *Journal of Nutrition* 122 (1992): 796–801; H. Kiltgaard, M. Mantoni, S. Schiaffino, et al., "Function, Morphology and Protein Expression of Aging Skeletal Muscle: A Cross Sectional Study of Elderly Men with Different Training Backgrounds," *Acta Physiologica Scandinavica* 140 (1990): 41–54; S. L. Charette, L. McEvoy, G. Pyka, et al., "Muscle Hypertrophy Response to Resistance Training in Older Women," *Journal of Applied Physiology* 70 (1991): 1912–16.

15. M. Elaine Cress, D. Paul Thomas, Jill Johnson, et al., "Effect of Training on VO$_2$Max, Thigh Strength, and Muscle Morphology in Septuagenarian Women," *Medicine and Science in Sports and Exercise* 23 (1991): 752–58; R. H. Whipple, L. I. Wolfson, and P. M. Amerman, "The Relationship of Knee and Ankle Weakness to Falls in Nursing Home Residents: An Isokinetic Study," *Journal of the American Geriatric Society* 35 (1987): 13–20; E. J. Bassey, M. A. Fiatarone, E. F. O'Neill, et al., "Leg Extensor Power and Functional Performance in Very Old Men and Women," *Clinical Science* 82 (1992): 321–27.

16. W. R. Frontera, C. N. Meredith, K. P. O'Reilly, et al., "Strength Conditioning in Older Men: Skeletal Muscle Hypertrophy and Improved Function," *Journal of Applied Physiology* 64 (1988): 1038–44; A. Aniansson and E. Gustafsson, "Physical Training in Elderly Men with Special Reference to Quadriceps Muscle Strength and Morphology," *Clinical Physiology* 1 (1981): 87–98; L. Larsson, "Physical Training Effects on Muscle Morphology in Sedentary Males at Different Ages," *Medicine and Science in Sports and Exercise* 14 (1982): 203–6.

17. Maria A. Fiatarone, Elizabeth C. Marks, Nancy D. Ryan, et al., "High-Intensity Strength Training in Nonagenarians: Effects on Skeletal Mass," *Journal of the American Medical Association* 263 (1990): 3029–34.

18. L. Larsson and T. Ansved, "Effects of Long-Term Physical Training and Detraining on Enzyme Histochemical and Functional Skeletal Muscle Characteristics in Man," *Muscle and Nerve* 8 (1985): 714–22; A. Thorstensson, "Observation on Strength Training and Detraining," *Acta Physiologica Scandinavica* 100 (1977): 491–93; R. S. Staron, M. J. Leonardi, D. L. Karapondo, et al., "Strength and Skeletal Muscle Adaptations in Heavy-Resistance-Trained Women After Detraining and Retraining," *Journal of Applied Physiology* 70 (1991): 631–40.

19. American College of Sports Medicine, "Position Stand: The Recommended Quantity and Quality of Exercise for Developing and Maintaining Cardiorespiratory and Muscular Fitness in Healthy Adults," *Medicine and Science in Sports and Exercise* 22 (1990): 265–74.

20. Paul L. McHenry, Myrvin H. Ellestad, Gerald F. Fletcher, et al. (American Heart Association Scientific Council), "Statement on Exercise: A Position Statement for Health Professionals by the Committee on Exercise and Cardiac Rehabilitation of the Council on Clinical Cardiology, American Heart Association," *Circulation* 81 (1990): 396–98.

21. "Vigorous Physical Activity Among High School Students—United States, 1990," *Morbidity and Mortality Weekly Report* 31 (1992): 33–35.

22. "Coronary Heart Disease Attributable to Sedentary Lifestyle—Selected States, 1988," *Morbidity and Mortality Weekly Report* 39 (1990): 541–44.

23. Y. Atomi, K. Ito, H. Iwasaki, and M. Miyashita, "Effects of Intensity and Frequency of Training on Aerobic Work Capacity of Young Females," *Journal of Sports Medicine* 18 (1978): 3–9; L. R. Gettman, M. L. Pollock, J. L. Durstine, et al., "Physiological Responses of Men to 1, 3, and 5 Day Per Week Training Programs," *Research Quarterly* 47 (1976): 638–46; R. C. Hickson and M. A. Rosenkoetter, "Reduced Training Frequencies and Maintenance of Aerobic Power," *Medicine and Science in Sports and Exercise* 13 (1981): 13–16; T. R. Crews and J. A. Roberts, "Effects of Interaction of Frequency and Intensity of Training," *Research Quarterly* 47 (1976): 48–55; M. L. Pollock, T. K. Cureton, and L. Greninger, "Effects of Frequency of Training on Working Capacity, Cardiovascular Function, and Body Composition of Adult Men," *Medicine and Science in Sports and Exercise* 1 (1969): 70–74; R. L. Terjung, K. M. Baldwin, J. Cooksey, et al., "Cardiovascular Adaptation to Twelve Minutes of Mild Daily Exercise in Middle-Aged Sedentary Men," *Journal of the American Geriatric Society* 21 (1973): 164–68; H. A. Wenger and G. J. Bell, "The Interactions of Intensity, Frequency, and Duration of Exercise Training in Altering Cardiorespiratory Fitness," *Sports Medicine* 3 (1986): 346–56.

24. B. J. Whipp and K. Wasserman, "Oxygen Uptake Kinetics for Various Intensities of Constant-Load Work," *Journal of Applied Physiology* 33 (1972): 351–56.

25. R. C. Hickson, J. M. Hagberg, A. A. Ehsani, and J. O. Holloszy, "The Course of the Adaptive Responses of Aerobic Power and

Heart Rate to Training," *Medicine and Science in Sports and Exercise* 13 (1981): 17–20.

26. Robert F. DeBusk, Ulf Stenestrand, Mary Sheehan, and William L. Haskell, "Training Effects of Long Versus Short Bouts of Exercise in Healthy Subjects," *American Journal of Cardiology* 65 (1990): 1010–13.

27. Dalynn T. Badenhop, Patrick A. Cleary, Stephen F. Schaal, et al., "Physiological Adjustments to Higher- or Lower-Intensity Exercise in Elders," *Medicine and Science in Sports and Exercise* 15 (1983): 496–502; Carmen C. Cononie, James E. Graves, Michael L. Pollock, et al., "Effect of Exercise Training on Blood Pressure in 70- to 79-Year-Old Men and Women," *Medicine and Science in Sports and Exercise* 23 (1991): 505–11; James M. Hagberg, James E. Graves, M. Limacher, et al., "Cardiovascular Responses to 70–79-Year-Old Men and Women to Exercise Training," *Journal of Applied Physiology* 66 (1989): 2589–94; Herbert A. De Vries, "Exercise Intensity Threshold for Improvement of Cardiovascular-Respiratory Function in Older Men," *Geriatrics* (April 1971): 94–101.

28. C. N. Meredith, W. R. Frontera, E. C. Fisher, et al., "Peripheral Effects of Endurance Training in Young and Old Subjects," *Journal of Applied Physiology* 66 (1989): 2844–49; Jerome L. Fleg and Edward G. Lakatta, "Role of Muscle Loss in the Age-Associated Reduction in VO_2Max," *Journal of Applied Physiology* 65 (1988): 1147–51; Bengt Saltin and Søren Strange, "Maximal Oxygen Uptake: "Old" and "New" Arguments for a Cardiovascular Limitation," *Medicine and Science in Sports and Exercise* 24 (1992): 30–37.

29. E. L. Smith, W. Reddan, and P. E. Smith, "Physical Activity and Calcium Modalities for Bone Mineral Increase in Aged Women," *Medicine and Science in Sports and Exercise* 13 (1981): 60–64; R. K. Chow, J. E. Harrison, and C. Notarius, "Effects of Two Randomized Programs on Bone Mass of Healthy Postmenopausal Women," *British Medical Journal* 295 (1987): 1441–44; G. P. Dalsky, K. S. Stocke, A. A. Ehsani, et al., "Weight–Bearing Exercise Training and Lumbar Bone Mineral Content in Postmenopausal Women," *Annals of Internal Medicine* 108 (1988): 824–28; Katie A. Grove and Ben R. Londeree, "Bone Density in Post Menopausal Women: High Impact versus Low Impact Exercise," *Medicine and Science in Sports and Exercise* 24 (1992): 1190–94; M. E. Nelson, E. C. Fisher, F. A. Dilmanian, et al., "A 1-Year Walking Program and Increased Dietary Calcium in Postmenopausal Women: Effects on Bone," *American Journal of Clinical Nutrition* 53 (1991): 1304–11; C. Snow-Harter,

M. L. Bouxsein, B. T. Lewis, et al., "Effects of Resistance and Endurance Exercise on Bone Mineral Status of Young Women: A Randomized Exercise Intervention Trial," *Journal of Bone Mineral Research* 7 (1992): 761–69.

30. JoAnn E. Manson, David M. Nathan, Andrzej S. Krolewski, et al., "A Prospective Study of Exercise and Incidence of Diabetes Among U.S. Male Physicians," *Journal of the American Medical Association* 268 (1992): 63–67; Susan P. Helmrich, David R. Ragland, Rita W. Leung and Ralph S. Paffenbarger, Jr., "Physical Activity and Reduced Occurrence of Non-Insulin-Dependent Diabetes Mellitus," *New England Journal of Medicine* 325 (1991): 147–52.

31. J. M. Hagberg, S. J. Montain, W. H. Martin 3d, and A. A. Ehsani, "Effect of Exercise Training in 60- to 69-Year-Old Persons with Essential Hypertension," *American Journal of Cardiology* 64 (1989): 348–53.

32. K. Kukkonen, R. Rauramaa, O. Siitonen, et al., "Physical Training of Obese Middle-Aged Persons," *Annals of Clinical Research* 14 (1982): 80–85; C. N. Meredith, M. J. Zackin, W. R. Frontera, and W. J. Evans, "Body Composition and Aerobic Capacity in Endurance-Trained Men," *Medicine and Science in Sports and Exercise* 19 (1987): 557–63.

33. John J. Duncan, Neil F. Gordon, and Chris B. Scott, "Women Walking for Health and Fitness: How Much Is Enough?" *Journal of the American Medical Association* 266 (1991): 3295–99; A. L. Hicks, J. D. MacDougall, and T. J. Muckle, "Acute Changes in High-Density Lipoprotein Cholesterol with Exercise of Different Intensities," *Journal of Applied Physiology* 63 (1987): 1956–60.

34. Wojtek J. Chodzko-Zajko, "Physical Fitness, Cognitive Performance, and Aging," *Medicine and Science in Sports and Exercise* 23 (1991): 868–72.

35. Robert J. Sonstroem and William P. Morgan, "Exercise and Self-Esteem: Rationale and Model," *Medicine and Science in Sports and Exercise* 21 (1989): 329–37.

36. E. F. Coyle, A. R. Coggan, M. K. Hopper, et al., "Determinants of Endurance in Well-Trained Cyclists," *Journal of Applied Physiology* 64 (1988): 2622–30.

37. Carl Foster, Nancy N. Thompson, and Ann C. Synder, *Physiology of Speed Skating* (Milwaukee: University of Wisconsin Medical School, February 1990). These values of V-Dot-O_2-Max are in conventional metric units of "milliliters of oxygen per minute per kilogram body weight." To convert to calories per hour per pound (or CHPs, as I have called them), divide by 7.33. Thus,

the V-Dot-O_2-Maxes of some champion endurance athletes can exceed 10 CHPs.

38. Leiv Sandvik, Jan Erikssen, Erik Thaulow, et al., "Physical Fitness as a Predictor of Mortality Among Healthy, Middle-Aged Norwegian Men," *New England Journal of Medicine* 328 (1993): 533–37; Steven N. Blair, Harold W. Kohl III, Ralph S. Paffenbarger, et al., "Physical Fitness and All-Cause Mortality: A Prospective Study of Healthy Men and Women," *Journal of the American Medical Association* 262 (1989): 2395–2410; Lars-Göran Ekelund, William L. Haskell, Jeffrey L. Johnson, et al., "Physical Fitness as a Predictor of Cardiovascular Mortality in Asymptomatic North American Men: The Lipid Research Clinics Mortality Follow–Up Study," *New England Journal of Medicine* 319 (1988): 1379–84.

39. Barbara E. Ainsworth, William L. Haskell, Arthur S. Leon, et al., "Compendium of Physical Activities: Classification of Energy Costs of Human Physical Activities," *Medicine and Science in Sports and Exercise* 25 (1993): 71–80.

40. Michele Scharff Olson, Henry N. Williford, Daniel L. Blessing, and Roy Greathouse, "The Cardiovascular and Metabolic Effects of Bench Stepping Exercise in Females," *Medicine and Science in Sports and Exercise* 23 (1991): 1311–18.

41. Bruce Arroll and Robert Beaglehole, "Potential Misclassification in Studies of Physical Activity," *Medicine and Science in Sports and Exercise* 23 (1991): 1176–78.

CHAPTER 4: BODY MASS INDEX

1. NIH Technology Assessment Conference Panel, "Methods for Voluntary Weight Loss and Control," *Annals of Internal Medicine* 116 (1992): 942–49.

2. The BMI is formally defined as a person's weight (in kilograms) divided by the square of her height (in squared meters). Here, I shall say that Eve's BMI is 23 "points," although it would be more accurate to say 23 "kilograms per squared meter." The chart is my attempt to work in pounds and inches rather than the less familiar metric units. To compute the BMI conversion factor for heights outside the range of the chart, divide the squared height (in squared inches) by 704.547. For example, a 7' tall man has a height of 84 inches, and thus a squared height of 84 × 84, which equals 7,056 squared inches. His BMI conversion factor would thus be 7056 ÷ 704.547, or 10.01.

3. To go backward from BMI to weight in pounds, multiply the BMI by the height-specific conversion factor in the chart. Thus,

for Eve, a BMI of 35 would correspond to a weight of 35 × 6 = 210 pounds.

4. Matthew F. Najjar and Michael Rowland, "Anthropomorphic Reference Data and Prevalence of Overweight," *Vital & Health Statistics*, ser. 11, no. 238 (Hyattsville, Md.: National Center for Health Statistics, October 1987), DHHS Publication no. (PHS) 87–1688, table 11.

5. Andrew W. Brotman, Nancy Rigotti, and David B. Herzog, "Medical Complications of Eating Disorders: Outpatient Evaluation and Management," *Comprehensive Psychiatry* 26 (1985): 258–72.

6. Najjar and Rowland, "Anthropomorphic Reference Data," tables 10 and 11. See also R. J. Kuczmarski, "Prevalence of Overweight and Weight Gain in the United States," *American Journal of Clinical Nutrition* 55 (1992, suppl. 2): 495S–502S.

7. U.S. Department of Agriculture, U.S. Department of Health and Human Services, *Nutrition and Your Health: Dietary Guidelines for Americans* (Washington, D.C.: U.S. Government Printing Office, 1990).

8. See Walter C. Willett, Meir Stampfer, JoAnn Manson, and T. Van Itallie, "New Weight Guidelines for Americans: Justified or Injudicious," *American Journal of Clinical Nutrition* 53 (1991): 1102–3; Walter C. Willett, Meir Stampfer, JoAnn Manson, and T. Van Itallie, "Reply to G. A. Bray and R. L. Atkinson," *American Journal of Clinical Nutrition* 55 (1992): 482–83; Walter C. Willett, Meir Stampfer, and JoAnn Manson, "Reply to R. P. Abernathy," *American Journal of Clinical Nutrition* 56 (1992): 1066–67.

9. A. J. Hartz, M. E. Fischer, G. Bril, et al., "The Association of Obesity with Joint Pain and Osteoarthritis in the HANES Data," *Journal of Chronic Diseases* 39 (1986): 311–19; M. A. Davis, W. H. Ettinger, and J. M. Neuhaus, "Obesity and Osteoarthritis of the Knee: Evidence from the National Health and Nutrition Examination Survey (NHANES I)," *Seminars in Arthritis and Rheumatology* 20 (1990, suppl.1): 34–41; D. T. Felson, "The Epidemiology of Knee Osteoarthritis: Results from the Framingham Osteoarthritis Study," *Seminars in Arthritis and Rheumatology* 20 (1990, suppl. 1): 42–50.

10. M. Modan, H. Halkin, S. Almog, et al., "Hyperinsulinemia: A Link Between Hypertension, Obesity, and Glucose Intolerance," *Journal of Clinical Investigation* 75 (1985): 809–17; W-H. Pan, S. Nanas, A. Dyer, et al., "The Role of Weight in the Positive Association Between Age and Blood Pressure," *American Journal of Epidemiology* 124 (1986): 612–23; R. N. Baumgartner, A. F. Roche, W. C. Chumlea, et al., "Fatness and Fat Patterns: Associations with Plasma Lipids and Blood Pressures in Adults,

18 to 57 Years of Age," *American Journal of Epidemiology* 126 (1987): 614–28; A. P. Rocchini, V. Katch, A. Schork, and R. P. Kelch, "Insulin and Blood Pressure During Weight Loss in Obese Adolescents," *Hypertension* 10 (1987): 267–73; Norman M. Kaplan, "The Deadly Quartet: Upper-Body Obesity, Glucose Intolerance, Hypertriglyceridemia, and Hypertension," *Archives of Internal Medicine* 149 (1989): 1514–20; Xiaozhang Jiang, Sathanur R. Srinivasan, Weihang Bao, and Gerald S. Berenson, "Association of Fasting Insulin with Blood Pressure in Young Individuals: The Bogalusa Heart Study," *Archives of Internal Medicine* 153 (1993): 323–28.

11. Society of Actuaries and Association of Life Insurance Medical Directors of America, *Body Build Study 1979* (Chicago: Society of Actuaries and Association of Life Insurance Medical Directors of America, 1980); Society of Actuaries, Committee on Mortality, *Build and Blood Pressure Study*, 2 vols. (Chicago: Society of Actuaries, 1979); "New Weight Standards for Men and Women," *Statistical Bulletin of the Metropolitan Life Insurance Company* 40 (1959): 1–4; "1983 Metropolitan Height and Weight Tables," *Statistical Bulletin of the Metropolitan Life Insurance Company* 64 (1983): 2–9.

12. JoAnn E. Manson, Graham A. Colditz, Meir J. Stampfer, et al., "A Prospective Study of Obesity and Risk of Coronary Heart Disease," *New England Journal of Medicine* 322 (1990): 882–89. See also JoAnn E. Manson, Graham A. Colditz, Meir J. Stampfer, et al., "A Prospective Study of Obesity and Risk of Stroke in Women" (abstract), *American Journal of Epidemiology* 130 (1989): 833.

13. The underlying data for figure 4.2 are given below. The statistical error ranges are shown in parentheses. (Thus, for currently smoking nurses with BMIs less than 21.00, the risk of heart attack or coronary death was 60 cases per 100,000, with a statistical error range of 43 to 81 cases per 100,000.)

BMI Range	Never Smoked	Past Smokers	Current Smokers
Less than 21.00	18 (9–32)	18 (7–38)	60 (43–81)
21.00 to 24.99	19 (13–27)	27 (17–40)	79 (64–98)
25.00 to 28.99	31 (19–47)	36 (19–64)	106 (77–141)
29.00 or more	44 (27–66)	76 (46–119)	209 (156–274)

For clarity, I have not shown the statistical error ranges in the figure, as I did for the Harvard Alumni Study in chapter 3. At each level of BMI, the error ranges for current smokers do not overlap those of the other two groups.

14. Xavier Pi-Sunyer, "Health Implications of Obesity," *American Journal of Clinical Nutrition* 53 (1991): 1595S–1603S; A. Rissanen, "Weight and Mortality of Finnish Men," *Journal of Clinical Epidemiology* 42 (1989): 781–89; S. P. Tsai, "Obesity and Morbidity Prevalence in a Working Population," *Journal of Occupational Medicine* 30 (1988): 589–91; E. A. Lew and L. Garfinkel, "Variations in Mortality by Weight Among 750,000 Men and Women," *Journal of Chronic Diseases* 32 (1979): 563–76; T. Harris, E. F. Cook, R. Garrison, et al., "Body Mass Index and Mortality Among Nonsmoking Older Persons: The Framingham Heart Study," *Journal of the American Medical Association* 259 (1988): 1520–24; M. D. A. F. Hoffmans, D. Kromhour, and C. de Lezenne Coulandar, "The Impact of Body Mass Index of 78,612 18-Year-Old Dutch Men on 32-Year Mortality from All Causes," *Journal of Clinical Epidemiology* 41 (1988): 749–56; T. Wilcosky, J. Hyde, J. J. B. Anderson, et al., "Obesity and Mortality in the Lipid Research Clinics Program Follow-Up Study," *Journal of Clinical Epidemiology* 43 (1990): 743–52; L. V. Sjostrom, "Morbidity of Severely Obese Subjects," *American Journal of Clinical Nutrition* 55 (1992, suppl.): 508S–515S; H. T. Waaler, "Height, Weight and Mortality: The Norwegian Experience," *Acta Medica Scandinavica Supplementum* 679 (1984): 1–56.

15. I-Min Lee, Ralph Seal Paffenbarger, Jr., and Chung-Cheng Hsieh, "Time Trends in Physical Activity Among College Alumni, 1962–1988," *American Journal of Epidemiology* 135 (1992): 915–25.

16. Graham A. Colditz, Walter C. Willett, M. J. Stampfer, et al., "Weight as a Risk Factor for Clinical Diabetes in Women," *American Journal of Epidemiology* 132 (1990): 501–13.

17. David F. Williamson, Jennifer Madans, Robert F. Anda, et al., "Smoking Cessation and Severity of Weight Gain in a National Cohort," *New England Journal of Medicine* 324 (1991): 739–45.

18. See also K. Lindsted, S. Tonstad, and J. W. Kuzman, "Body Mass Index and Patterns of Mortality Among Seventh-Day Adventist Men," *International Journal of Obesity* 15 (1991): 397–406; Aviva Must, Paul F. Jacques, Gerard E. Dallal, et al., "Long-Term Morbidity and Mortality of Overweight Adolescents: A Follow-Up of the Harvard Growth Study of 1922 to 1935," *New England Journal of Medicine* 327 (1992): 1350–57; T. I. A. Sorensen and

S. Sonne-Holm, "Mortality in Extremely Overweight Young Men," *Journal of Chronic Diseases* 30 (1977): 359–67.

19. Ralph S. Paffenbarger, Jr., Robert T. Hyde, Alvin L. Wing, et al., "The Association of Changes in Physical-Activity Level and Other Lifestyle Characteristics with Mortality Among Men," *New England Journal of Medicine* 328 (1993): 538–45, table 3.

20. June Stevens, Julian E. Keil, Philip F. Rust, et al., "Body Mass Index and Body Girths as Predictors of Mortality in Black and White Women," *Archives of Internal Medicine* 152 (1992): 1257–62; J. Wienpahl, D. R. Ragland, and S. Sidney, "Body Mass Index and 15-Year Mortality in a Cohort of Black Men and Women," *Journal of Clinical Epidemiology* 43 (1990): 949–60.

21. Claude Bouchard, "Heredity and the Path to Overweight and Obesity," *Medicine and Science in Sports and Exercise* 23 (1991): 285–91.

22. The Working Group on Eating Disorders of the American Psychiatric Association has proposed a new diagnosis of "binge-eating disorder" for the fourth edition of its *Diagnostic and Statistical Manual of Mental Disorders,* forthcoming in 1993 or 1994. See R. Spitzer, M. Devlin, B. T. Walsh, et al., "Binge-Eating Disorder: A Multisite Field Trial of the Diagnostic Criteria," *International Journal of Eating Disorders* 11 (1992): 192–203; Susan Zelitch Yanovski, Melissa Leet, Jack A. Yanovski, et al., "Food Selection and Intake of Obese Women with Binge-Eating Disorder," *American Journal of Clinical Nutrition* 56 (1992): 975–80.

23. Kelly D. Brownell and Thomas A. Wadden, "The Heterogeneity of Obesity: Fitting Treatments to Individuals," *Behavior Therapy* 22 (1991):153–77; Beatrice S. Kanders, R. Armour Forse, and George L. Blackburn, "Obesity," in *Conn's Current Therapy,* ed. R. E. Rakel (Philadelphia: Saunders, 1991), pp. 524–31; George L. Blackburn and Beatrice S. Kanders, "Medical Evaluation and Treatment of the Obese Patient with Cardiovascular Disease," *American Journal of Cardiology* 60 (1987): 55G–58G.

24. T. A. Wadden, T. B. Van Itallie, and G. L. Blackburn, "Responsible and Irresponsible Use of Very Low Calorie Diets in the Treatment of Obesity," *Journal of the American Medical Association* 263 (1990): 83–85.

25. "Gastrointestinal Surgery for Severe Obesity," NIH Consensus Development Conference Statement, March 25–27, 1991.

26. Thomas A. Wadden, Gary D. Foster, Kathleen A. Letizia, and Albert J. Stunkard, "A Multicenter Evaluation of a Proprietary Weight Reduction Program for the Treatment of Marked Obesity," *Archives of Internal Medicine* 152 (1992): 961–66.

27. Sharon Alger, Karen Larson, Vicky L. Boyce, et al., "Effect of Phenylpropanolamine on Energy Expenditure and Weight Loss in Overweight Women," *American Journal of Clinical Nutrition* 57 (1993): 120–26; George A. Bray, "Barriers to the Treatment of Obesity" (editorial), *Annals of Internal Medicine* 115 (1991): 152–53.

28. George A. Bray, "Lipogenesis in Human Adipose Tissue: Some Effects of Nibbling and Gorging," *Journal of Clinical Investigation* 51 (1972): 537–48.

29. Dietary surveys suggest that after white bread, rolls, and crackers, and doughnuts, cookies and cakes, alcoholic beverages are the largest source of fuel in the American diet. See *Edell Health Letter* 12 (March 1993): 5.

30. William M. Sherman, J. Andrew Doyle, David R. Lamb, and Richard H. Strauss, "Dietary Carbohydrate, Muscle Glycogen, and Exercise Performance During 7 Days of Training," *American Journal of Clinical Nutrition* 57 (1993): 27–31; Edward F. Coyle and Effie Coyle, "Carbohydrates That Speed Recovery from Training," *The Physician and Sportsmedicine* 21 (February 1993): 11–123.

31. C. Bouchard, A. Tremblay, J.-P. Després, "The Response to Long-Term Overfeeding in Identical Twins," *New England Journal of Medicine* 322 (1990): 1477–82.

32. D. M. Dreon, B. Frey-Hewitt, N. Ellsworth, et al., "Dietary Fat: Carbohydrate Ratio and Obesity in Middle-Aged Men," *American Journal of Clinical Nutrition* 47 (1988): 995–1000.

33. Steven W. Lichtman, Krystyna Pisarska, Ellen Raynes Berman, et al., "Discrepancy Between Self-Reported and Actual Caloric Intake and Exercise in Obese Subjects," *New England Journal of Medicine* 327 (1992): 1893–98.

34. Wayne C. Miller, "Diet Composition, Energy Intake, and Nutritional Status in Relation to Obesity in Men and Women," *Medicine and Science in Sports and Exercise* 23 (1991): 280–84.

35. E. Ravussin, S. Lillioja, W. C. Knowler, et al., "Reduced Rate of Energy Expenditure as a Risk Factor for Body-Weight Gain," *New England Journal of Medicine* 318 (1988): 467–72.

36. E. A. H. Sims and E. Danforth, Jr., "Expenditure and Storage of Energy in Man," *Journal of Clinical Investigation* 79 (1987): 1019–25.

37. E. Ravussin, S. Lillioja, T. E. Anderson, et al., "Determinants of 24-Hour Energy Expenditure in Man: Methods and Results Using a Respiratory Chamber," *Journal of Clinical Investigation* 78 (1986): 1568–78.

38. George A. Bray, "Effect of Caloric Restriction on Energy Expenditure in Obese Patients," *Lancet* 2 (1969): 397–98.

39. Françoise Froidevaux, Yves Schutz, Laurent Christin, and Eric Jéquier, "Energy Expenditure in Obese Women Before and During Weight Loss, After Refeeding, and in the Weight-Relapse Period," *American Journal of Clinical Nutrition* 57 (1993): 35–42.

40. Konstantin N. Pavlou, Suzanna Krey, and William P. Steffee, "Exercise as an Adjunct to Weight Loss and Maintenance in Moderately Obese Subjects," *American Journal of Clinical Nutrition* 49 (1989): 1115–23; Stephen D. Phinney, Betty M. LaGrange, Maureen O'Connell, and Elliott Danforth, Jr., "Effects of Aerobic Exercise on Energy Expenditure and Nitrogen Balance During Very Low Calorie Dieting," *Metabolism* 37 (1988): 758–65; Konstantin N. Pavlou, Janet E. Whatley, Peter W. Jannace, et al., "Physical Activity as a Supplement to a Weight-Loss Dietary Regimen," *American Journal of Clinical Nutrition* 49 (1989): 1110–14; Konstantin N. Pavlou, William P. Steffee, Robert H. Lerman, and Belton A. Burrows, "Effects of Dieting and Exercise on Lean Body Mass, Oxygen Uptake, and Strength," *Medicine and Science in Sports and Exercise* 17 (1985): 466–71; J. E. Lindsay Carter and William H. Phillips, "Structural Changes in Exercising Middle-Aged Males During a Two-Year Period," *Journal of Applied Physiology* 27 (1969): 787–94; Mary Ellen Sweeney, James O. Hill, Patricia A. Heller, et al., "Severe vs. Moderate Energy Restriction with and Without Exercise in the Treatment of Obesity: Efficiency of Weight Loss," *American Journal of Clinical Nutrition* 57 (1993): 127–34; A. D. Lemmons, S. N. Kreitzman, A. Coxon, and A. Howard, "Selection of Appropriate Exercise Regimens for Weight Reduction During VLCD and Maintenance," *International Journal of Obesity* 13 (1989): 119–23.

41. Douglas L. Ballor and Eric T. Poehlman, "Resting Metabolic Rate and Coronary-Heart-Disease Risk Factors in Aerobically and Resistance-Trained Women," *American Journal of Clinical Nutrition* 56 (1992): 968–74.

42. G. A. Gaesser and G. A. Brooks, "Muscular Efficiency During Steady-Rate Exercise: Effects of Speed and Work Rate," *Journal of Applied Physiology* 38 (1975): 1132–39; Douglas L. Ballor, John P. McCarthy, and E. Joan Wilterdink, "Exercise Intensity Does Not Affect the Composition of Diet- and Exercise-Induced Body Mass Loss," *American Journal of Clinical Nutrition* 51 (1990): 142–46.

43. J. L. Herring, P. A. Molé, C. N. Meredith, and J. S. Stern, "Effect of Suspending Exercise Training on Resting Metabolic Rate in Women," *Medicine and Science in Sports and Exercise* 24 (1992): 59–65; Angelo Tremblay, Jean-Pierre Després, Claude Leblanc, et al., "Effect of Intensity of Physical Activity on Body Fatness and Fat Distribution," *American Journal of Clinical Nutrition* 51 (1990): 153–57; D. Lennon, F. Nagle, F. Stratman, et al., "Diet and Exercise Training Effects on Resting Metabolic Rate," *International Journal of Obesity* 9 (1985): 39–47; S. Maehlum, M. Grandmontagne, E. A. Newsholme, and O. M. Sejersted, "Magnitude and Duration of Excess Postexercise Oxygen Consumption in Healthy Young Subjects," *Metabolism* 35 (1986): 425–49; E. T. Poehlman, "A Review: Exercise and Its Influence on Resting Energy Metabolism in Man," *Medicine and Science in Sports and Exercise* 21 (1989): 515–25; R. Bahr and O. M. Sejersted, "Effect of Intensity of Exercise on Excess Postexercise O_2 Consumption," *Metabolism* 40 (1991): 836–41; C. J. Gore and R. T. Withers, "Effect of Exercise Intensity and Duration on Postexercise Metabolism" (and erratum), *Journal of Applied Physiology* 68 (1990): 2362–68, and 69 (1990): 1934; C. E. Broeder, K. A. Burrhus, L. S. Svanevik, and J. H. Wilmore, "The Effects of Aerobic Fitness on Resting Metabolic Rate" and "The Effects of Either High-Intensity Resistance or Endurance Training on Resting Metabolic Rate," *American Journal of Clinical Nutrition* 55 (1992): 795–801; 802–10.

CHAPTER 5: THE GOOD MINUS THE BAD

1. *Lipid Research Clinics Population Studies Data Book, vol. 1, The Prevalence Study*. NIH Publication No. 80–1527. (Washington, D.C.: U.S. Government Printing Office, July 1980).
2. I. Jialal and S. M. Grundy, "Preservation of the Endogenous Antioxidants in Low Density Lipoprotein by Ascorbate But Not Probucol During Oxidative Modification," *Journal of Clinical Investigation* 87 (1991): 597–601.
3. N. E. Miller, "Raising High Density Lipoprotein Cholesterol. The Biochemical Pharmacology of Reverse Cholesterol Transport," *Biochemistry and Pharmacology* 40 (1990): 403–10.
4. Dr. Redford Williams, quoted in Ann Landers, "Curb Anger, Live Longer," *Boston Globe,* 17 Jan. 1990, p. 66.
5. Lawrence K. Altman, "A Bald Spot on Top May Predict Heart Risk," *New York Times,* 24 Feb. 1993, p. 1.
6. Samuel M. Lesko, Lynn Rosenberg, and Samuel Shapiro, "A

Case-Control Study of Baldness in Relation to Myocardial Infarction in Men," *Journal of the American Medical Association* 269 (1993): 998–1003.

7. Cf. Christopher J. Georges, "Studies Find a Link Between Aggressiveness and Cholesterol Levels," *New York Times,* 11 Sept. 1990, and Gina Kolata, "Cholesterol's New Image: High Is Bad; So Is Low," *New York Times,* 11 Aug. 1992, p. C1, with Jane E. Brody, "Study Seems to Ease Fear on Low Cholesterol Level," *New York Times,* 21 March 1993, p. 25.

8. I measure total cholesterol, as well as LDL, HDL, and VLDL cholesterol, in units of "milligrams per deciliter," which is standard for U.S. clinical laboratories. The total cholesterol cutoffs come from "Report of the National Cholesterol Education Program Expert Panel on Detection, Evaluation, and Treatment of High Blood Cholesterol in Adults," *Archives of Internal Medicine* 148 (1988): 36–69; National Cholesterol Education Program, *Report of the Expert Panel on Population Strategies for Blood Cholesterol Reduction: Executive Summary* (Washington, D.C.: U.S. Department of Health and Human Services, November 1990), NIH publication no. 90–3047. In new guidelines from the National Cholesterol Education Program, to be issued in June 1993, these total cholesterol cutoffs will remain unchanged.

9. M. Miller, L. A. Mead, P. O. Kwiterovich, Jr., and T. A. Pearson, "Dyslipidemias with Desirable Plasma Cholesterol Levels and Angiographically Demonstrated Coronary Artery Disease," *American Journal of Cardiology* 65 (1990): 1–5; M. Miller, A. Seidler, P. O. Kwiterovich, Jr., and T. A. Pearson, "Long-Term Predictors of Subsequent Cardiovascular Events with Coronary Artery Disease and 'Desirable' Levels of Plasma Total Cholesterol," *Circulation* 86 (1992): 1165–70.

10. In the Lipid Research Clinics Prevalence Mortality Follow-up Study, each one-point increase in LDL cholesterol raised coronary risk by 1.3 percent in men and 1.0 percent in women. In the Coronary Primary Prevention Trial, each one-point increase in LDL cholesterol raised coronary risk by 1.1 percent in men. The corresponding LDL-cholesterol effects in other major U.S. trials were: the Multiple Risk Factor Intervention Trial, 1.0 percent for men; and the Framingham Heart Study, 0.6 percent for men and 1.2 percent for women. See David J. Gordon, "Is HDL a Risk Factor?" in NIH Consensus Development Conference, *Triglyceride, High Density Lipoprotein, and Coronary Heart Disease* (Bethesda, Md.: National Institutes of Health, February 26–28, 1992): 21–24; and David J. Gordon, communi-

cation to author, April 12, 1993. In the text, I have given a range of 1.0 to 1.5 percent to take into account statistical uncertainty in the estimated LDL-cholesterol-effects. In one statistical "meta-analysis" of the major studies of cholesterol and coronary heart disease, the authors estimated that each 1 percent decline in L was estimated to produce a 2 percent decline in coronary risk. But that study related percentage changes in L, not LDL cholesterol points, to coronary risk. In the major studies, the average L was about 190, so a 1 percent change in L would correspond to 1.9 points. That means each 1.9-point decline in LDL cholesterol would result in a 2 percent decline in coronary risk, which is consistent with my estimates. See M. F. Muldoon, S. B. Manuck, and K. A. Matthews, "Lowering Cholesterol Concentrations and Mortality: A Quantitative Review of Primary Prevention Trials," *British Medical Journal* 301 (1990): 309–14.

11. "Report of the National Cholesterol Education Program Expert Panel on Detection, Evaluation, and Treatment of High Blood Cholesterol in Adults."

12. NIH Consensus Development Panel on Triglyceride, High-Density Lipoprotein, and Coronary Heart Disease, "Triglyceride, High-Density Lipoprotein, and Coronary Heart Disease," *Journal of the American Medical Association* 269 (1993): 505–10. See also: *Triglyceride, High-Density Lipoprotein, and Coronary Heart Disease.*

13. D. J. Gordon, J. L. Probstfield, R. J. Garrison, et al., "High-Density Lipoprotein Cholesterol and Cardiovascular Disease. Four Prospective American Studies," *Circulation* 79 (1989): 8–15.

14. In the process of triglyceride unloading, VLDL can assume a transitional form called IDL (Intermediate-Density Lipoprotein). IDL Transport Trucks, which are only partially stripped of triglyceride, can then go on to become LDL Trucks, or they can return directly to IDL Unloading Docks in the liver's Grand Central Truck Station.

15. Lipid Research Clinics Investigators, "The Lipid Research Clinics Coronary Primary Prevention Trial: Results of 6 Years of Post-Trial Follow-Up," *Archives of Internal Medicine* 152 (1992): 1399–1410; Lipid Research Clinics Investigators, "The Lipid Research Clinics Coronary Primary Prevention Trial Results: II. The Relationship of Reduction in Incidence of CHD to Cholesterol Lowering," *Journal of the American Medical Association* 251 (1984): 365–74.

16. P. L. Canner, K. G. Berge, N. K. Wenger, et al., "Fifteen-Year

Mortality in Coronary Drug Project Patients: Long-Term Benefit with Niacin," *Journal of the American College of Cardiology* 8 (1986): 1245–55.

17. M. Heikki Frick, Olli Elo, Kauko Haapa, et al., "Helsinki Heart Study: Primary-Prevention Trial with Gemfibozil in Middle-Aged Men with Dyslipidemia," *New England Journal of Medicine* 317 (1987): 1237–45.

18. R. I. Levy, J. F. Brensike, S. E. Epstein, et al., "The Influence of Changes in Lipid Values Induced by Cholestyramine and Diet on Progression of Coronary Artery Disease: Results of NHLBI Type II Coronary Intervention Study," *Circulation* 69 (1984): 325–37.

19. D. H. Blankenhorn, S. A. Nessim, R. L. Johnson, et al., "Beneficial Effects of Combined Colestipol-Niacin Therapy on Coronary Atherosclerosis and Coronary Venous Bypass Grafts," *Journal of the American Medical Association* 257 (1987): 3233–40; D. H. Blankenhorn, S. P. Azen, D. W. Crawford, et al., "Effects of Colestipol-Niacin Therapy on Human Femoral Atherosclerosis," *Circulation* 83 (1991): 438–47.

20. Greg Brown, John J. Albers, Lloyd D. Fisher, et al., "Regression of Coronary Artery Disease as a Result of Intensive Lipid-Lowering Therapy in Men with High Levels of Apolipoprotein B," *New England Journal of Medicine* 323 (1990): 1289–98.

21. Yaakov Henkin, David W. Garber, Laura C. Osterlund, and Betty E. Darnell, "Saturated Fats, Cholesterol, and Dietary Compliance," *Archives of Internal Medicine* 152 (1992): 1167–74.

22. D. Ornish, S. E. Brown, L. W. Scherwitz, et al., "Can Lifestyle Changes Reverse Coronary Heart Disease? The Lifestyle Heart Trial," *Lancet* 336 (1990): 129–33. See Sandra Blakeslee, "Arteries Are Unblocked Without Drugs in Study," *New York Times,* 21 July 1990.

23. In the Helsinki Heart Study, the drug-treated group achieved a 16-point drop in L and a 5-point rise in H. This would mean a 26-point drop in my J index. If every 1-point drop in J were associated with a 1.0 to 1.5 percent decline in coronary risk, then the drug-treated group would have a predicted 26 to 39 percent decline in coronary rates. In fact, the drug-treated group had a 34 percent lower CHD incidence rate, which is right on target. See table 2 and text in Frick, et al., "Helsinki Heart Study." Some specialists may argue that we already have other compound cholesterol-lipoprotein indices, such as the $C{:}H$ ratio and the $L{:}H$ ratio. I have found these ratio-type indices worse than useless in general medical practice. Sometimes they

are quite misleading. In any case, they don't fit the data as well as *J* does.

24. C. E. Davis, D. Gordon, J. LaRosa, et al, "Correlations of Plasma High Density Lipoprotein Cholesterol Levels with Other Plasma Lipid and Lipoprotein Concentrations," *Circulation* 62 (1980, suppl. IV): IV24–IV30. In men, the correlation between *H* and *L* is less than 0.1. There is a slightly greater correlation in women who are treated with postmenopausal estrogens.

25. Carlos A. Dujovne and William S. Harris, "Variabilities in Serum Lipid Measurements: Do They Impede Proper Diagnosis and Treatment of Dyslipidemia?" *Archives of Internal Medicine* 150 (1990): 1583–85; Lisa Bookstein, Samuel S. Gidding, Mark Donovan, and Frederick A. Smith, "Day-to-Day Variability of Serum Cholesterol, Triglyceride, and High-Density Lipoprotein Cholesterol Levels," *Archives of Internal Medicine* 150 (1990): 1653–57; Michael Mogadam, Susan W. Ahmed, Arthur H. Mensch, and Ira D. Godwin, "Within-Person Fluctuations of Serum Cholesterol and Lipoproteins," *Archives of Internal Medicine* 150 (1990): 1645–48.

26. A rather striking example is the Helsinki Heart Study, where *C, L, H,* and *T* values varied seasonally even among people taking cholesterol-lowering drugs. See Frick et al., "Helsinki Heart Study." See also D. J. Gordon, D. C. Trost, J. Hyde, et al., "Seasonal Cholesterol Cycles: The Lipid Research Clinics Coronary Primary Prevention Trial Placebo Group," *Circulation* 76 (1987): 1224–31.

27. Matthew F. Muldoon, Elizabeth A. Bachen, Stephen B. Manuck, et al., "Acute Cholesterol Responses to Mental Stress and Change in Posture," *Archives of Internal Medicine* 152 (1992): 775–80.

28. T. A. Gerace, J. Hollis, J. K. Ockene, and K. Svendsen, "Smoking Cessation and Change in Diastolic Blood Pressure, Body Weight, and Plasma Lipids," *Preventive Medicine* 20 (1991): 602–20; Michael Criqui, L. D. Cowan, H. A. Tyroler, et al., "Lipoproteins as Mediators for the Effects of Alcohol Consumption and Cigarette Smoking on Cardiovascular Mortality: Results from the Lipid Research Clinics Follow-up Study," *American Journal of Epidemiology* 126 (1987): 629–37; R. J. Moffatt, "Normalization of High Density Lipoprotein Cholesterol Following Cessation from Cigarette Smoking," *Advances in Experimental Medicine and Biology* 273 (1990): 267–72; A. G. Olsson and J. Molgaard, "Relations Between Smoking, Food Intake, and Plasma Lipoproteins," *Advances in Experimental Medicine and Biology* 273 (1990): 237–43; M. Quensel, A. Soderstrom, C. D.

Agardh, and P. Nilsson-Ehle, "High Density Lipoprotein Concentrations After Cessation of Smoking: The Importance of Alterations in Diet," *Atherosclerosis* 75 (1989): 189–93.

29. M. Higuchi, K. Iwaoka, T. Fuchi, et al., "Relation of Running Distance to Plasma HDL-Cholesterol Level in Middle-Aged Male Runners," *Clinical Physiology* 9 (1989): 121–30; B. F. Hurley, "Effects of Resistive Training on Lipoprotein-Lipid Profiles: A Comparison to Aerobic Exercise Training," *Medicine and Science in Sports and Exercise* 21 (1989): 689–93; P. D. Reaven, J. B. McPhillips, E. L. Barrett-Connor, and M. H. Criqui, "Leisure Time Exercise and Lipid and Lipoprotein Levels in an Older Population," *Journal of the American Geriatric Society* 38 (1990): 847–54; R. M. Schieken, "Effect of Exercise on Lipids," *Annals of the New York Academy of Sciences* 623 (1991): 269–74; R. A. Stein, D. W. Michielli, M. D. Glantz, et al., "Effects of Different Exercise Training Intensities on Lipoprotein Cholesterol Fractions in Healthy Middle-Aged Men," *American Heart Journal* 119 (1990): 277–83; H. R. Superko, "Exercise Training, Serum Lipids, and Lipoprotein Particles: Is There a Change Threshold?" *Medicine and Science in Sports and Exercise* 23 (1991): 677–685; J. Stray-Gundersen, M. A. Denke, and S. M. Grundy, "Influence of Lifetime Cross-Country Skiing on Plasma Lipids and Lipoproteins," *Medicine and Science in Sports and Exercise* 23 (1991): 695–702.

30. E. Barrett-Connor and T. L. Bush, "Estrogen Replacement and Coronary Heart Disease," *Cardiovascular Clinics* 30 (1989): 159–72; T. L. Bush, E. Barrett-Connor, L. D. Cowan, et al., "Cardiovascular Mortality and Noncontraceptive Use of Estrogen in Women: Results from the Lipid Research Clinics Program Follow-up Study," *Circulation* 75 (1987): 1102–9; P. L. Colvin, Jr., B. J. Auerbach, L. D. Case, et al., "A Dose-Response Relationship Between Sex Hormone-Induced Change in Hepatic Triglyceride Lipase and High-Density Lipoprotein Cholesterol in Postmenopausal Women," *Metabolism* 40 (1991): 1052–56; R. A. Lobo, "Clinical Review 27: Effects of Hormonal Replacement on Lipids and Lipoproteins in Postmenopausal Women," *Journal of Clinical Endocrinology and Metabolism* 73 (1991): 925–30; M. J. Stampfer and G. A. Colditz, "Estrogen Replacement Therapy and Coronary Heart Disease: A Quantitative Assessment of the Epidemiological Evidence," *Preventive Medicine* 20 (1991): 47–63.

31. Criqui, et al., "Lipoproteins as Mediators for the Effects of Alcohol Consumption and Cigarette Smoking on Cardiovascular Mortality"; J. A. Cauley, L. H. Kuller, R. E. LaPorte, et al.,

"Studies on the Association Between Alcohol and High Density Lipoprotein Cholesterol: Possible Benefits and Risks," *Advances in Alcohol and Substance Abuse* 6 (1987): 53–67; R. A. Hegele, "Alcohol and Atherosclerosis Risk," *Canadian Medical Association Journal* 145 (1991): 317; G. Weidner, S. L. Connor, M. A. Chesney, et al., "Sex Differences in High Density Lipoprotein Cholesterol Among Low-level Alcohol Consumers" (and erratum), *Circulation* 83 (1991): 176–80, 1461; M. Hagiage, C. Marti, D. Rigaud, et al., "Effect of a Moderate Alcohol Intake on the Lipoproteins of Normotriglyceridemic Obese Subjects Compared with Normoponderal Controls," *Metabolism* 41 (1992): 856–61; I. Suh, B. J. Shaten, J. Cutler, and L. H. Kuller, "Alcohol Use and Mortality from Coronary Heart Disease: The Role of High-Density Lipoprotein Cholesterol," *Annals of Internal Medicine* 116 (1992): 881–87; R. D. Langer, M. H. Criqui, and D. M. Reed, "Lipoproteins and Blood Pressure as Biological Pathways for Effect of Moderate Alcohol Consumption on Coronary Heart Disease," *Circulation* 85 (1992): 910–15.

32. Some researchers have suggested that French wine may also keep blood clots from forming atop atherosclerotic plaques in coronary arteries. See S. Renaud and M. de Lorgeril, "Wine, Alcohol, Platelets, and the French Paradox for Coronary Heart Disease," *Lancet* 339 (1992): 1523–26; D. Sharp, "When Wine is Red," *Lancet* 341 (1993): 27–28; M. Nestle, "Wine and Coronary Heart Disease" (letter), *Lancet* 340 (1992): 314–15; S. C. Renaud, A. D. Beswick, A. M. Fehily, et al., "Alcohol and Platelet Aggregation: The Caerphilly Prospective Heart Disease Study," *American Journal of Clinical Nutrition* 55 (1992): 1012–17.

33. Henkin et al., "Saturated Fats, Cholesterol, and Dietary Compliance."

34. U.S. Food and Drug Administration, "Food Labeling; General Provisions; Nutrition Labeling; Label Format; Nutrient Content Claims; Health Claims; Ingredient Labeling; State and Local Requirements; and Exemptions; Final Rules," *Federal Register* 58 (two books, January 6, 1993): 467–2300, 2301–2964; U.S. Food and Drug Administration, "New Food Labeling Regulations Issued," *FDA Medical Bulletin* 23 (March 1993): 3–4, 10.

35. Kaj N. Seidelin, Søren Meisner, and Klaus Bukhave, "Percentage Distribution of Fatty Acids in Subcutaneous Adipose Tissue of Patients with Peptic Ulcer Disease," *American Journal of Clinical Nutrition* 57 (1993): 70–72.

36. Actually, about 7 out of 10 LDL Trucks dock at the Grand Central Truck Station in the liver. Some of the remaining LDL Trucks dock at the adrenal glands, where the cholesterol is used to make the body's internal steroids. The scientific name for the LDL Truck Docking Stations is the "LDL Receptor." See: M.S. Brown and J.L. Goldstein, "A Receptor-Mediated Pathway for Cholesterol Homeostasis," *Science* 234 (1986): 34–47.

37. G. L. Vega, M. A. Denke, and S. M. Grundy, "Metabolic Basis of Primary Hypercholesterolemia," *Circulation* 84 (1991): 118–28.

38. D. K. Spady and L. A. Woollett, "Interaction of Dietary Saturated and Polyunsaturated Triglycerides in Regulating the Processes That Determine Plasma Low-Density Lipoprotein Concentrations in the Rat," *Journal of Lipid Research* 31 (1990): 1809–19.

39. D. M. Hegsted, "Serum Cholesterol Response to Dietary Cholesterol: A Re-Evaluation," *American Journal of Clinical Nutrition* 44 (1986): 299–305; D. M. Hegsted, R. D. McGandy, M. L. Myers, and F. J. Stare, "Quantitative Effects of Dietary Fat on Serum Cholesterol in Man," *American Journal of Clinical Nutrition* 17 (1965): 237–42; D. M. Hegsted, "Egg Consumption and Serum Cholesterol" (letter), *American Journal of Clinical Nutrition* 57 (1993): 87–88.

40. K. C. Hayes, A. Pronczuk, S. Lindsey, et al., "Dietary Saturated Fatty Acids (12:0, 14:0, 16:0) Differ in Their Impact on Plasma Cholesterol and Lipoproteins in Nonhuman Primates," *American Journal of Clinical Nutrition* 53 (1991): 491–98; S. M. Grundy and M. A. Denke, "Dietary Influences on Serum Lipids and Lipoproteins," *Journal of Lipid Research* 31 (1990): 1149–72; K. Sundram, A. H. Hassan, O. H. Siru, and K. C. Hayes, "Dietary Palmitate Lowers Cholesterol Relative to Laurate and Myristate in Humans" (abstract), *Arteriosclerosis and Thrombosis* 11 (1991): 1614; T. K. W. Ng, K. C. Hayes, G. F. DeWitt, et al., "Dietary Palmitic and Oleic Acids Exert Similar Effects on Serum Cholesterol and Lipoprotein Profiles in Normocholesterolemic Men and Women," *Journal of the American College of Nutrition* 11 (1992): 383–90.

41. A. Bonanome and S. M. Grundy, "Effect of Dietary Stearic Acid on Plasma Cholesterol and Lipoprotein Levels," *New England Journal of Medicine* 318 (1988): 1244–48.

42. S. M. Grundy, L. Florentin, D. Nix, and M. F. Whelan, "Comparison of Monounsaturated Fatty Acids and Carbohydrates for Reducing Raised Levels of Plasma Cholesterol in Man," *Ameri-*

can Journal of Clinical Nutrition 47 (1988): 965–69; S. M. Grundy, "Monounsaturated Fatty Acids and Cholesterol Metabolism: Implications for Dietary Recommendations," *Journal of Nutrition* 119 (1989): 529–33; J. C. Shepherd, C. J. Packard, J. R. Patsch, et al., "Effects of Dietary Polyunsaturated and Saturated Fat on the Properties of High-Density Lipoprotein and the Metabolism of Apolipoprotein A-I," *Journal of Clinical Investigation* 60 (1978): 1582–92.

43. S. M. Grundy and G. L. Vega, "Plasma Cholesterol Responsiveness to Saturated Fatty Acids," *American Journal of Clinical Nutrition* 47 (1988): 822–24.

44. During the process of partial hydrogenation, some of the "double-bonds" of the unsaturated fatty acids are resaturated. But other double-bonds are converted from the natural *cis* configuration to an artificial *trans* configuration. M. C. Linder, *Nutritional Biochemistry and Metabolism with Clinical Applications* (New York: Elsevier, 1985).

45. R. P. Mensink and M. B. Katan, "Effect of Dietary Trans Fatty Acids on High-Density and Low-Density Lipoprotein Cholesterol Levels in Healthy Subjects," *New England Journal of Medicine* 323 (1990): 439–45; S. M. Grundy, "Trans Monounsaturated Fatty Acids and Serum Cholesterol Levels" (editorial), *New England Journal of Medicine* 323 (1990): 480–81.

46. R. M. Reves, "Effect of Dietary Trans Fatty Acids on Cholesterol Levels," *New England Journal of Medicine* 324 (1991): 338–39.

47. Rebecca Troisi, Walter C. Willett, and Scott T. Weiss, "Trans Fatty Acid Intake in Relation to Serum Lipid Concentrations in Adult Men," *American Journal of Clinical Nutrition* 56 (1992): 1019–24.

48. Walter C. Willett, Meier J. Stampfer, JoAnn E. Mason, et. al., "Intake of Trans Fatty Acids and Risk of Coronary Heart Disease in Women," *Lancet* 341 (1993): 581–85.

49. G. J. Hopkins, T. G. Kennedy, and K. K. Carroll, "Polyunsaturated Fatty Acids as Promoters of Mammary Carcinogenesis Induced in Sprague-Dawley Rats by 7,12-Dimethylbenz[a]anthracene," *Journal of the American Cancer Insitute* 66 (1981): 517–22; Catherine E. Woteki and Paul R. Thomas, *Eat for Life: The Food and Nutrition Board's Guide to Reducing Your Risk of Chronic Disease* (Washington, D.C.: National Academy Press, 1992).

50. Frank M. Sacks and Walter W. Willett, "More on Chewing the Fat: The Good Fat and the Good Cholesterol" (editorial), *New England Journal of Medicine* 325 (1991): 1740–42.

51. J. T. Knuiman, C. E. West, M. B. Katan, et al., "Total Choles-

terol and High Density Lipoprotein Cholesterol Levels in Populations Differing in Fat and Carbohydrate Intake," *Arteriosclerosis* 7 (1987): 612–19.

52. H. Lee-Han, M. Cousins, M. Beaton, et al., "Compliance in a Randomized Clinical Trial of Dietary Fat Reduction in Patients with Breast Dysplasia," *American Journal of Clinical Nutrition* 48 (1988): 575–86.

53. Edward P. Havranek, "Lipid Levels and 'Affluent' Diets" (letter), *New England Journal of Medicine* 327 (1992): 53.

54. H. H. Vorster, A. J. S. Benade, H. C. Barnard, et al., "Egg Intake Does Not Change Plasma Lipoproteins and Coagulation Profiles," *American Journal of Clinical Nutrition* 55 (1992): 400–410. See also D. M. Hegsted, "Egg Consumption and Serum Cholesterol" (letter), and Hester H. Vorster, "Reply to Hegsted" (letter), *American Journal of Clinical Nutrition* 57 (1993): 87–89.

55. D. Kromhout, E. B. Bosschieter, C. Coulander, et al., "The Inverse Relationship Between Fish Consumption and 20-Year Mortality from Coronary Heart Disease," *New England Journal of Medicine* 312 (1985): 1205–9; S. E. Norell, A. Ahlbom, M. Feychting, and N. L. Pederson, "Fish Consumption and Mortality from Coronary Heart Disease," *British Medical Journal* 293 (1986): 426–40; D. J. Hunter, I. Kazda, A. Chockalingam, and J.G. Fodor, "Fish Consumption and Cardiovascular Mortality in Canada: An Inter-regional Comparison," *American Journal of Preventive Medicine* 4 (1988): 5–10.

56. Joan Sabaté, Gary E. Fraser, Kenneth Burke, et al., "Effects of Walnuts on Serum Lipid Levels and Blood Pressure in Normal Men," *New England Journal of Medicine* 328 (1993): 603–7.

57. Gary E. Fraser, Joan Sabaté, W. Lawrence Beeson, and T. Martin Strahan, "A Possible Protective Effect of Nut Consumption on Risk of Coronary Heart Disease. The Adventist Health Study," *Archives of Internal Medicine* 152 (1992): 1416–24.

58. I. K. Crombie, W. C. Smith, R. Tavendale, et al., "Geographical Clustering of Risk Factors and Lifestyle for Coronary Heart Disease in the Scottish Heart Health Study," *British Heart Journal* 64 (1990): 199–203; W. C. Smith, M. C. Shewry, H. Tunstall-Pedoe, et al., "Cardiovascular Disease in Edinburgh and North Glasgow—A Tale of Two Cities," *Journal of Clinical Epidemiology* 43 (1990): 637–43; A. J. Lee, W. C. Smith, G. D. Lowe, and H. Tunstall-Pedoe, "Plasma Fibrinogen and Coronary Risk Factors: The Scottish Heart Health Study," *Journal of Clinical Epidemiology* 43 (1990): 913–19.

59. Blossom H. Patterson, Gladys Block, and William F. Rosenberger, "Fruit and Vegetables in the American Diet: Data from the NHANES II Survey," *American Journal of Public Health* 80 (1992): 1443–49.

CHAPTER 6: SMOKING AND NOTHINGNESS

1. "Cigarette Smoking Among Adults—United States, 1991," *Morbidity and Mortality Weekly Report* 42 (1993): 230–33.
2. In the 1987 National Health Interview Survey (NHIS), 31.6 percent of current smokers had temporarily quit smoking for at least one day during the past year. See U.S. Department of Health and Human Services, *The Health Benefits of Smoking Cessation: A Report of the Surgeon General* (Washington, D.C.: U.S. Government Printing Office, 1990), DHHS publication no. (CDC) 90–8416, vol. app., table 5. I multiplied the latter percentage by the total number of current smokers (46.3 million in 1991) in order to obtain my estimate of 15 million unsuccessful quitters each year. Other surveys, however, suggest that a higher proportion of smokers may try unsuccessfully to quit. In the 1989 CMA Survey, for example, 41 percent of Canadian smokers tried unsuccessfully to quit during the past year. See Jeffrey E. Harris, "Cigarette Advertising and Promotion in Canada: Effects on Cigarette Smoking and Public Health," Expert Report in *RJR-MacDonald Inc. vs Attorney General of Canada* (Montréal, Québec: Department of Justice, Canada, August 7, 1989), table 9.
3. In the 1987 NHIS, 81.3 percent of current smokers had tried to quit smoking at some time in the past. See U.S. Department of Health and Human Services, *The Health Benefits of Smoking Cessation,* vol. app., table 5. I multiplied the latter percentage by the total number of current smokers in order to obtain my estimate that 38 million current smokers had tried to stop at one time or another.
4. T. J. Glynn, M. W. Manley, and T. F. Pechacek, "Physician-Initiated Smoking Cessation Program: The National Cancer Institute Trials," in *Advances in Cancer Control: Screening and Prevention Research,* ed., P. F. Engstrom, B. Rimer, and L. E. Mortenson (New York: Wiley-Liss, 1990), pp. 11–25; T. E. Kottke, R. N. Battista, G. H. Defriese, and M. L. Brekke, "Attributes of Successful Smoking Cessation Interventions in Medical Practice. A Meta-Analysis of 39 Controlled Trials," *Journal of the American Medical Association* 259 (1988): 2882–89; R. Y. Demers,

A. V. Neale, R. Adams, et al., "The Impact of Physicians' Brief Smoking Cessation Counseling: A MIRNET Study," *Journal of Family Practice* 31 (1990): 625–29; L. I. Solberg, P. L. Maxwell, T. E. Kottke, et al., "A Systematic Primary Care Office-Based Smoking Cessation Program," *Journal of Family Practice* 30 (1990): 647–54; L. M. Nett, "The Physician's Role in Smoking Cessation: A Present and Future Agenda," *Chest* 97 (1990, suppl. 2): 28S–32S; S. R. Cummings, T. J. Coates, R. J. Richard, et al., "Training Physicians in Counseling About Smoking Cessation. A Randomized Trial of the 'Quit for Life' Program," *Annals of Internal Medicine* 110 (1989): 640–47; D. M. Wilson, D. W. Taylor, J. R. Gilbert, et al., "A Randomized Trial of a Family Physician Intervention for Smoking Cessation," *Journal of the American Medical Association* 260 (1988): 1570–74.

5. J. E. Seely, E. Zuskin, and A. Bouhys, "Cigarette Smoking: Objective Evidence for Lung Damage in Teenagers," *Science* 172 (1971): 741–43; G. J. Beck, C. A. Doyle, and E. N. Schachter, "Smoking and Lung Function," *American Review of Respiratory Diseases* 123 (1981): 149–55; U.S. Department of Health and Human Services, *The Health Consequences of Smoking—Chronic Obstructive Lung Disease: A Report of the Surgeon General, 1984* (Washington, D.C.: U.S. Government Printing Office, 1984), DHHS publication no. (PHS) 84–50205.

6. D. E. Niewoehner, J. Kleinerman, and D. B. Rice, "Pathologic Changes in the Peripheral Airways of Young Cigarette Smokers," *New England Journal of Medicine* 291 (1974): 755–58.

7. R. J. Knudson and M.D. Lebowitz, "Comparison of Flow-Volume and Closing Volume Variables in a Random Population," *American Review of Respiratory Disease* 116 (1977): 1039–45; J. Manfreda, N. Nelson, and R. M. Cherniack, "Prevalence of Respiratory Abnormalities in a Rural and an Urban Community," *American Review of Respiratory Disease* 117 (1978): 215–26; B. Nemery, N. E. Moavero, L. Brasseru, and D. C. Stanescu, "Significance of Small Airways Tests in Middle-Aged Smokers," *American Review of Respiratory Disease* 124 (1982): 232–38.

8. A. S. Buist, H. Shezzo, N. R. Anthonisen, et al., "Relationship Between the Single-Breath N_2 Test and Age, Sex, and Smoking Habit in Three North American Cities," *American Review of Respiratory Disease* 120 (1979): 305–18.

9. D. W. Dockery, F. E. Speizer, B. G. Ferris, Jr., et al., "Cumulative and Reversible Effects of Lifetime Smoking on Simple Tests of Lung Function in Adults," *American Review of Respiratory Disease* 137 (1988): 286–92.

10. M. P. Rosen, A. J. Greenfield, T. G. Walker, et al., "Cigarette Smoking: An Independent Risk Factor for Atherosclerosis in the Hypogastric-Cavernous Arterial Bed of Men with Arteriogenic Impotence," *Journal of Urology* 145 (1991): 759–63.

11. L. Lissner, C. Bengtsson, L. Lapidus, and C. Bjorkelund, "Smoking Initiation and Cessation in Relation to Body Fat Distribution Based on Data from a Study of Swedish Women," *American Journal of Public Health* 82 (1992): 273–75; R. J. Moffatt and S. G. Owens, "Cessation from Cigarette Smoking: Changes in Body Weight, Body Composition, Resting Metabolism, and Energy Consumption," *Metabolism* 40 (1991): 465–70; R. J. Troisi, J. W. Heinold, P. S. Vokonas, and S. T. Weiss, "Cigarette Smoking, Dietary Intake, and Physical Activity: Effects on Body Fat Distribution—The Normative Aging Study," *American Journal of Clinical Nutrition* 53 (1991): 1104–11; J. C. Seidell, M. Cigolini, J.-P. Deslypere, et al., "Body Fat Distribution in Relation to Physical Activity and Smoking Habits in 38-year-old European Men. The European Fat Distribution Study," *American Journal of Epidemiology* 133 (1991): 257–65; W. Y. Fujimoto, D. L. Leonetti, R. W. Bergstrom, et al., "Cigarette Smoking, Adiposity, Non-Insulin-Dependent Diabetes, and Coronary Heart Disease in Japanese-American Men," *American Journal of Medicine* 89 (1990): 761–71; E. Barrett-Connor and K. T. Khaw, "Cigarette Smoking and Increased Central Adiposity," *Annals of Internal Medicine* 111 (1989): 783–87.

12. Lynn Rosenberg, David W. Kaufman, Susan P. Helmrich, and Samuel Shapiro, "The Risk of Myocardial Infarction After Quitting Smoking in Men Under 55 Years of Age," *New England Journal of Medicine* 313 (1985): 1511–14; Lynn Rosenberg, Julie R. Palmer, and Samuel Shapiro, "Decline in the Risk of Myocardial Infarction Among Women Who Stop Smoking," *New England Journal of Medicine* 322 (1990): 213–17; Judith K. Ockene, Lewis H. Kuller, Kenneth H. Svendsen, and Elain Meilahn, "The Relationship Between Smoking Cessation to Coronary Heart Disease and Lung Cancer in the Multiple Risk Factor Intervention Trial (MRFIT)," *American Journal of Public Health* 80 (1990): 954–58; U.S. Department of Health and Human Services, *The Health Benefits of Smoking Cessation,* chap. 6, table 2; Walter C. Willett, Adele Green, Meir J. Stampfer, et al., "Relative and Absolute Excess Risks of Coronary Heart Disease Among Women Who Smoke Cigarettes," *New England Journal of Medicine* 317 (1987): 1303–9.

13. W. C. Krupski, G. C. Olive, C. A. Weber, and J. H. Rapp, "Comparative Effects of Hypertension and Nicotine on Injury-Induced Myointimal Thickening," *Surgery* 102 (1987): 409–15; M. Zimmerman and J. McGeachie, "The Effect of Nicotine on Aortic Endothelium: A Comparative Study," *Atherosclerosis* 63 (1987): 33–41. Antioxidants may also reduce lung cancer risk in smokers. See Marylin S. Menkes, George W. Comstock, Jean P. Vuilleumier, et al., "Serum Beta-Carotene, Vitamins A and E, Selenium, and the Risk of Lung Cancer," *New England Journal of Medicine* 315 (1986): 1250–54.

14. R. M. Pittilo, J. M. Clarke, D. Harris, et al., "Cigarette Smoking and Platelet Adhesion," *British Journal of Haematology* 58 (1984): 627–32.

15. U.S. Department of Health and Human Services, *The Health Benefits of Smoking Cessation*, chap. 4, tables 4 and 7.

16. Jeffrey E. Harris, "Changes in Smoking-Attributable Mortality," chap. 3 in U.S. Department of Health and Human Services, *Reducing the Health Consequences of Smoking: 25 Years of Progress. A Report of the Surgeon General* (Washington, D.C.: U.S. Government Printing Office, 1989), DHHS publication no. (CDC) 89–8411, pp. 117–69.

17. Ralph S. Paffenbarger, Jr., Robert T. Hyde, Alvin L. Wing, et al., "The Association of Changes in Physical-Activity Level and Other Lifestyle Characteristics with Mortality Among Men," *New England Journal of Medicine* 328 (1993): 538–45, table 4.

18. U.S. Department of Health and Human Services, *The Health Benefits of Smoking Cessation*, chap. 3, tables 3 and 8. These estimates apply to male smokers of more than one pack daily, such as Andrew. The statistical error ranges are continuing smokers, 67 to 70 percent; quitters, 77 to 82 percent; and men who never smoked, 88 to 89 percent.

19. T. A. Gerace, J. Hollis, J. K. Ockene, and K. Svendsen, "Smoking Cessation and Change in Diastolic Blood Pressure, Body Weight, and Plasma Lipids," *Preventive Medicine* 20 (1991): 602–20.

20. U.S. Department of Health and Human Services, *The Health Consequences of Smoking: Nicotine Addiction* (Washington, D.C.: U.S. Government Printing Office, 1988), DHHS publication no. (CDC) 88–8406; U.S. Department of Health and Human Services, *The Health Benefits of Smoking Cessation*.

21. American Psychological Association, *Diagnostic and Statistical Manual of Mental Disorders*, 3rd ed., rev. (Washington, D.C.:

American Psychiatric Association, 1987), pp. 165–68.

22. Jerome R. Head, "The Effects of Smoking," *Illinois Medical Journal* 76 (1939): 283–87.

23. Jeffrey E. Harris, "Experts' Report on Risk-Utility Analysis," in *Cipollone v. Liggett Group, et al.* (Newark, N.J.: U.S. District Court, January 17, 1986). See also J. H. Jaffe, "Trivializing Dependence," *British Journal of Addiction* 85 (1990): 1425–31.

24. J. R. Hughes, S. T. Higgins, and D. Hatsukami, "Effects of Abstinence from Tobacco: A Critical Review," in *Research Advances in Alcohol and Drug Problems*, vol. 10, ed. L. T. Kozlowski, H. Annis, H. D. Cappell, et al. (New York: Plenum Press, 1990), pp. 317–98.

25. J. C. Barefoot and M. Girodo, "The Misattribution of Smoking Cessation Symptoms," *Canadian Journal of Behavioral Science* 4 (1972): 358–63.

26. K. M. Cummings, G. Giovino, G. Jaèn, and L. J. Emrich, "Reports of Smoking Withdrawal Symptoms over a 21-Day Period of Abstinence," *Addictive Behaviors* 10 (1985): 373–81; Saul M. Shiffman and Murray E. Jarvik, "Smoking Withdrawal Symptoms in Two Weeks of Abstinence," *Psychopharmacology* 50 (1976): 35–39.

27. J. Gross and M. L. Stitzer, "Nicotine Replacement: Ten-Week Effects on Tobacco Withdrawal Symptoms," *Psychopharmacology* 98 (1989): 334–41; F. R. Snyder and J. E. Henningfield, "Effects of Nicotine Administration Following 12 Hours of Tobacco Deprivation: Assessment on Computerized Performance Tasks," *Psychopharmacology* 97 (1989): 17–22; J. R. Hughes, S. W. Gust, and T. F. Pechacek, "Prevalence of Tobacco Dependence and Withdrawal," *American Journal of Psychiatry* 144 (1987): 205–8.

28. J. R. Hughes, S. W. Gust, K. Skoog, et al., "Symptoms of Tobacco Withdrawal. A Replication and Extension," *Archives of General Psychiatry* 48 (1991): 52–59.

29. R. J. West, P. Hajek, and M. Belcher, "Severity of Withdrawal Symptoms as a Predictor of Outcome of an Attempt to Quit Smoking," *Psychological Medicine* 19 (1989): 981–85; E. R. Gritz, C. R. Carr and A. C. Marcus, "The Tobacco Withdrawal Syndrome in Unaided Quitters," *British Journal of Addiction* 86 (1991): 57–69.

30. To statisticians: Former smokers reported the last date that they smoked. Current smokers reported the starting and ending dates of their last unsuccessful attempt to quit. Accordingly, the reported intervals in the current state (that is, the time since

relapsing for current smokers and time since quitting for non-smokers) are subject to length-biased sampling, and the reported interval in the prior state (that is, the duration of the last failed attempt among current smokers) may also be biased. The chart is derived from nonparametric, maximum-likelihood estimates of the joint distribution function for quit and relapse intervals under the stationarity assumptions that: the joint distribution of quit and relapse intervals within an arbitrarily chosen cycle is invariant to a translation along the time axis; and the sequence of successive quit events adheres to the length-biased sampling property, that is, the probability that a cycle of length X overlaps a preselected time origin is proportional to X. See D. R. Cox and P. A. W. Lewis, *The Statistical Analysis of Series of Events* (London: Chapman & Hall, 1966), p. 61; G. E. Dinse and S. W. Lagakos, "Nonparametric Estimation of Lifetime and Disease Onset Distributions from Incomplete Observations," *Biometrics* 38 (1982): 921–32; B. W. Turnbull and T. J. Mitchell, "Nonparametric Estimation of the Distribution of Time to Onset for Specific Diseases in Survival/Sacrifice Experiments," *Biometrics* 40 (1984): 41–50; J. S. Williams and S. W. Lagakos, "Models for Censored Survival Analysis: Constant-Sum and Variable-Sum Models," *Biometrika* 64 (1977): 215–24.

31. J. R. Hughes, S. W. Gust, R. M. Keenan, and J. W. Fenwick, "Effect of Dose on Nicotine's Reinforcing, Withdrawal-Suppression, and Self-Reported Effects," *Journal of Pharmacology and Experimental Therapeutics* 252 (1990): 1175–83.

32. S. Chapman, "Stop-Smoking Clinics: A Case for Their Abandonment," *Lancet* 2 (1985): 918–20.

33. Jeffrey E. Harris, "Cigarette Smoking in the United States, 1950–1978," in U.S. Department of Health, Education, and Welfare, *Smoking and Health. A Report of the Surgeon General* (Washington, D.C.: U.S. Government Printing Office, 1979), DHEW publication no. (PHS) 79–50066, pp. A1–A29; Jeffrey E. Harris, "Patterns of Cigarette Smoking," in *The Health Consequences of Smoking for Women. A Report of the Surgeon General* (Washington, D.C.: U.S. Government Printing Office, 1980), pp. 17–42.

34. Jeffrey E. Harris, "The 1983 Increase in the Federal Excise Tax on Cigarettes," in *Tax Policy and the Economy*, vol. 1, ed. Lawrence R. Summers (Cambridge, Mass.: MIT Press, 1987), pp. 87–111.

35. M. C. Fiore, T. E. Novotny, J. P. Pierce, et al., "Methods Used to Quit Smoking in the United States: Do Cessation Programs

Help?" *Journal of the American Medical Association* 263 (1990): 2760–65; "Public Health Focus: Effectiveness of Smoking-Control Strategies—United States," *Morbidity and Mortality Weekly Report* 41 (1992): 645–53.

36. K. Battig, R. Buzzi, R. Nil, "Smoke Yield of Cigarettes and Puffing Behavior in Men and Women," *Psychopharmacology* 76 (1982): 139–48; R. B. Bridges, J. G. Combs, J. W. Humble, et al., "Puffing Topography as a Determinant of Smoke Exposure," *Pharmacology Biochemistry and Behavior* 37 (1990): 29–39; R. Nil, R. Buzzi, and K. Battig, "Effects of Different Cigarette Smoke Yields on Puffing and Inhalation: Is the Measurement of Inhalation Volumes Relevant for Smoke Absorption?" *Pharmacology Biochemistry and Behavior* 24 (1986): 587–95; M. A. H. Russell, M. Jarvis, R. Iyer, and C. Feyerabend, "Relation of Nicotine Yield of Cigarettes to Blood Nicotine Concentrations in Smokers," *British Medical Journal* 280 (1980): 972–76; A. R. Guyatt, A. J. T. Kirkham, A. G. Baldry, et al., "How Does Puffing Behavior Alter During the Smoking of a Single Cigarette?" *Pharmacology Biochemistry and Behavior* 33 (1988) :189–95; A. R. Guyatt, J. T. Kirkham, D. C. Mariner, et al., "Long-Term Effects of Switching to Cigarettes with Lower Tar and Nicotine Yields," *Psychopharmacology* 99 (1989): 80–86.

37. K. O. Fagerstrom, "Efficacy of Nicotine Chewing Gum: A Review," in *Nicotine Replacement: A Critical Evaluation,* ed. O. F. Pomerleau, K. O. Fagerstrom, et al. (New York: Alan R. Liss, 1988), pp. 109–28; W. L. Lam, P. C. Sze, H. S. Sacks, and T. C. Chalmers, "Meta-Analysis of Randomized Controlled Trials of Nicotine Chewing Gum," *Lancet* 2 (1987): 27–29; M. Kornitzer, F. Kittel, M. Dramaix, and P. Bourdoux, "A Double Blind Study of 2 mg vs. 4 mg Nicotine Gum in an Industrial Setting," *Journal of Psychosomatic Research* 31 (1987): 171–76.

38. D. M. Daughton, S. A. Heatley, J. J. Prendergast, et al., "Effect of Transdermal Nicotine Delivery as an Adjunct to Low-Intervention Smoking Cessation Therapy," *Archives of Internal Medicine* 151 (1991): 749–52; Transdermal Nicotine Study Group, "Transdermal Nicotine for Smoking Cessation. Six-Month Results from Two Multicenter Controlled Clinical Trials," *Journal of the American Medical Association* 266 (1991): 3133–38; T. Abelin, A. Buehler, P. Muller, et al., "Controlled Trial of Transdermal Nicotine Patch in Tobacco Withdrawal," *Lancet* 1 (1989): 7–10; R. D. Hurt, G. G. Laugher, K. P. Offord, et al., "Nicotine-Replacement Therapy with Use of a Transdermal Nicotine Patch: A Randomized Doubleblind Placebo-

Controlled Trial," *Mayo Clinic Proceedings* 65 (1990): 1529–37; G. Buchkremer, H. Bents, M. Horstman, et al., "Combination of Behavioral Smoking Cessation with Transdermal Nicotine Substitution," *Addictive Behaviors* 14 (1989): 229–38; P. Tønnesen, J. Nørregaard, K. Simonsen, and U. Säwe, "A Double–Blind Trial of a 16-Hour Transdermal Nicotine Patch in Smoking Cessation," *New England Journal of Medicine* 325 (1991): 311–15.

39. N. L. Benowitz, "Pharmacodynamics of Nicotine: Implications for Rational Treatment of Nicotine Addiction," *British Journal of Addiction* 86 (1991): 495–99.

40. Tønnesen et al., "A Double-Blind Trial of a 16-Hour Transdermal Nicotine Patch"; Basel, "Habitrol Nicotine Transdermal System," Marion Merrell Dow, "Nicoderm Nicotine Transdermal System," Parke-Davis, "Nicotrol Nicotine Transdermal System," and Lederle, "Prostep Nicotine Transdermal System," in *Physicians' Desk Reference,* 47th edition (Montvale, N.J.: Medical Economics Data, 1993).

41. J. Gorsline, S. K. Gupta, D. Dye, and C. N. Rolf, "Nicotine Dose Relationship for Nicoderm (Nicotine Transdermal System) at Steady State," *Pharmacology Research* 10 (1991, suppl.): S299; M. A. Russell, M. Raw, and M. J. Jarvis, "Clinical Use of Nicotine Chewing-Gum," *British Medical Journal* 280 (1980): 1599–1602; O. F. Pomerleau, "Nicotine and the Central Nervous System: Biobehavioral Effects of Cigarette Smoking," *American Journal of Medicine* 93 (1992, suppl. 1A): 2S–7S; S. C. Mulligan, J. G. Masterson, J. G. Devane, and J. G. Kelly, "Clinical and Pharmacokinetic Properties of a Transdermal Nicotine Patch," *Clinical Pharmacology and Therapeutics* 47 (1990): 331–37.

42. M. C. Fiore, D. E. Jorenby, T. B. Baker, and S. L. Kenford, "Tobacco Dependence and the Nicotine Patch. Clinical Guidelines for Effective Use," *Journal of the American Medical Association* 268 (1992): 2687–94.

43. Marion Merrell Dow, "Nicorette (nicotine polacrilex)," in *Physicians' Desk Reference,* 47th edition, 1993. Four-milligram nicotine chewing gum is likely to be available in 1993 or 1994.

44. J. Hughes, "Dependence Potential and Abuse Liability of Nicotine Replacement Therapies," *Biomedicine and Pharmacotherapy* 43 (1989): 11–17.

45. N. L. Benowitz, P. Jacob III, and C. Savanapridi, "Determinants of Nicotine Intake While Chewing Nicotine Polacrilex Gum," *Clinical Pharmacology and Therapeutics* 41 (1987): 467–73; M. E. McNabb, R. V. Ebert, and K. McCusker, "Plasma Nicotine Lev-

els Produced by Chewing Nicotine Gum," *Journal of the American Medical Association* 248 (1982): 865–68; M. E. McNabb, "Chewing Nicotine Gum for 3 Months: What Happens to Plasma Nicotine Levels," *Canadian Medical Association Journal* 131 (1984): 589–92; P. Tønnesen, V. Fryd, M. Hansen, et al., "Two and Four mg Nicotine Chewing Gum and Group Counseling in Smoking Cessation: An Open Randomized Controlled Trial with a 22-Month Follow-Up," *Addictive Behaviors* 13 (1988): 17–27.

46. W. M. Fee and M. J. Stewart, "A Controlled Trial of Nicotine Chewing Gum in a Smoking Withdrawal Clinic," *Practitioner* 226 (1982): 148–151; K. Jamrozik, G. Fowler, M. Vessey, and N. Wald, "Placebo Controlled Trial of Nicotine Chewing Gum in General Practice," *British Medical Journal* 287 (1983): 1782–85.

47. M. Kornitzer, F. Kittel, M. Dramaix, and P. Bourdoux, "A Double Blind Study of 2 mg vs. 4 mg Nicotine Gum in an Industrial Setting," *Journal of Psychosomatic Research* 31 (1987): 171–76; Tønnesen et al., "Two and Four mg Nicotine Chewing Gum and Group Counseling."

48. R. E. Johnson, V. J. Stevens, J. F. Hollis, G. T. Woodson, "Nicotine Chewing Gum Use in the Outpatient Care Setting," *Journal of Family Practice* 34 (1992): 61–65.

49. M. Hasenfratz and K. Battig, "Nicotine Absorption and the Subjective and Physiologic Effects of Nicotine Toothpicks," *Clinical Pharmacology and Therapeutics* 50 (1991): 456–61; M. A. Russell, "The Future of Nicotine Replacement," *British Journal of Addiction* 86 (1991): 653–58.

50. G. Sutherland, J. A. Stapleton, M. A. H. Russell, et al., "Randomised Controlled Trial of Nasal Nicotine Spray in Smoking Cessation," *Lancet* 340 (1992): 324–29; M. J. Jarvis, P. Hajek, M. A. H. Russell, et al., "Nasal Nicotine Solution as an Aid to Cigarette Withdrawal: A Pilot Clinical Trial," *British Journal of Addiction* 82 (1987): 83–88.

51. Philip Tønnesen, Jesper Nørregaard, Kim Mikkelsen, et al., "A Double-Blind Trial of a Nicotine Inhaler for Smoking Cessation," *Journal of the American Medical Association* 269 (1993): 1268–71.

52. A. I. M. Hjalmarson, "Effect of Nicotine Chewing Gum in Smoking Cessation," *Journal of the American Medical Association* 252 (1984): 2835–38.

53. A. H. Glassman, W. K. Jackson, B. T. Walsh, et al., "Cigarette Craving, Smoking Withdrawal, and Clonidine," *Science* 226 (1984): 864–66; Alexander H. Glassman, Fay Stetner, B. Timo-

thy Walsh, et al., "Heavy Smokers, Smoking Cessation, and Clonidine. Results of a Double-Blind, Randomized Trial," *Journal of the American Medical Association* 259 (1988): 2863–66; John R. Hughes, "Clonidine, Depression, and Smoking Cessation," *Journal of the American Medical Association* 259 (1988): 2901–2; S. A. Ornish, S. Zisook, and L. A. McAdams, "Effects of Transdermal Clonidine Treatment on Withdrawal Symptoms Associated with Smoking Cessation. A Randomized, Controlled Trial," *Archives of Internal Medicine* 148 (1988): 2027–31; R. Davison, K. Kaplan, D. Fintel, et al., "The Effect of Clonidine on the Cessation of Cigarette Smoking," *Clinical Pharmacology and Therapeutics* 44 (1988): 265–67.

54. J. Walinder, J. Balldin, K. Bokstrom, et al., "Clonidine Suppression of the Alcohol Withdrawal Syndrome," *Drug and Alcohol Dependence* 8 (1981): 345–48.

55. D. R. Jasinski, R. E. Johnson, and T. R. Kocher, "Clonidine in Morphine Withdrawal: Differential Effect on Signs and Symptoms," *Archives of General Psychiatry* 42 (1985): 1063–66.

56. P. Franks, J. Harp, B. Bell, "Randomized, Controlled Trial of Clonidine for Smoking Cessation in a Primary Care Setting," *Journal of the American Medical Association* 262 (1989): 3011–13; A. V. Prochazka, T. L. Petty, L. Nett, et al., "Transdermal Clonidine Reduced Some Withdrawal Symptoms But Did Not Increase Smoking Cessation," *Archives of Internal Medicine* 152 (1992): 2065–69.

57. M. D. Robinson, W. A. Smith, E. A. Cederstrom, D. E. Sutherland, "Buspirone Effect on Tobacco Withdrawal Symptoms: A Pilot Study," *Journal of the American Board of Family Practice* 4 (1991): 89–94; M. D. Robinson, Y. L. Pettice, W. A. Smith, et al., "Buspirone Effect on Tobacco Withdrawal Symptoms: A Randomized Placebo-Controlled Trial," *Journal of the American Board of Family Practice* 5 (1992): 1–9; D. E. Hilleman, S. M. Mohiuddin, M. G. Del Core, and M. H. Sketch, Sr., "Effect of Buspirone on Withdrawal Symptoms Associated with Smoking Cessation," *Archives of Internal Medicine* 152 (1992): 350–52.

58. N. B. Edwards, J. K. Murphy, A. D. Downs, et al., "Doxepin as an Adjunct to Smoking Cessation: A Double-Blind Pilot Study," *American Journal of Psychiatry* 146 (1989): 373–76.

59. P. B. Clarke, "Nicotinic Receptor Blockade Therapy and Smoking Cessation," *British Journal of Addiction* 86 (1991): 501–5.

60. S. J. Leischow and M. L. Stitzer, "Smoking Cessation and Weight Gain," *British Journal of Addiction* 86 (1991): 577–81.

61. R. C. Klesges, L. M. Klesges, A. W. Meyers, et al., "The Effects of

Phenylpropanolamine on Dietary Intake, Physical Activity, and Body Weight after Smoking Cessation," *Clinical Pharmacology and Therapeutics* 47 (1990): 747–54.

62. Bonnie Spring, Judith Wurtman, Ray Gleason, et. al., "Weight Gain and Withdrawal Symptoms After Smoking Cessation: A Preventive Intervention Using d-Fenfluramine," *Health Psychology* 10 (1991): 216–223.

CHAPTER 7: BREAST CANCER

1. Jeff M. Hall, Ming K. Lee, Beth Newman, et al., "Linkage of Early-Onset Familial Breast Cancer to Chromosome 17q21," *Science* 250 (1990): 1684–89.

2. E. B. Claus, N. J. Risch, and W. D. Thompson, "Age at Onset as an Indicator of Familial Risk of Breast Cancer," *American Journal of Epidemiology* 131 (1990): 961–72.

3. These estimates are based on the tables in Mitchell H. Gail, Louise A. Brinton, David P. Byar, et al., "Projecting Individual-ized Probabilities of Developing Breast Cancer for White Females Who Are Being Examined Annually," *Journal of the National Cancer Institute* 81 (1989): 1879–86. The statistical margins of error are: ten-year probability of breast cancer, 5 to 18 percent; twenty-year probability, 11 to 31 percent; and thirty-year probability, 16 to 42 percent.

4. Leslie Roberts, "Genetic Counseling: A Preview of What's in Store," *Science* 259 (1993): 624; idem, "Zeroing In on a Breast Cancer Susceptibility Gene," *Science* 259 (1993): 622–25.

5. Jay R. Harris, Marc E. Lippman, Umberto Veronesi, and Walter Willett, "Breast Cancer," *New England Journal of Medicine* 327 (1992): 319–28, 390–98, 473–80.

6. J. B. Kampert, A. S. Whittemore, and R. S. Paffenbarger, Jr., "Combined Effect of Child-Bearing, Menstrual Events, and Body Size on Age-Specific Breast Cancer Risk," *American Journal of Epidemiology* 128 (1988): 962–79.

7. G. Wyshak and R. E. Frisch, "Evidence for Secular Trend in Age of Menarche," *New England Journal of Medicine* 306 (1982): 1033–35.

8. E. White, "Projected Changes in Breast Cancer Incidence Due to the Trend Toward Delayed Childbearing," *American Journal of Public Health* 77 (1987): 495–97; B. MacMahon, P. Cole, T. M. Lin, et al., "Age at First Birth and Breast Cancer Risk," *Bulletin of the World Health Organization* 43 (1970): 209–21; D. Trichopoulos, C. C. Hsieh, B. Macmahon, et al., "Age at Any Birth

and Breast Cancer Risk," *International Journal of Cancer* 31 (1983): 701–4; M. Ewertz, S. W. Duffy, H. O. Adami, et al., "Age at First Birth, Parity and Risk of Breast Cancer: A Meta-Analysis of 8 Studies from the Nordic Countries," *International Journal of Cancer* 46 (1990): 597–603.

9. S. A. Narod, J. Feunteun, H. T. Lynch, et al., "Familial Breast–Ovarian Cancer Locus on Chromosome 17a12–q23," *Lancet* 338 (1991): 82–83.

10. Brian E. Henderson, Ronald K. Ross, and Malcolm C. Pike, "Hormonal Chemoprevention of Cancer in Women," *Science* 259 (1993): 633–38; Susan G. Nayfield, J. E. Karp, L. G. Ford, et al., "Potential Role of Tamoxifen in Prevention of Breast Cancer," *Journal of the National Cancer Institute* 83 (1991): 1450–59; N. E. Davidson, "Tamoxifen—Panacea or Pandora's Box?" *New England Journal of Medicine* 326 (1992): 885–86.

11. M. A. Kirschner, G. Schneider, N. H. Ertel, and E. Worton, "Obesity, Androgen, Estrogens and Cancer Risk," *Cancer Research* 42 (1982, suppl.): 3281S–3282S; P. F. Bruning, J. M. Bonfrer, and A. A. Hart, "Non-protein Bound Estradiol, Sex Hormone Binding Globulin, Breast Cancer and Breast Cancer Risk," *British Journal of Cancer* 51 (1985): 479–84.

12. S. Tretli, "Height and Weight in Relation to Breast Cancer Incidence and Mortality: A Prospective Study of 570,000 Women in Norway," *International Journal of Cancer* 44 (1989): 23–30; F. deWaard, J. Poortman, and B. J. Collette, "Relationship of Weight to the Promotion of Breast Cancer After Menopause," *Nutrition and Cancer* 2 (1981): 237–40.

13. M. P. Longnecker, J. A. Berlin, M. J. Orza, T. C. Chalmers, "A Meta-Analysis of Alcohol Consumption in Relation to Risk of Breast Cancer," *Journal of the American Medical Association* 260 (1988): 652–56.

14. Maureen Henderson, "Current Approaches to Breast Cancer Prevention," *Science* 259 (1993): 630–31.

15. G. J. van Oortmarssen, J. D. F. Habbema, and P. J. van der Maas, "A Model for Breast Cancer Screening," *Cancer* 66 (1990): 1601–12; S. H. Fox, M. Moskowitz, E. L. Saenger, et al., "Benefit/Risk Analysis of Aggressive Mammographic Screening," *Radiology* 128 (1978): 359–65.

16. Gina Kolata, "Big New Study Finds No Link Between Fat and Breast Cancer," *New York Times,* 21 Oct. 1992; Dolores Kong, "Diet's Link to Breast Cancer Is Downplayed," *Boston Globe,* 21 Oct. 1992, p. 1.

17. Gina Kolata, "Studies Say Mammograms Fail to Help Many

Women: New Data Show No Benefit for Women Under 50," *New York Times,* 26 Feb. 1993, p. A1; Elizabeth Neus, "Mammogram Guidelines Face Scrutiny," *USA Today,* 25 Feb. 1993, p. 1A.

18. Eliot Marshall, "Search for a Killer: Focus Shifts from Fat to Hormones," *Science* 259 (1993): 618–21.

19. Jay R. Harris et al., "Breast Cancer."

20. Barry A. Miller, Eric J. Feuer, and Benjamin F. Hankey, "The Increasing Incidence of Breast Cancer Since 1982: Relevance of Early Detection," *Cancer Causes and Control* 2 (1991): 67–74; Barry A. Miller, Eric J. Feuer, and Benjamin F. Hankey, "Breast Cancer" (letter), *New England Journal of Medicine* 327 (1992): 1756–57.

21. Computed from figures 1A and 1B in Miller, Feuer, and Hankey, "Breast Cancer."

22. Janet B. Henrich, "The Postmenopausal Estrogen/Breast Cancer Controversy," *Journal of the American Medical Assocation* 268 (1992): 1900–1902; K. K. Steinberg, S. B. Thacker, S. J. Smith, et al. "A Meta-Analysis of the Effect of Estrogen Replacement Therapy on the Risk of Breast Cancer," *Journal of the American Medical Assocation* 265 (1991): 1985–90.

23. Gabe Mirkin, "Statistics on Breast and Prostate Cancer," *Mirkin Report* 3 (Nov. 1992): 2.

24. See, for example, Susan M. Love and Karen Lindsey, *Dr. Susan Love's Breast Book* (Reading, Mass.: Addison-Wesley, 1990), p. 139.

25. Jeffrey E. Harris, "Social and Economic Causes of Cancer," in *Pathways to Health: The Role of Social Factors,* ed. John Bunker, Diana S. Gomby, and Barbara H. Kehrer (Menlo Park: Henry J. Kaiser Family Foundation, 1989), pp. 165–216.

26. Breast cancer diagnosis rates for women in their eighties appear to be lower than those of women in their seventies. This is probably because many elderly women die with undetected breast cancer. Whatever the reason for the anomaly, it casts further doubt on the accuracy of estimates of lifetime breast cancer risk. See figure 2 in "Breast and Cervical Cancer Surveillance, United States, 1973–1987," *Morbidity and Mortality Weekly Report* 41 (1992, SS–2): 1–15.

27. A. B. Miller, C. J. Baines, T. To, and C. Wall, "Canadian National Breast Screening Study: 1. Breast Cancer Detection and Death Rates Among Women Aged 40 to 49 Years," *Canadian Medical Association Journal* 147 (1992): 1459–76.

28. Neus, "Mammogram Guidelines Face Scrutiny."

29. Kolata, "Studies Say Mammograms Fail to Help Many Women."

30. Jeffrey E. Harris, "Environmental Policy Making: Act Now or Wait for More Information?" in *Valuing Health Risks, Costs, and Benefits for Environmental Decision Making,* ed. P. B. Hammond and R. Coppock (Washington, D.C.: National Academy Press, 1990), pp. 107–33.

31. S. W. Fletcher, R. P. Harris, J. J. Gonzalez, et al., "Increasing Mammography Utilization: A Controlled Study," *Journal of the National Cancer Institute* 85 (1993): 112–20; National Center for Health Statistics, "Breast Cancer Risk Factors and Screening: United States, 1987," *Vital and Health Statistics,* ser. 10, no. 172 (Hyattsville, Md.: U.S. Department of Health and Human Services, Jan. 1990).

32. R. P. Harris, S. W. Fletcher, J. J. Gonzalez, et al., "Mammography and Age: Are We Targeting the Wrong Women? A Community Survey of Women and Physicians," *Cancer* 67 (1991): 2010–14; "Use of Mammography—United States, 1990," *Morbidity and Mortality Weekly Report* 39 (1990): 621–30; "Cancer Screening Behaviors Among U.S. Women: Breast Cancer, 1987–1989, and Cervical Cancer, 1988–1989," *Morbidity and Mortality Weekly Report* 41 (1992, suppl. SS–2): 17–25.

33. Daniel B. Kopans, "Evaluation of a Breast Mass" (letter), *New England Journal of Medicine* 328 (1993): 810–11.

34. D. B. Kopans, J. E. Meyer, A. M. Cohen, and W. C. Wood, "Palpable Breast Masses: The Importance of Preoperative Mammography," *Journal of the American Medical Association* 246 (1981): 2819–22.

35. See table 2 in "Breast and Cervical Cancer Surveillance, United States, 1973–1987," *Morbidity and Mortality Weekly Report* 41 (1992, SS–2): 1–15.

36. S. W. Duffy, L. Tabar, G. Fagerberg, et al., "Breast Screening, Prognostic Factors and Survival—Results from the Swedish Two-County Study," *British Journal of Cancer* 64 (1991): 1133–88.

37. D. M. Ikeda, I. Andersson, C. Wattsgard, et al., "Interval Carcinomas in the Malmö Mammographic Screening Trial: Radiographic Appearance and Prognostic Considerations," *American Journal of Roentgenology* 159 (1992): 287–94.

38. Miller et al., "Canadian National Breast Screening Study: 1"; A. B. Miller, C. J. Baines, T. To, and C. Wall, "Canadian National Breast Screening Study: 2. Breast Cancer Detection and Death Rates among Women Aged 50 to 59 Years," *Canadian Medical Association Journal* 147 (1992): 1477–88.

39. M. M. Roberts, F. E. Alexander, T. J. Anderson, et al., "Edinburgh Trial of Screening for Breast Cancer: Mortality at Seven Years," *Lancet* 335 (1990): 241–46.

40. P. P. Glasziou, "Meta-Analysis Adjusting for Compliance: The Example of Screening for Breast Cancer," *Journal of Clinical Epidemiology* 45 (1992): 1251–56.

41. C. J. Baines, A. B. Miller, D. B. Kopans, et al., "Canadian National Breast Screening Study: Assessment of Technical Quality by External Review (with Discussion)," *American Journal of Roentgenology* 155 (1990): 743–49.

42. Miller et al., "Canadian National Breast Screening Study: 1," and "Canadian National Breast Screening Study: 2."

43. A. Stacey-Clear, K. A. McCarthy, D. A. Hall, et al., "Breast Cancer Survival Among Women Under Age 50: Is Mammography Detrimental?" *Lancet* 340 (1992):991–94.

44. Walter C. Willett, David J. Hunter, Meir Stampfer, et al., "Dietary Fat and Fiber in Relation to Risk of Breast Cancer: An 8-Year Follow-Up," *Journal of the American Medical Association* 268 (1992): 2037–44.

45. W. C. Willett, M. J. Stampfer, G. A. Colditz, et al., "Relation of Meat, Fat, and Fiber Intake to the Risk of Colon Cancer in a Prospective Study Among Women," *New England Journal of Medicine* 323 (1990): 1664–72.

46. Brian E. Henderson, Ronald K. Ross, and Malcolm Pike, "Toward the Primary Prevention of Cancer," *Science* 254 (1991): 1131–38.

Index